Strategic Choices
for America's Hospitals

Managing Change
in Turbulent Times

Stephen M. Shortell
Ellen M. Morrison
Bernard Friedman

with the assistance of

Susan L. Hughes
Edward F. X. Hughes

Strategic Choices
for America's Hospitals

Managing Change
in Turbulent Times

Jossey-Bass Publishers

San Francisco   •   Oxford   •   1990

STRATEGIC CHOICES FOR AMERICA'S HOSPITALS
Managing Change in Turbulent Times
by Stephen M. Shortell, Ellen M. Morrison, and Bernard Friedman

Copyright © 1990 by: Jossey-Bass Inc., Publishers
350 Sansome Street
San Francisco, California 94104
&
Jossey-Bass Limited
Headington Hill Hall
Oxford, OX3 0BW

Library of Congress Cataloging-in-Publication Data

Shortell, Stephen M. (Stephen Michael), date.
    Strategic choices for America's hospitals : managing change in
turbulent times / Stephen M. Shortell, Ellen M. Morrison, Bernard
Friedman. — 1st ed.
        p.   cm. — (Jossey-Bass health series) (Jossey-Bass
management series)
    Includes bibliographical references.
    ISBN 1-55542-188-1 (alk. paper)
    1. Hospitals—Administration.   2. Organizational change.
I. Morrison, Ellen M., date.   II. Friedman, Bernard, date.
III. Series.   IV. Series: Jossey-Bass management series.
RA971.S49   1989
362.1'1'068—dc20   89-45605
                                                                        CIP

JACKET DESIGN BY WILLI BAUM

FIRST EDITION

Code 8961

A joint publication in
The Jossey–Bass Health Series
and
The Jossey–Bass Management Series

Contents

Preface   xiii

Acknowledgments   xxi

The Authors   xxv

**Part One: Change and Adaptation
in the Hospital Industry**   **1**

1. Examining the Hospital's Turbulent Environment   3

2. Understanding How Hospitals Respond to
Change: A Model of Strategic Adaptation   27

3. Strategic Change, Corporate Goals, and
Management Processes   46

4. Structuring the Relationship Between the
Corporation and the Hospital   90

ix

**Part Two: Managing Change and Adaptation:
Four Strategic Orientations**   **111**

5. The Four Orientations: Their Environments,
    Performance, and Management Processes   113

6. Managing the Prospector Orientation   133

7. Managing the Defender Orientation   161

8. Managing the Analyzer Orientation   183

9. Managing the Reactor Orientation   207

**Part Three: Ensuring Hospital Success:
Lessons and Future Directions**   **227**

10. Sustaining a Competitive Advantage   229

11. Key Requirements for Success in a
    Changing Health Care Environment   254

12. The Model Revisited: Directions
    for Further Research   280

13. Crafting Health Policy in the 1990s:
    Strengthening the Ties Between Industry
    Leaders and Policymakers   301

Resources   **329**

A. The Strategic Planning Survey   331

B. Interview Questionnaires   350

C. Research Variables and Measures   358

D. Availability and Profitability of
    Hospital Services   363

Contents

E. Analyses of Performance: Profitability and Market Share   365

F. Related Study Publications   367

References   369

Index   389

Preface

What do organizations do when their environments change radically?

Why do some organizations change their strategies while others stand pat?

In what direction are changes made?

Why do some changes succeed and others fail?

What are the implications of strategic adaptation for the larger society of which the organization is a member?

These questions seem simple and straightforward, but they open the door to a variety of complex and subtle issues that challenge both managers and students of organizations. There is a growing body of literature on how strategy influences performance, but little is known about how a *change* in strategy affects performance. In fact, many are skeptical that organizations *can* change their strategies, given the amount of effort and skill required to recognize the need to change, to formulate "correct" new strategies, and to implement the changes required. This is the *structural inertia* view of organizations (see, for example, Hannan and Freeman, 1984). Others argue that organizations do have the capacity to change, to adapt to their environment, and even, to influence it actively — the *strategic choice* school of thinking (see, for example, Child, 1972). More recently, we have recognized that elements of both inertia and choice are present in organizational life (see, for example, Drazin and Van de Ven, 1985; Hrebiniak and Joyce, 1985).

There is a need to study the conditions and circumstances under which strategic change does or does not occur, and with what results — for both the organization and the larger environment of which it is a part. *Strategic Choices for America's Hospitals* is one of the first attempts to address these issues empirically within the context of a strategic adaptation model. The book has three purposes: (1) to advance knowledge about the basic processes of strategic adaptation, (2) to advance the strategic thinking and behavior of executives in the hospital industry, and (3) to suggest ways in which greater knowledge of how hospitals adapt strategically can contribute to more effective health care policies. Toward these ends, we examined the strategic adaptation processes of eight leading hospital systems from 1983 through 1987, with some extension to 1988.

The dramatic changes occurring within the hospital industry provide an excellent setting for the study of strategic adaptation. Hospitals, the largest component of an approximately $600-billion health care industry, are in a state of flux. In 1988 alone, eighty-one hospitals closed and hundreds of others were divested through employee stock ownership plans or sale to other investors. Significant financial and organizational restructuring is occurring, from leveraged buyouts, to megasystems, to "hospitals without walls." The ferment is not unlike what is happening among financial institutions or airlines, but the changes in health care take on added significance because of the firmly entrenched interests of professional groups and the deeply personal nature of the service rendered.

Miles and Cameron's Study

In important ways this book builds on Miles and Cameron's seminal study (1982) of strategic adaptation among the big six tobacco companies. Like Miles and Cameron, we focus on how a single industry (hospitals) responds to a significant environmental change — in this case predetermined fixed payment rates for Medicare patients rather than cost-based payment. We examine in detail the adaptation strategies used and their effect on efficiency and organizational legitimacy (that is, credibility with the public and with important stakeholders), and we suggest important implications for hospital management and for public policy.

Our study, however, differs from Miles and Cameron's in important ways. First, while Miles and Cameron focused on an industry that is highly concentrated — essentially, the top six firms *are* the industry — we examine a highly fragmented industry (there are nearly 7,000 hospitals) in which the concept of industrywide market share has little meaning.

Second, we examine strategic adaptation from the perspective of both the system's corporate office and the individual hospitals that make up the system. This enables us to provide some insights on strategic adaptation in multidivisional organizations in which individual divisions have varying degrees of autonomy.

Third, in studying hospitals we can focus on an industry with different ownership orientations: investor-owned, for-profit hospital companies and voluntary, not-for-profit hospital systems. This adds a degree of richness unavailable in previous work and allows us to extend the findings to not-for-profit organizations.

Fourth, by selecting hospitals we are able to study an industry dominated by largely autonomous professionals (physicians) and explore their role in the strategic adaptation process. We believe the lessons learned are applicable to other fields undergoing increased professionalization (for example, law offices, architectural firms, and advertising agencies) and to not-for-profit service organizations, such as museums, universities, churches, and arts organizations.

Finally, our study differs somewhat from that of Miles and Cameron in its method and emphasis. Miles and Cameron use a longer time frame (twenty-five years) and give greater attention to the historical method. We use a shorter time frame (three years) immediately surrounding a major environmental jolt. We give more attention to quantifying strategic orientations, measuring the degree of change over time, and examining the managerial implications of implementing various strategies. Reflecting the nature of the hospital industry, we also examine a somewhat broader range of performance measures. By noting these similarities as well as differences, we hope to increase the understanding of strategic adaptation as it occurs in different industries and distinguish factors that may promote successful strategic adaptation across different industries from those that may be idiosyncratic to specific industrial settings (Hirsch, 1975, 1984).

Audience for the Book

This is a book for those who study strategy making (academicians), those who do it (executives), and those who try to promote it (makers of public policy). For the academic community, we attempt to shed light on the extent to which strategic change occurs, the direction of change, and its effects on a wider variety of performance dimensions than considered in previous work. Based on existing literature and the study findings, we develop a model of strategic adaptation that can be used to guide further research. In particular, we give attention to the important role of an organization's current strategy in deciding whether to change to a new strategy. We advance the notion of a strategic comfort zone and give special attention to the strategy-making relationship between the corporate office and individual hospitals as business units.

For executives, the book provides lessons and guidelines for managing strategic adaptation in turbulent times and for weighing choices between a new strategy and a current one. We provide guidelines for organizations actively engaged in widespread diversification activities (called *prospectors*), for those trying to become more efficient in current product or market domains (called *defenders*), for those with a mix of both (called *analyzers*), and for those that have difficulty developing a consistent, coherent strategic orientation (called *reactors*). The book is likely to be particularly useful for executives faced with managing strategic change in organizations dominated by professionals.

For policymakers, whether at the local, state, or national level, the book highlights the importance of recognizing and understanding the likely strategic responses of an industry to changes in public policy. We offer suggestions that will help policymakers implement policies that are more likely to be positively accepted. We make some predictions about the future evolution of the hospital industry and its implications for management, public policy, and social welfare. In the process, we present some ideas for developing more effective interaction between the industry and policymakers.

Overview of the Contents

Part One, "Change and Adaptation in the Hospital Industry," describes the setting for the study and develops the model of strategic adaptation. In the first chapter we describe the important "frame-breaking" change represented by the Medicare prospective payment system established in 1983, particularly the shift from a production mentality to a marketing mentality, from a caretaking mind set to a risk-taking mind set, and from an operations orientation to a strategic orientation. We also highlight other significant changes and describe the eight hospital systems that served as the focus of the study. The chapter concludes with a brief summary of the major data sources and measures of the key concepts associated with the model.

In Chapter Two we present the model of strategic adaptation, which permits us to understand and predict the nature of change. The notion of a *strategic comfort zone* serves as a unifying concept for considering the issues involved. In this chapter we examine the full model, setting the stage for applying it to the dynamic changes occurring in the hospital industry.

Chapter Three describes the eight systems: their missions, their philosophies and goals, their strategic orientations, and the quality of their strategic planning and control processes. We discuss the extent to which hospitals have changed their strategies in response to the environmental jolts in the industry, the direction of the change, and the roles played by boards and physicians. The chapter tells a story of experimentation, trial-and-error learning, and recognizing the importance of local markets.

In Chapter Four we examine the relationship between the corporate office and individual hospitals in regard to overall structure and the strategic planning and control process, highlighting similarities and differences.

Part Two, "Managing Change and Adaptation," contains five chapters. Chapter Five provides an overview of the characteristics of four strategic archetypes — prospector, defender, analyzer, and reactor — including performance indicators for both "doing good" (community service) and "doing well" (financial strength), and ownership differences (investor-owned versus not-for-profit). The next four chapters (Chapters Six through Nine) examine in depth the dynamics involved in managing each type, providing lessons and guidelines for managing strategic adaptation using examples drawn from multiple study materials and the industry at large.

In Part Three, "Ensuring Hospital Success," we explore the implications of the lessons learned from our study for the future of strategic management and of the hospital industry. In Chapter Ten we draw together the major findings from Part Two and discuss generic lessons, strategy-specific lessons, and some "switching rules" for successful adaptation.

Chapter Eleven presents some key attributes that are likely to facilitate success in the health care environment of the future: creating integrated continuums of care, behaving as a true corporate system, establishing effective hospital-physician partnerships, and engaging in strategic leadership development. A brief questionnaire is included for those interested in assessing their hospitals on a variety of dimensions.

In Chapter Twelve we summarize the contributions of our study to the field of strategic management in general and to strategic adaptation in particular, and we highlight several areas for further research.

Chapter Thirteen suggests the need for a closer relationship between the industry and policymakers. We present a specific proposal for an ongoing interface that would promote greater mutual understanding, along with a scenario of how the health care system might be organized over the coming decade.

We conclude the book with a series of resources that include the strategic planning survey, corporate office interview protocols, and a listing of related study publications.

Because the book is far ranging, different chapters will be of greater interest to some readers than to others. For the academic community, Chapters One, Two, Five, and Twelve will be of greatest interest, although Chapters Six through Nine contain many qualitative findings that will also be of interest. For practicing executives, Chapters Three through Eleven will be of greatest interest. For policymakers, Chapters Ten, Eleven, and Thirteen are of greatest importance; the remaining chapters might be skimmed.

Notes on the Text

Throughout the book, two sets of terms are used interchangeably: (1) *strategic adaptation* and *strategic change,* and (2) *strategic archetype* and *strategic orientation.* We generally view strategic adaptation as the overall process by which an organization adapts to its environment. This adaptation process may or may not involve significant change in strategy. In general, we use the term *adaptation* when speaking of the overall process and the term *change* when discussing whether specific changes in strategic orientation were made. The term *archetype* refers to an organization's specific strategic predisposition toward the environment, a predisposition made up of certain characteristics and behaviors that reinforce each other. The term *orientation* is meant to connote the same idea. Using both terms interchangeably provides some variety to the mind and eye.

We also note that while the eight systems (with their permission) are identified by name, individual hospitals are not. Executives in all the hospitals were guaranteed confidentiality so that they could express their judgments candidly. The hospital names used here are fictitious. In the unlikely event that we have struck upon the name of a "real" hospital, we can only say, "It is not *that* hospital."

There is little doubt that the corporation has come to

American health care (Starr, 1982). Renée Fox has highlighted the great need for studies that deal with the "forms that this ostensible growth of corporate medicine is taking and of its planned and unplanned, manifest and latent, anticipated and unanticipated consequences" (1985, p. 10). *Strategic Choices for America's Hospitals* is one attempt to fill that need. But we believe this need goes well beyond American health care, to encompass issues of strategic adaptation faced by organizations in many industries. It is our hope that this book provides further understanding of how organizations and industries change in both shaping and being shaped by society's demands.

September 1989   Stephen M. Shortell
                                          Evanston, Illinois

                                          Ellen M. Morrison
                                          San Francisco, California

                                          Bernard Friedman
                                          Chicago, Illinois

Acknowledgments

A project of this scope requires the cooperation and support of many groups and individuals. The research on which the book is based was supported by a three-year grant from the National Center for Health Services Research and Health Care Technology Assessment (grant number HS05159) and a two-year grant from the Robert Wood Johnson Foundation (grant number 9181). We are deeply grateful for their support. Important assistance was also received from the American Hospital Association and many state hospital associations in endorsing survey instruments, from the Health Care Financing Administration in providing Medicare patient mortality data, and from the Joint Commission on Accreditation of Healthcare Organizations in providing data on the structure and process of patient care. Daniel Longo, James Prevost, and James Roberts from the Joint Commission on Accreditation of Healthcare Organizations were particularly helpful in facilitating use of the commission data.

This study would not have been possible without the outstanding support and cooperation received from individuals in the eight hospital systems, ranging from top corporate board members, executives, and staff to hospital CEOs and their staffs. Their willingness to be studied and their openness in sharing information have made a significant contribution to our understanding of how hospital systems are adapting to the growing demands of the health care environment. They have provided insights that could not otherwise have been obtained, and for that they deserve the appreciation of all. Throughout the study, we were struck by two traits: the pride each system takes in its many accomplishments, and the humility with which it acknowledges its shortcomings.

Among the many people involved, special appreciation is owed the executive officers who granted permission for the study. These include Royce Diener, John Moxley, and Walter Weisman of American Medical International; Thomas Frist, Jr., and the late David Williamson of the Hospital Corporation of America; Richard Eamer, John Bedrosian, and Leonard Cohen of National Medical Enterprises; John King of Evangelical Health Systems; Donald Wegmiller and William Kreykes of Health Central (now called Health One); Scott Parker, David Jeppson, and Kenneth Johnson of Intermountain Health Care; Edward Connors of the Sisters of Mercy Health Corporation; and Richard Barr of Southwest Community Health Services. We are greatly in their debt.

Another group "lived" the study with us in a special way— our advisory committee. Their many valuable suggestions helped guide us through a maze of data-collection challenges, and they also contributed their own considerable expertise and insights. Members included Penelope Roeder of American Medical International; Robert Lane and Robert Vraciu of the Hospital Corporation of America; Harold Ting and Sidney Tyler of National Medical Enterprises; Richard Risk and Carl Zimmerman of Evangelical Health Systems; Rebecca Bloom and Lynda Seasley of Health Central (Health One); Jeanne Fitzgerald, Nancy Giunto, and Kurt Reitjes of Intermountain Health Care; Joseph Lovett and Stephanie McCutcheon of Sisters of Mercy Health Corporation; and Peter Snow of Southwest Community Health Services.

Special recognition is due Daniel Ermann, our project officer at the National Center for Health Services Research and Health Care Technology Assessment, who served as a member of the advisory committee and provided many helpful suggestions throughout the study. The suggestions of Robert Blendon and Alan Cohen of the Robert Wood Johnson Foundation were particularly helpful in designing our instruments to measure the diversification of services. The research also benefited from the comments and suggestions of our site visitors, Alan Detsky, Joel May, and Donald Steinwachs; from our financial consultants, Robert Derzon and Frank Skala; from the expertise of Robert Dewar in helping to construct the functional and divisional measures; and from the advice of Robert Duncan when the study was in its early formative stages. James Begun, Michael Bice, and John Grant provided outside reviews that were immensely helpful in integrating various sections of the book and helping us clarify our arguments. The book also benefited from the insightful comments of Alain Enthoven, Brad Gray, Brad Kirkman-Liff, Joel Shalowitz, and Edward Zajac. A special note of appreciation is due our colleague Walter McNerney, who provided important advice, counsel, and encouragement throughout the study.

Many research associates, research assistants, and support staff worked on the study over the years. Among these, special recognition is due Tracey Camp, Robert J. Humphery, Lori Messerschmidt, Joan Nockels, and Jeff Orrok. We also express our appreciation to Lee Berg, James E. Coverdill, Binne Douglas, Mary P. Erdmans, Brian R. Golden, Susan Harris, Laura Honzel, Glynis James, Britta Jenkins, Yong June Kim, Kathy Lee, Maida Lerman, Anne Malczewski, John Messerschmidt, Bridget O'Hara, Shelley Robbins, Juliana Shortell, Sonya Thomas, Hollis W. Tibbets, Joan L. Vitek, and James Wolter. Special acknowledgment is due Alice Schaller and Cathy Ver Halen for their excellent work in manuscript preparation.

The overall research project also benefited greatly from the efforts of our colleagues, Edward F. X. Hughes and Susan

L. Hughes. Susan assisted in developing our diversification questionnaire and in the site visits, and Edward helped in developing our patient outcome measures. Their contributions are also
reflected in the related publications of the study presented in
Appendix F.

Finally, we want to express our appreciation to Alis Valen-
cia, health editor at Jossey-Bass; her suggestions had an important influence in shaping the organization and style of the book
to appeal to multiple audiences. Appreciation is also expressed
to the Jossey-Bass staff for their work in producing the book
on schedule.

The Authors

Stephen M. Shortell is A. C. Buehler Distinguished Professor of hospital and health services management and professor of organization behavior at the J. L. Kellogg Graduate School of Management, Northwestern University. He also holds appointments in the medical school and the Department of Sociology and is director of the Program on Organization Behavior in Health at the university's Center for Health Services and Policy Research. Shortell received his B.B.A. degree (1966) from the University of Notre Dame; his M.P.H. degree (1968) from the University of California, Los Angeles; and his M.B.A. degree (1970) from the University of Chicago. He received his Ph.D. degree (1972) from the Graduate School of Business, University of Chicago, in the behavioral sciences. He taught at the University of Chicago and the University of Washington before joining the Northwestern University faculty in 1982.

Shortell's main interests in recent years have been studying the performance of health care organizations, exploring the processes associated with strategic adaptation, and examining the relationship between professionals and organizations. He has published extensively in these and related areas. Among his previous books are *Hospital-Physician Joint Ventures: A National Demonstration in Primary Care* (1984, with T. Wickizer and J. Wheeler) and *Health Care Management: A Text in Organization Theory and Behavior* (2nd ed., 1988, with A. Kaluzny). He is the recipient of the 1986 Dean Conley Article of the Year Award from the American College of Health Care Executives for his article "The Medical Staff of the Future: Replanting the Garden" (published in *Frontiers of Health Service Management,* Fall 1985).

Shortell has been a visiting lecturer and fellow at several universities, is a frequent presenter at academic and professional meetings; has served on the editorial boards of several professional journals, including *The Academy of Management Review, The Academy of Management Journal, Health Services Research, Medical Care,* and *The Journal of Health and Social Behavior,* among others; and is an adviser and consultant to many private and public organizations. He is a member of the Institute of Medicine of the National Academy of Sciences, past president of the Association for Health Services Research, and chairman of the Accrediting Commission for Graduate Education in Health Services Administration.

Ellen M. Morrison is a postdoctoral fellow in health services research at the San Francisco and Berkeley campuses of the University of California. Her fellowship is a National Research Service Award funded by the Public Health Service. She received her B.A. degree (1977) from the University of California, Los Angeles, and her M.A. (1982) and Ph.D. degrees (1987) from the University of Chicago, all in sociology.

Drawing on her expertise in interview methodology, Morrison took primary responsibility for the analysis of hospital system executives interviews reported in Chapters Three and Four. She also served as project director, overseeing all aspects of the study. At the University of California, San Francisco, Morrison collaborates with faculty at the Institute for Health Policy Studies and the Institute for Health and Aging on several research projects related to her methodological interests in qualitative data collection and analysis and her conceptual interests in health care organizations and their environments. She is particularly interested in research efforts that closely integrate qualitative and quantitative methods and in studying the development and policy implications of managed care systems.

Bernard Friedman is former vice-president for research at the Hospital Research and Educational Trust, American Hospital Association. He received his B.A. degree (1966) from Northwestern University and his Ph.D. degree (1971) from Massachusetts Institute of Technology, both in economics. Friedman has taught economics at Brown University and Northwestern University. His studies of health insurance, hospital cost containment, and the incentive effects of public programs have been published in leading journals and textbooks.

In the last several years, he has been engaged with issues of competition and reimbursement models in health care, under grants sponsored by the Health Care Financing Administration, the Veterans Administration (VA), the National Center for Health Services Research, the Johnson Foundation, and the Retirement Research Foundation. He has worked to analyze the effects of a Medicare voucher system, the deceleration of Medicaid expenses after the Omnibus Budget Reconciliation Act of 1981, effects and costs of state catastrophic health insurance programs, and the trends of budget and workload pressures at the VA in dealing with a growing elderly veteran population.

Strategic Choices
for America's Hospitals

Managing Change
in Turbulent Times

Part One

Change and Adaptation in the Hospital Industry

1

Examining the Hospital's Turbulent Environment

For the past fifty years health care, particularly hospitals, has been a growth industry. The 1930s saw the introduction and rise of private health insurance coverage. With passage of the Hill-Burton Act, the 1940s and 1950s brought significant postwar expansion in the number of hospitals. Medicare and Medicaid legislation of the 1960s increased financial access to health services for the elderly and the poor. Throughout these decades, health manpower legislation greatly expanded the supply of providers. The dominant themes were increasing the public's access to health care services and incorporating the latest advances in medical technology.

During this period health care expenditures as a percentage of the gross national product grew from 4.4 percent in 1950 to 11.1 percent in 1987. If they continue to increase at the present rate, costs will reach $1.5 trillion by the year 2000, or 15 percent of the gross national product. Hospitals represent the largest portion of these expenditures—44 percent, or about $200 billion of personal health care expenditures in 1987. These increases outpaced growth in the consumer price index by a significant margin, causing growing concern about the rising cost of health care.

In response, the federal government introduced the Health Planning and Resource Development Act in 1974, giving state and local agencies the authority to review hospital capital expenditures through approving or disapproving requests called "certificates of need." The goal was to reduce duplication of services and encourage hospitals to share costly technologies. At approximately the same time, a number of states introduced rate review programs designed to control hospital operating revenues. Although the evidence on the effect of the certificate of need programs is ambiguous, it is the general consensus that state rate review programs slowed the rate of increase in hospital costs by about 2 to 3 percent (Morrisey, Conrad, Shortell, and Cook, 1984; Dranove and Cone, 1985).

Nonetheless, the overall effect of these cost-containment efforts was disappointing; the cost of medical care continued to increase faster than the consumer price index through the 1980s (see Figure 1.1). Of particular significance was the growth in federal expenditures; Medicare expenditures increased sixteen-fold between 1966 and 1986 and Medicaid sixfold (Health Insurance Association of America and Health Care Financing Administration, 1988). A growing number of policymakers, employers (who pay the premiums for their employees), and other third-party payors, concerned about the dramatic increase in costs, began to wonder what they were getting for their money. It was against this backdrop that Congress, faced with rising budget deficits, established the Medicare Prospective Payment System (PPS) in 1983.

The Challenges of a Changed Environment

Before October 1983, most hospitals were reimbursed their full costs for patient care. The PPS legislation set predetermined fixed payment levels for 468 diagnosis-related groups of conditions for all Medicare patients (Office of Technology Assessment, 1985). Hospitals that could provide care within the price limit could pocket the savings. Those that could not had to absorb the losses. Since Medicare patients constitute approximately 40 percent of an average hospital's inpatients, the payment

**Figure 1.1. Medical Care Inflation
Versus the Overall Consumer Price Index.**

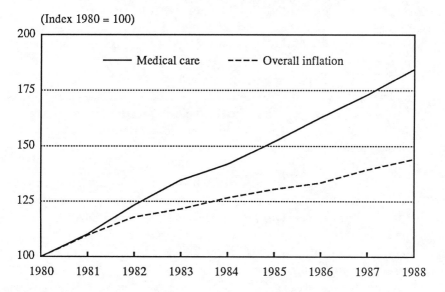

(Index 1980 = 100)

Note: The Consumer Price Index (CPI) measures the effect of medical care price changes only. It does not measure changes in the total amount Americans spend.

Source: U.S. Bureau of Labor Statistics, 1988.

change represented a significant environmental change for the industry. For the first time there existed a national systematic incentive for hospitals to contain costs and provide services as efficiently as possible.

The 1983 legislation was a major jolt in the hospital environment, and it triggered a number of aftershocks. The legislation itself was designed to be phased in over a three-year period, moving from payment based on a hospital's own history of medical costs to regionally and nationally determined rates. Thus, while many hospitals' profit margins actually increased in the first year or two of the program, margins have since declined as payment rates tightened (operating profit margins dropped from .7 percent in 1984 to – .7 percent in 1987, and median total profit margins from 4.6 to 3.0 percent; Health Care Financial Management Association, 1988). Hospital credit ratings have also declined; between 1983 and 1987, 22 percent of audited hospitals' ratings dropped, and only 5 percent increased. It is estimated that 50 percent of hospitals will lose money on their Medicare patients in 1989. Rural hospitals have been particularly hard hit, because of lower reimbursement rates in comparison with urban hospitals.

Private insurance companies and Blue Cross and Blue Shield plans feared that hospitals would cross-subsidize their costs to private paying patients to make up for their losses from Medicare patients. Many, therefore, developed their own versions of prospective payment programs, with strict review of hospital utilization.

By 1984, health care expenditures for the big three auto companies—Chrysler, Ford, and General Motors—had risen to $3.2 billion. Nearly $600 of the price of every Chrysler car was directly attributable to medical care costs. These manufacturers, and others, began to look for more cost-effective alternatives: health maintenance organizations (HMOs), preferred provider organizations (PPOs), and related "managed care" programs. These programs negotiated hospital rate discounts of up to 50 percent in some areas. From 1980 to 1987 the number of HMOs tripled (from approximately 230 to over 700) and enrollment also tripled (from 10 million to 30 million; Interstudy, 1988). The number of PPOs has shown even more dramatic growth, increasing from 13 in 1980 to 454 in 1987 (American Hospital Association, 1988). Some industry forecasts suggest that during the 1990s, 90 percent of Americans will receive care under some form of managed program (Bernstein and Associates, 1985).

In recent years, Congress has also established peer review organizations (PROs, successors to the earlier professional standards review organizations) designed to help ensure appropriate hospital use as well as to make sure that necessary services were being rendered. The continued evolution of new technologies, the AIDS epidemic, the aging of the population, the growing number of Americans without health insurance coverage (37 million in 1988), the redefinition of the roles of physicians and allied health professionals, the acute shortage of nurses in many sections of the country, and, of course, the increased competition among hospitals and between hospitals and physicians have all been a part of the changing health care environment. Conflicting demands were being placed on hospitals to respond to new responsibilities while conserving resources.

Considering New Strategies. The introduction of PPS and these associated events represent an example of frame-breaking change encompassing a sharp departure from the past (Tushman, Newman, and Romanelli, 1987). Such changes frequently require concurrent shifts in an organization's strategies, structures, people, and decision-making processes, often within a relatively short period. There is evidence that hospitals responded strongly to the new incentives (Schramm and Gabel, 1988; Feder, Hadley, and Zuckerman, 1987). For example, the average length of stay, which had been declining by 1 to 2 percent a year for more than a decade, dropped by 9 percent in the first year of PPS; overall hospital occupancy rates fell by 12 percent (Guterman and Dobson, 1986). The total number of days Americans spent in hospitals declined nearly 20 percent between 1980 and 1986, with an offsetting sharp increase in outpatient visits (Health Insurance Association of America and Health Care Financing Administration, 1988). Ambulatory surgery grew dramatically—from 16 percent of all hospital operations in 1980 to 40 percent in 1986 (Prospective Payment Assessment Commission, 1987).

To contain costs and offset the decline in patient days, hospitals reduced their work force by 2.3 percent during the first year of PPS, with continued reductions the second year. Expenses for supplies and equipment increased at only half the rate of previous years (Health Care Financing Administration, 1985). The number of routine tests ordered dropped significantly, as did the use of such well-established procedures as electrocardiography and occupational and physical therapy (Sloan, Morrisey, and Valvona, 1988).

At a broader level, the increased financial and competitive pressures have led more hospitals to join systems (defined as two or more hospitals with a common form of ownership) or alliances (see Figure 1.2) and to pursue a variety of diversifica-

Figure 1.2. Growth in System Hospitals, 1979–2000.

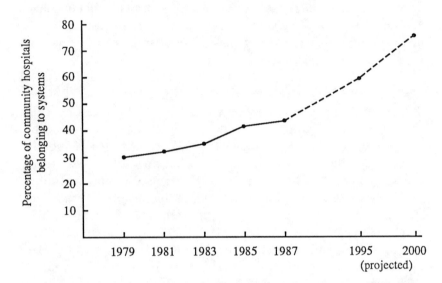

Sources: Directory of Multihospital Systems, 1980–87 editions, published by
the American Hospital Association, copyright 1980–1987; *American Hospital Association Guide to the Health Care Field,* 1988 edition, published by the American Hospital
Association, copyright 1988; *Multi-Hospital Systems: Perspectives and Trends,* published by Arthur Andersen & Co. and the American Hospital Association, copyright 1987.

tion initiatives (Coyne and Cobbs, 1988). Hoping to achieve
economies of scale, increase access to capital, and provide a competitive advantage, approximately 45 percent of the nation's community hospitals now belong to systems. This figure is expected
to grow to 60 percent by 1995 (Arthur Andersen & Co. and
the American College of Hospital Administrators, 1984) and
possibly 80 percent by the end of the century (Shortell, 1988).
In addition to the hospitals in systems, 1,774 others (31 percent) belong to more loosely structured alliances, networks, and
consortia constituting "quasi firms" (Luke, Begun, and Pointer,
1989). Some observers have referred to the growth of systems
and alliances (particularly investor-owned systems) as the most
important development of the day (Relman, 1980); others suggest it is likely to accelerate development of "an entirely new
system of corporate medical enterprise" (Starr, 1982, p. 419).

At the same time, there has been a marked increase in the number of hospital closures. Between 1980 and 1987, 519 of the nation's hospitals closed, with a steady increase from 35 in 1983 to 96 in 1987 (American Hospital Association, 1988).

Developing New Mind Sets. The frame-breaking change associated with PPS requires three fundamental reorientations for hospital executives and their organizations:

1. The need to move from a product orientation (we provide services to patients brought to us by the medical staff) to a market orientation (we must define market needs and preferences and actively develop programs to meet these needs).
2. The need to move from a caretaking mentality (our job is to be stewards of the hospital's assets) to a risk-taking mentality (our job is to increase the hospital's assets).
3. The need to move from operational management (we run a good shop) to strategic management (we must position the organization to seize future opportunities).

Before PPS and the forces associated with it, hospitals were primarily passive recipients of patients brought to them by the hospitals' medical staffs. Physicians were the primary customers, and hospitals competed to keep them happy by expanding and updating plant and equipment. The focus was on the "product." Since PPS, hospitals have had to assume a more proactive, market-oriented stance that recognizes multiple market segments including selected employer groups, managed care plans, HMOs and PPOs, and targeted consumer groups such as women and children, health promotion advocates, and the elderly. Rather than passively waiting for patients to come to their doorstep, hospitals have had to conduct systematic market research to assess needs and then design a portfolio of services to meet those needs. Competition and marketing are foreign to traditional hospital and physician cultures. This first change means giving up old ways and adopting a distinctly new mind set.

Before PPS, hospital executives were largely rewarded for being caretakers, for providing a good "doctors' workshop."

Hospital board members, in their stewardship role of safeguarding the hospital's assets, reinforced the basic caretaking mentality. A premium was placed on keeping physicians happy; above all, the board strove to avoid conflict with the medical staff. In today's environment, with constraints placed on inpatient revenues, the need to discharge patients sooner, declining admissions, increased competition from new forms of providers, and declining profit margins, hospitals need to become prudent risk takers — another fundamentally new mind set. Rather than merely safeguarding the hospital's assets, board members must be actively involved in expanding the hospital's revenue base. Rather than simply preserving the "doctors' workshop," hospital executives find themselves involved in diversification and new venture activities — sometimes in cooperation with their physicians and sometimes in direct competition.

The challenges posed by PPS have also meant a shift from an internal, operational management focus to a broader external, strategic management orientation. Before PPS, hospitals, being paid on a cost-plus basis, did not need to think or behave strategically. Now, strategy making is essential for survival. Not only the performance of hospitals is being threatened but their social legitimacy as well (Seay and Sigmond, 1989). This is reflected in attempts to repeal the tax-exempt status of not-for-profit hospitals on the grounds that some do not provide adequate uncompensated care and other services to the community. Adopting a broader external strategic focus is difficult for many hospital executives. Most intellectually recognize the need for such a shift, but many are emotionally and psychologically unable to make it. This is reflected in growing CEO turnover, approaching 25 percent in 1988 (American College of Health Care Executives, American Hospital Association, and Heidrick and Struggles, 1988). Even those who have successfully made the transition have done so with difficulty. As the CEO of one study system commented: "The most difficult thing for me to do as I took on the broadened responsibilities was to not only see the big picture but to try to make sense out of it strategically. The skills and orientations needed are very different from operational management. I still struggle with it."

The degree to which these shifts were made, how they were made, and what impact they had on performance are the central issues of this book. Our focus is on eight hospital systems and their member hospitals from 1983 to 1987.

Study Methods

Sample

Assisted by previous research (Lewis and Alexander, 1986), we selected eight systems for study. Given the fragmented nature of the industry, we deliberately chose a sample that reflected differences in ownership, system size, hospital size, geographical location and concentration, and degree of centralization of decision making. Table 1.1 highlights selected characteristics of the eight systems. Three of the eight were investor-owned for-profit corporations, three were not-for-profit secular systems, and two were not-for-profit religiously affiliated systems. They ranged in size from 4 owned and managed hospitals to more than 200. The hospitals were located in forty-five states with good geographical spread among urban, suburban, and rural areas.

Overall, 63 percent of all investor-owned hospitals in the country and 7 percent of all not-for-profit hospitals are included in the study. Compared to other U.S. investor-owned system hospitals, those in the study were less likely to be under ninety-nine beds (37 versus 51 percent), more likely to have some teaching involvement (6.7 versus 2.0 percent), and slightly less likely to be located in central-city urban areas (37 versus 47 percent) and had higher occupancy rates (53 versus 47 percent).

Compared to the country as a whole, the not-for-profit system hospitals in the study were less likely to have teaching involvement (16 versus 31 percent), to be located in a non-central-city urban area (19 versus 45 percent), and more likely to be located in rural areas (33 versus 16 percent) and had somewhat lower occupancy rates (54 versus 60 percent). The findings, therefore, cannot be strictly generalized to other system hospitals or hospitals at large. But the sample is large enough

Table 1.1. Characteristics of the Eight Systems in the Study.

	Ownership	System Size[a]	Average Hospital Bed Size (Range)	Location Distribution			
				Central City Urban	Non-Central-City Urban	Collar County	Rural
American Medical International	Investor-owned	55	165 (52–601)	50.9%	18.2%	25.5%	5.5%
Hospital Corporation of America	Investor-owned	227	144 (36–547)	30.2	19.1	31.6	19.1
National Medical Enterprises	Investor-owned	30	163 (33–341)	48.3	20.7	24.1	6.9
Evangelical Health System	Not-for-profit, religious	4	378 (166–873)	50.0	25.0	25.0	0
Health Central (Health One)	Not-for-profit, secular	12	134 (21–282)	10.0	20.0	20.0	50.0
Intermountain Health Care	Not-for-profit, secular	16	130 (15–472)	25.0	18.8	18.8	37.5
Sisters of Mercy	Not-for-profit, religious	19	218 (26–520)	21.1	26.3	15.8	36.8
Southwest Community Health Services	Not-for-profit, secular	7	109 (25–413)	14.3	14.3	42.8	28.6

[a]Number of hospitals participating in the study over the entire time period.

and heterogenous enough that the substantive lessons on strategic adaptation are relevant for the entire industry.

Major Data Sources

Table 1.2 summarizes the data sources for each of the concepts measured in the study. The overall study approach is that of triangulation (Denzin, 1970), where multiple data-collection strategies are used to capture the dynamics of a complex process. The focus is on both process and variance (Mohr, 1982). The process approach, relying primarily on qualitative research, focuses on the dynamics of change and examines how change is accomplished. The variance approach focuses on explaining the differences in performance outcomes (what worked and what did not) as a result of the change; it relies mostly on quantitative analysis.

Local environmental characteristics were measured using existing secondary data sources such as the Area Resource File and preexisting measures of regulatory stringency (Chapko

Table 1.2. Major Concepts and Data Sources for the Study.

Major Concepts	Data Sources
Environmental munificence and hostility	Area Resource File; zip code tape; Intergovernmental Health Policy Project; legislative updates
Strategic orientation, strategic change, and strategic comfort zone	Strategic planning survey questionnaire, 1984 and 1987 (see Resource A)
Services diversification, profitability, and charity care	Corporate office interviews (see Resource B); scope of services questionnaire (available on request)
Management processes: strategic planning and control	Strategic planning survey questionnaire, 1987; corporate office interviews
Hospital costs, productivity, profitability, and uncompensated care	American Hospital Association data tapes, 1983, 1985; system-furnished audited cost reports; Medicare cost reports
Patient outcomes	Health Care Financing Administration data files, 1983–84

and others, 1984; Shortell, Morrisey, and Conrad, 1985). Strategic orientations and changes were identified through a strategic planning survey questionnaire administered in 1984 and 1987; personal interviews in 1984 and 1987; and analysis of archival data involving annual reports, news clippings, and the trade literature. Completed strategic planning questionnaires were received from 94 percent of the hospitals ($N = 525$) in 1984 and 87 percent in 1987 ($N = 487$). Services diversification and profitability data were collected through a scope-of-services questionnaire administered in both 1984 and 1987. Completed questionnaires were received from 96 percent of the hospitals ($N = 550$) in 1984 and 92 percent ($N = 525$) in 1987. Data on management processes involving strategic planning and control activities and relationships were collected through the 1987 strategic planning questionnaire and through the corporate office interviews. Hospital cost, productivity, profitability, and uncompensated care data were obtained directly from audited financial statements (standardized for differences in accounting practices; see Friedman and Shortell, 1988), and further checked against American Hospital Association data, Medicare cost reports, and selected state health facility data. Data on patient outcome in terms of case mix and severity-adjusted mortality rates for Medicare patients were obtained from the Health Care Financing Administration. Additional data related to hospital accreditation requirements were obtained from the Joint Commission on Accreditation of Health Care Organizations.

The data were collected at points corresponding as close as possible to the time period of the study: 1983–1987. Completely validated data for this time period were available for 370 hospitals, and they served as the focal point of the analysis. Details about measures of the key concepts are highlighted below and also included in the Resources.

Key Measures

Environmental Munificence and Hostility. We measured two dimensions of each hospital's local environment: *munificence* (see Dess and Beard, 1984; Rasheed and Prescott, 1987) and *hostility* (see Aldrich, 1979). Munificence, or favorable market demands, includes resources to purchase health care services (for example, per capita income adjusted for the manufacturing wage index, poverty rate per 1,000 population, median home value, and education) and resources to provide care, or favorable resource supply (for example, number of physicians per capita, central-city location, and the percentage of white-collar and health professionals in the labor force).

Hostility includes both competition and regulation. Competition was measured by the number of competing hospitals in the market area of the study hospitals (using zip code data; Luft, Robinson, Garnick, Maerki, and McPhee, 1987; and determinations by hospital CEOs), the CEOs' perceived intensity of competition (on a 1–5 scale, 1 = low and 5 = high), the presence or absence of competing ambulatory surgery or urgent care centers, the number of HMOs in a hospital's market area, and the percentage of a state's population enrolled in HMOs. The degree of regulation was measured by the stringency of state rate-review programs designed to control operating revenues and certificate-of-need programs designed to control capital expenditures. The stringency measures are based on previous research (Chapko and others, 1984; Shortell, Morrisey, and Conrad, 1985). They include such dimensions as whether the rate-review program was mandatory or voluntary, whether hospitals were required to repay excess revenue, whether department screens were used in reviewing budgets, and whether cross subsidies were allowed by department or payor. For certificate of need, criteria included the dollar threshold levels established for new programs, equipment, and facilities, the extent of penalties for violation, and the number of different kinds of health care organizations (for example, ambulatory surgery centers, outpatient diagnostic centers) covered by the legislation.

Strategic Orientation and Strategic Change. The Miles and Snow (1978) typology of prospectors, defenders, analyzers, and reactors was used to measure each hospital's strategic orientation. Miles and Snow define a *prospector* as an organization that makes relatively frequent changes in and additions to its set of services and markets. It consistently attempts to be first to provide new services or develop new markets, even if some ultimately prove unsuccessful. A prospector responds rapidly to early signals of market needs or opportunities. A *defender* is an organization that offers a relatively stable set of services to defined markets. It is generally not at the forefront of new service or market development. It tends to ignore changes that have no direct impact on current areas of operation and concentrates instead on doing the best job possible in its existing arena. It emphasizes internal technical efficiency. An *analyzer* maintains a relatively stable base of services, as does a defender, while at the same time developing selected, promising new services and markets, as does a prospector. The analyzer is seldom first to provide new services or expand into new markets. However, by carefully monitoring the actions of others, analyzers attempt to follow with a more cost-effective or well-conceived service. Finally, a *reactor* is an organization that does not appear to have a consistent response to market changes. At times, the reactor will make no change unless forced to by external events; at other times, it will move into new fields only after considerable evidence of potential success; and at still other times, it will be an early entrant into new fields of opportunity. Overall, it appears to lack a coherent strategy.

These definitions reflect the organization's orientation to the marketplace, or what Miles and Snow term the *entrepreneurial problem.* But the typology also addresses two other problems that organizations must resolve: the engineering and the administrative problems. The engineering problem deals with the production and distribution of goods and services. Prospectors need to maintain as much flexibility as possible in their production process and not become overly wedded to existing technologies. Defenders tend to emphasize a single cost-efficient technology and strive to make continuous improvements in it. Analyzers must have both stable and flexible components, with emphasis given to a strong applied research group. Reactors are difficult to categorize on any of these dimensions.

The administrative problem addresses issues of organizational control. The prospector's challenge lies in facilitating and coordinating numerous and diverse activities. This requires extensive market research, broad-based rather than intensive planning, decentralized control, and more complex coordination and conflict management. Defenders emphasize strict control to maximize efficiency. They have more limited environmental scanning, intensive cost-oriented planning, centralized control, and relatively simple coordination and conflict-management mechanisms. Analyzers need to deal with both stable and dynamic aspects of their operation. They emphasize marketing and applied research, coordination between marketing and production, a moderately centralized control system, and very complex and expensive coordination mechanisms. Again, reactors are difficult to designate because of their lack of a consistent strategic orientation.

As the people most knowledgeable about the hospitals' strategic plans, the CEOs were asked to place their hospitals on a seven-point scale in which response categories 1 and 2 represented defender positions; categories 3, 4, and 5 were analyzers; 6 and 7 were prospectors; and the residual "off-scale" category represented the reactors (see Resource A). In some analyses the collapsed categories were used, and in others the entire scale (from 1 to 7) was used. For both 1984 and 1987 questionnaires, the CEOs were asked to respond in terms of their current situation, two years earlier, and two years hence. This permitted us to assess changes in strategic orientation over time and to compare intended and realized strategies (see Mintzberg, 1978).

The CEO measures were validated in both 1984 and 1987 using data on the number of diversified services offered, the number of new services initiated in the most recent three years, the number of new services planned for the future, and the degree of emphasis given to new service and new market development strategies (Zajac and Shortell, 1989). We expected that prospectors would score highest on each of these measures, defenders lowest, and analyzers in between. As shown in Table 1.3, our predictions were largely confirmed. Test-retest reliability conducted on a subsample of nineteen CEOs across the eight systems indicated agreement within one point of the seven-point scale (defender to prospector) in 71 percent of the cases. Thus, considerable confidence can be placed in the measures of strategic orientation.

Table 1.3. Miles and Snow Typology:
Tests of Validity (One-Way Analysis of Variance).

	1984	1987
1. Number of diversified services offered (bed size adjusted)		
Prospectors	8.2	10.0
Analyzers	7.2	9.3
Defenders	5.7	7.9
	$F = 2.65; p \leq .07$	$F = 2.66; p \leq .07$
2. Number of new services offered in past three years		
Prospectors	3.1	4.2
Analyzers	2.7	3.9
Defenders	1.5	3.4
	$F = 3.38; p \leq .03$	$F = .93; p \leq .39$
3. Number of new services planned		
Prospectors	3.0	1.6
Analyzers	2.0	1.1
Defenders	1.7	.7
	$F = 4.19; p \leq .016$	$F = 3.12; p \leq .045$
4. Emphasis given to new service and new market development activities (diversification)		
Prospectors	46.5[a]	79.0[b]
Analyzers	37.5	72.5
Defenders	26.4	59.4
	$F = 21.7; p \leq .001$	$F = 6.99; p \leq .001$

[a] 0 to 100 points.
[b] 0 to 200 points.

Strategic Comfort Zone. The collapsed categories of the strategic orientation continuum were used in measuring each hospital's strategic comfort zone. (As discussed further in Chapter Two, a *strategic comfort zone* is the level of confidence an organization has in switching from one strategy to another. We suggest that most organizations will switch to strategies that are not radically different from their current strategy.) Prospectors that remained prospectors, prospectors that became analyzers, analyzers that remained analyzers, analyzers that became prospectors, analyzers that became defenders, defenders that remained defenders, defenders that became analyzers, reactors that remained reactors, and reactors that became analyzers were all defined as being *within* their strategic comfort zone. Prospectors that became defenders or reactors, analyzers that became reactors, defenders that became prospectors or reactors, and reactors that became prospectors or defenders were all defined as operating *outside* their strategic comfort zone. The underlying assumption behind these classifications was that an organization that switched farther than the closest adjacent category was extending itself beyond its capabilities and experiences.

The major exception was the reactor category, which was viewed as having some characteristics of both a prospector and a defender domain, similar to an analyzer. Thus, a reactor attempting to become a focused analyzer was considered a more comfortable strategic state than a reactor attempting to become a "pure" prospector or defender. In addition, any organization falling into the reactor category from any of the other strategic states was defined as operating outside its comfort zone.

The assumptions underlying these classifications are consistent with the characteristics of the four strategic orientations discussed further in Chapter Two. For example, an organization with a defender strategy — which is difficult to reverse — would have many more problems trying to make the jump to a prospector strategy, which is characterized by high diversity of products and markets, than it would switching to an analyzer strategy, which attempts to balance current products and markets with more modest new-product undertakings. The extent to which the strategic comfort zone concept provides insights into the process of strategic adaptation is considered in Part Two, Chapters Five through Nine.

Services Diversification and Profitability. The extent of diversification activities was measured at two points through a scope-of-services questionnaire involving thirty-four out-of-hospital services. These included outpatient services (for example, outpatient chemotherapy and radiation therapy, urgent care centers); geriatric services (for example, geriatric day care, home-delivered meals to seniors); outpatient diagnostic services (for example, computerized tomography, or CT, scans; magnetic resonance imaging, which provides high-resolution images of internal organs and body structures); outpatient health promotion services (for example, health screening, fitness centers); and home health and extended care services (for example, durable medical equipment, in-home skilled nursing). The degree of charity care offered and the profitability of each service (operating revenues in excess of operating costs) were also collected.

Management Processes: Strategic Planning and Control.
We also examined the relationship of the corporate or regional office and the individual hospital units in strategic planning and control activities. The extent to which these activities were centralized was measured in three ways. First, we determined the degree of involvement of each group (corporate office, regional office, hospital CEO, hospital board, hospital management, and physician leaders) in initiating, formulating, and giving final approval of strategic plans (see Resource A). This is referred to as the *overall centralization of strategic planning.* Second, we determined which group (corporate office, regional office, or individual hospital) was primarily responsible for specific strategic planning tasks, such as environmental assessment, competitive analysis, market research, and business plan development (see Resource A). This was called *centralization of specific strategic planning functions.*

Third, we measured the degree to which each group had authority to make decisions involving twelve items, ranging from choosing a marketing plan for a new outpatient service at an individual hospital, to acquiring a new hospital, to appointing an individual hospital CEO (see Resource A). This was called *centralization of decision making.* These decisions were also subdivided into those involving strategic content (for example, buying a new hospital, deciding to add ambulatory surgery) versus those involving strategic implementation (for example, determining individual hospital budget levels and deciding to involve more physicians in individual hospital governance).

We also assessed the perceived quality or effectiveness of the strategic planning and control system (see Resource A). On the basis of factor analysis and the existing literature (Ramanujam and Venkatraman, 1987), we included five relevant dimensions: (1) the perceived quality of information systems, (2) the perceived quality of implementation processes, (3) the perceived effectiveness of market research, (4) the perceived quality of involvement of key stakeholders such as board members and physicians, and (5) the perceived quality of strategic planning assistance provided by corporate and/or regional offices.

In addition, we constructed a measure of the overall organizational structure of the corporate system, based on an analysis of organization charts. Three readers associated with the study evaluated each position as to whether it was a functional or a divisional orientation. The few differences among the readers were clarified through phone calls with corporate executives. Examples of functional areas of responsibility include finance, planning and business development, human resources, and marketing. Examples of divisional organization included vice-president positions created for geographical areas or vice-presidents of acute care, psychiatric, and rehabilitation hospitals. In these cases, functional responsibilities were typically included under each divisional head. On the basis of these distinctions, a ratio of functional to divisional organization was constructed for each system. The influence of this variable on the corporate office–individual hospital relationship is discussed further in Chapter Four.

Cost Containment and Financial Viability. The extent to which each hospital engaged in twenty-three specific cost-containment practices was also measured (see Resource A). On the basis of factor analysis, these items clustered into three scales, involving (1) staff reductions, (2) program or service consolidations, and (3) productivity and efficiency improvements. An overall cost-containment scale based on all twenty-three items was also used.

Factors influencing the continued viability of each hospital were also assessed (see Resource A). These items factored into five scales involving (1) economic survivability, (2) maintaining access to capital and new technology, (3) the importance of maintaining a high-quality image, (4) the importance of diversification, and (5) the importance of maintaining a strong marketing orientation.

Performance. The multiple performance measures are divided into two groups: those associated with "doing good" and those involved with "doing well." The "doing good" measures recognize the hospital's commitment to its community, particularly in regard to the provision of care to the poor and those with less ability to pay for their care. The "doing well" measures reflect the hospital's need for fiscal solvency. "Doing good" measures include (1) bad debt and charity care as a percentage of outpatient revenue, (2) Medicaid revenue as a percentage of total outpatient revenue, (3) uncompensated care (bad debt plus charity care) as a percentage of total hospital revenue, (4) the percentage of diversified services for which no charity care is provided, (5) the number of unprofitable services offered, based on a list of services that were essentially unprofitable for the majority of hospitals in the study (see Resource D), (6) whether the hospital had a formally organized quality assurance department (see question 9a, Resource A), (7) the quality assurance budget per admission (see question 9b, Resource A), (8) the severity-adjusted death rate for sixteen conditions (see Resource C), and (9) the number of contingency recommendations in the areas of medical staff, quality assurance, medical records, and nursing care plans made by the Joint Commission on Accreditation of Health Care Organizations (a contingency recommendation means that the hospital is not fully compliant with quality standards).

The "doing well" measures include (1) operating margin as a percentage of net revenue, (2) after-tax net income as a percentage of total income, (3) the percentage of diversified services that are profitable, (4) the percentage of fifteen specific services that are profitable (see Resource A), (5) market share across the fifteen services, adjusted for number of competitors (see Resource A), (6) the percentage of high-share and high-growth services (see Resource A), (7) the cost per adjusted admission, and (8) admissions per full-time–equivalent employee.

Given the diversity of strategic orientations examined, we considered it necessary to develop multiple performance measures that would be sensitive to the various orientations. Thus, we included measures such as the profitability of specific service lines and the profitability of diversification activities as well as more traditional measures, such as overall profitability and costs. This multifaceted approach helps to provide a more comprehensive and realistic assessment of the impact of specific strategic changes (see Fahey and Christensen, 1986; Chakravarthy, 1986).

The Ownership Issue

The hospital industry has both for-profit and not-for-profit ownership forms. These differences have been of considerable interest (Yoder, 1986; Hansmann, 1980). Critics of investor-owned hospitals contend that they neglect care of the poor and medically indigent in their pursuit of profits (Lewin, Eckels, and Miller, 1988; Schlesinger and Dorwart, 1984). Critics of not-for-profit hospitals maintain that they are inefficiently managed (Herzlinger and Krasker, 1987). Not-for-profit hospitals have also come under scrutiny for the amount of charity care provided in relation to their tax-exempt not-for-profit status (Seay and Sigmond, 1989).

From a strategic perspective, the most important distinctions between the two forms relate to the nondistribution constraint in not-for-profit hospitals (that is, they cannot distribute profits in any form to outside parties) and the differences in purposes and mission (for discussion of the reasons for the coexistence of for-profit and not-for-profit hospitals, see Yoder, 1986; Hansmann, 1980). The fact that not-for-profit hospitals are not subject to the discipline of Wall Street and the expectations of stockholders suggests that they may be less inclined to pursue profit-maximizing strategies and less aggressive in achieving low-cost production of services. At the same time, because their missions — education, community outreach, and the provision of charity care — have traditionally been defined more broadly, they might be expected to be more diversified. Further, because not-for-profit hospitals do not need to justify growth plans to stockholders or focus exclusively on short-run objectives, they may be able to take a longer view in developing their strategies and to stay with current strategies for a longer period (Gray, forthcoming).

Not-for-profit hospitals can be further differentiated according to whether they are church-affiliated or secular. Through the historical mission of service to the poor, church-affiliated hospitals might be expected to place greater emphasis on community outreach and provision of charity care than secular not-for-profit hospitals.

Others argue that the revolutionary changes occurring within the health care industry are causing these distinctions to blur (Institute of Medicine, 1986). Given the incentive to contain costs and growing competition within the industry, all hospitals — regardless of ownership form — must pay greater attention to bottom-line considerations. All hospitals must pursue strategies to both contain costs and seek additional revenue sources. Whether the environmental forces are driving both types of hospitals closer together in their strategic orientation and operating philosophy is ultimately an empirical question, which this book partially addresses. We suggest that ownership form is a proxy for hospital mission and that it may condition the *way* hospitals respond, if not the actual content of response.

Other Measures

Other measures were used in various analyses to control for differences in hospital characteristics and patient mix. These included hospital bed size, location, presence of an approved medical residency program, an index of hospital case mix developed by the Health Care Financing Administration to measure the severity of patient mix, the percentage of patient days involving use of intensive care beds, the number of years the hospital has been a system member, the age of the main physical building of the hospital, the total number of inpatient services and high-technology services offered by the hospital, and the ratio of registered nurses to full-time–equivalent personnel.

The Qualitative Approach

In addition to the data collected through questionnaires, existing data tapes, and source documents, we conducted 112 in-depth face-to-face interviews with corporate decision makers and staff in 1984–85 and 37 followup telephone interviews in 1987. In 1984, we interviewed each system's chief executive officer, chairman of the board, chief operating officer of the system's acute care hospitals, and individuals responsible for strategic planning, finance, marketing, human resources, information systems, development, and government relations. In 1987, we conducted interviews with the chief operating officer of each system's acute care hospitals and individuals responsible for strategic planning, finance, marketing, and human resources.

In both years, these individuals were asked to describe their system's mission, goals, philosophy, strengths and weaknesses, principal strategies, and issues involved in implementing their strategies. Additional questions were asked specific to each executive's responsibilities and expertise in planning, finance, marketing, and human resources. (See Resource B for sample interview protocols.)

The insights derived from these interviews complemented the quantitatively based measures and helped to provide a fuller understanding of the strategic adaptation process. They also facilitated a more holistic understanding of each system's strategies and of the relationship between the corporate office and individual hospital units. By treating each system as a whole, we could consider the relationship among the different quantitatively measured variables in combination with each other (see Ragin, 1987). The interviews also served as a rich source of specific examples, quotes, and "mini-cases" illustrating the major findings and lessons.

Summary

The profound changes taking place in the hospital industry triggered by the introduction of Medicare Prospective Payment System in 1983 provide a rich setting for examining the processes associated with strategic adaptation. By selecting eight leading hospital systems differing by ownership, size, geographical location, and related variables, it is possible to assess a wide range of potential responses to these changes. By following the eight systems and their hospitals over a four-year period (1983–1987), we have an opportunity to document the dynamics associated with the adaptation process. Using a combination of publicly available data, original questionnaires, and personal interviews provides an opportunity both to quantify the degree of strategic adaptation and its effects on performance and to obtain a deeper understanding of the underlying processes involved. The Miles and Snow typology of prospectors, defenders, analyzers, and reactors is used to characterize hospital strategies, and the associated measures are shown to be valid representations. Given this background, a model of the strategic adaptation process that served as a framework for the study is presented in Chapter Two.

2

Understanding How Hospitals Respond to Change: A Model of Strategic Adaptation

Strategic adaptation is the process by which an organization abandons its current core strategies for another set that it believes will provide a better position for continued viability. Although this book addresses strategic adaptation in the hospital industry, we develop a model of the process that we believe is useful to executives in any industry. In this sense, the hospital industry serves as a setting for understanding how managers go about initiating and implementing strategic change, particularly when faced with major environmental jolts (see Meyer, 1982).

Can organizations change in significant ways? Can managers recognize the need to change and then manage the implementation process successfully? On these questions, theorists and practitioners differ. Some argue that organizations are severely constrained in their ability to change (Aldrich, 1979; Quinn, 1980; Hannan and Freeman, 1984). Certain inertial forces tend to preserve the status quo: investments in current goals, policies, people, technology, structures, and reward systems. These are costly to change, not only financially but psychically as well. People's careers and identities are often linked to

27

preserving the status quo, particularly when the organization has enjoyed past success and has been rewarded for it. Sometimes just two or three key leaders with significant ego investment in preserving current directions are sufficient to create inertia. Frequently, this occurs where the owners are also the managers or where the top executive team has long tenure. Even when these factors are not present, the simple fear of the unknown may be enough to retard significant change. It is more comfortable to stay with the tried and familiar, even when they appear to be serving the organization poorly, than to venture into uncharted waters that might bring total doom.

Others argue that organizations can and do make significant change in response to their environment and to internal imperatives (Chandler, 1962; Child, 1972; Lawrence and Lorsch, 1967; Pfeffer and Salancik, 1978; Schendel and Hofer, 1979; Singh, Tucker, and House, 1986). They argue that managers play a key role in assessing environmental shifts and altering the organization's strategy and structure to meet the associated demands. Managers can also play a key role in anticipating future environmental shifts and in developing sufficient organizational slack (excess resources) to meet future demands. Further, managers can play an important role in developing collective strategies with other organizations to gain greater influence and control over environmental forces (Astley and Fombrun, 1983; Fombrun and Zajac, 1987; Jarillo, 1988; Nielsen, 1988).

As is often the case, neither perspective—inertia or strategic choice—provides a complete understanding. Both provide useful insights on the issue of strategic adaptation (Astley and Van de Ven, 1983; Hrebiniak and Joyce, 1985; Tushman and Romanelli, 1985; Hambrick and Finkelstein, 1987). The inertial school correctly notes that environmental forces pose some very important constraints that limit the amount of change possible and frame the boundaries and context of change. The strategic choice school reminds us that organizations are not lifeless black boxes, but collections of people who develop and implement strategies to promote organizational survival and growth. Every organization has some degree of flexibility and strives to expand its ability to control its own destiny. There is a strong argument for appreciating both perspectives.

What is largely missing, however, is the specification of the conditions and circumstances under which significant change occurs (Boeker, 1988; Child and Kieser, 1981; Grant, 1988). Toward this end, we briefly summarize what is known about significant strategic change and develop a model—which guides this book—for understanding the conditions and circumstances that facilitate or impede the adaptive process.

We define strategy as "the plans and activities developed by an organization in pursuit of its goals and objectives, particularly in regard to positioning itself to meet external demands relative to its competition" (Shortell, Morrison, and Robbins, 1985, p. 220). Any changes in plans and activities that have implications for the organization's position vis-à-vis its environment and its competition are, therefore, within the scope of strategic adaptation. The primary focus of this book is on change in an organization's basic strategic orientation in relation to the external environment. Attention is given to both the content and process dimensions of the change.

Existing Research

Most of the existing literature suggests that strategic change occurs infrequently but increases with significant environmental shifts (Ginsberg and Grant, 1985; Pettigrew, 1987). Even when basic strategic orientations persist, there is evidence that executive leaders play a key role in modifying the basic orientation to fit changes in the environment (Miles and Cameron, 1982).

Among more recent work, Thompson, Pettigrew, and Rubashow (1985), in a study of 190 British manufacturing companies, found that 33 percent of 1,000 middle- and senior-level executives reported "radical" strategic changes occurring since 1979 and an additional 56 percent acknowledged at least some degree of change; only 10 percent reported little or no change. Similar findings were reported in a recent study of fifteen U.S. manufacturing firms in which new-product development was seen as the primary indicator of a major strategic shift (Severance and Passino, 1986). This shift was accompanied by significant managerial turnover, substantial investment in plant equipment and research and development, and upgraded control systems. At the same time, formal strategic planning processes were downplayed, and greater attention was given to informal processes involving vision creation and team building.

A recent reanalysis of Rumelt's (1974) data involving 414 firms indicated that 18 percent had engaged in a major strategic reorientation, 20 percent had experienced a significant organizational reorientation, and 16 percent had experienced both. The remaining 46 percent had only fine tuned existing strategies and policies (Bhambri and Greiner, 1987).

A study of sixteen multinational companies undertaking significant change found that while strategic adaptation was possible, it was also fraught with considerable difficulty (Doz and Prahalad, 1987). Successful adaptation was possible in only eight firms, was occurring very slowly in two others, and had essentially failed in the remaining six. A key variable differentiating the successful from the unsuccessful appeared to be the ability of a single person to obtain a leadership position and to articulate a new vision that organizational members accepted.

Two studies provide some initial estimates of the frequency of strategic changes in the hospital industry. A study of ninety Texas hospitals in four metropolitan areas revealed that 30 percent had changed strategies from a placid environmental period (1976 to 1980) to the more turbulent environment experienced from 1981 through 1985 (Ginn and McDaniel, 1987). In a study precursor to that reported in this book, Zajac and Shortell (1989) found that 54 percent of hospitals belonging to eight hospital systems had changed strategies between 1982 and 1984.

While these studies provide evidence for the existence of strategic change, few investigators have explored the implications for performance. An exception is the work of Smith and Grimm (1987), who found that firms that changed their strategies when faced with deregulation in the railroad industry outperformed those who did not.

However, documenting the occurrence of strategic change fails to explain why some organizations change while others do not, particularly organizations operating in the same industry and presumably facing similar environmental forces. On the basis of the present study, we suggest that the answer lies in a model of strategic adaptation that focuses on factors associated with perceiving the *need* for change and factors associated with the *ability* to change. The organization's current strategy plays a key role in this process (Zajac and Shortell, 1989).

The Model

Any model of strategic adaptation must address the questions of whether, why, what, and how change occurs. Some organizations appear to change while others do not, even when faced with similar environmental conditions. Why is this so? Second, what is it that changes? What is the content of the change? Finally, how does it occur? How is it brought about? We are also interested in a further question: what is the impact of the change?

These questions embrace linear, adaptive, and interpretive perspectives of strategic change (Ginsberg and Grant, 1985). They recognize that strategies involve decisions and actions designed to achieve organizational goals (the linear model); that they also involve patterns of choices designed to align the organization with its environment (the adaptive model); and that it is a process in which leaders attempt to give meaning and legitimacy to those actions (the interpretive model).

The model of strategic adaptation that addresses these questions is shown in Figure 2.1. Its dimensions are described under three groupings: the perceived need to change, the perceived ability to change, and managing the change process.

Perceived Need to Change

The ability of executives to recognize the need for change is the starting point of the model. This recognition is likely to be a function of both the environment facing the organization

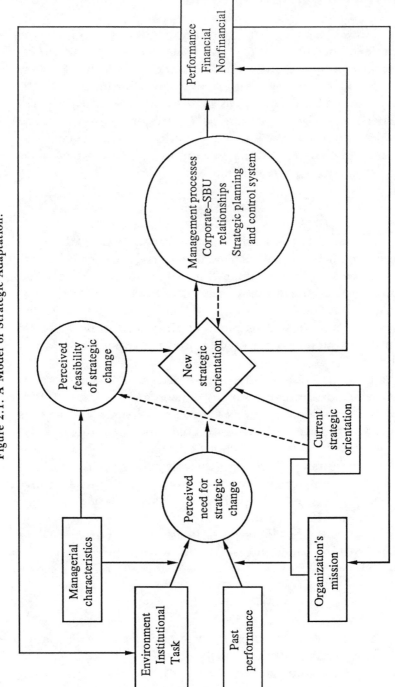

Figure 2.1. A Model of Strategic Adaptation.

and its performance in that environment. Consideration of these factors will also be influenced by characteristics of the managers themselves, the organization's mission, and its current strategic orientation.

Environment. Two important components are the institutional environment and the task environment. The *institutional environment* includes the larger political economy within which organizations function, including societal norms and expectations, industrial policy, degree of regulation, and related factors (DiMaggio and Powell, 1983; Lenz and Engledow, 1986; Scott, 1987). The *task environment* refers to more immediate factors that may influence performance, such as local market structure, degree of competition, resource availability, and the bargaining power of suppliers and buyers (Porter, 1980; Aldrich, 1979; Dess and Beard, 1984). While greater attention has been given to the task environment, changes in either one or both can affect managers' perception of the need for strategic change.

Institutional examples include changes in tax laws, foreign trade import and export policies, and large-scale demographic shifts in the population. Task environment examples include increases or decreases in competition, introduction of new technologies, and changes in union contracts. Any one change or combination may cause the organization to change its current strategies, if the change is considered important to the organization's mission and goals.

Past Performance. The other primary source of the perceived need for change is the organization's evaluation of its past performance in relation to either its own, competitors', or industrywide standards. Identifying such performance gaps can be an important motivator for strategic change (Boeker, 1988). The extent to which past performance has generated slack resources (that is, profits that can be used to hire additional staff or for investments in new products and services) can also influence the likelihood of change (Cheng and Kesner, 1988).

Managerial Characteristics. Environmental assessment and performance evaluation, however, are done most frequently by an organization's top management. Thus, their perception of changes and gaps, and what these mean for the organization, are an important part of the process (Dutton and Duncan, 1987; Pfeffer and Salancik, 1978; Weick, 1979). These in turn will be influenced by characteristics of these managers (Hambrick and Mason, 1984; Hambrick and Finkelstein, 1987; Hambrick, 1988). For example, a top management team with a primarily marketing background may be more sensitive to changes in market structure and performance data related to market share than a team with financial or production backgrounds, who may be more sensitive to changes in traditional financial performance indicators or tax and legal changes. Individuals pay selective attention to the environment according to interests and selectively interpret the information they receive.

Mission. Selective perception and interpretation of the environment also take place within the context of the organization's mission and current strategy, two additional factors that can influence the perceived need for strategic change. Top executives may perceive the organization's mission differently. One executive may perceive a change in international monetary policies as a significant threat because she views the company as a developing leader in international business. A second executive may view the same change as having little impact because he does not believe that international business is central to the company's mission.

Characteristics of the mission itself may play a role. Organizations with broad missions may be better able to adapt to environmental shifts. For example, a more diversified company may be better able to withstand an environmental threat to one of its business lines than a company that has concentrated most of its business in that single area. Some missions are also more flexible. Thus, a hospital with no specific commitment to serve the poor may have more strategic flexibility than a hospital whose basic mission includes serving the poor. Faced with reductions in third-party payment, the first hospital may have more alternatives than the second, which cannot abandon its basic mission without destroying its identity as an organization.

Current Strategic Orientation. Complex organizations generally do not have a single strategy but rather have multiple strategies reflecting different stakeholders, interests, business units, markets, competitive threats, and related factors. Nonetheless, these different strategies usually have a common thread or focus. We refer to this common focus as the organization's overall *strategic orientation,* or what others have termed "generic strategy" (Porter, 1980).

There are several typologies and taxonomies of generic strategies, including Miles and Snow's (1978) prospectors, analyzers, defenders, and reactors; Porter's (1980) cost leadership versus differentiation; and Miller and Friesen's (1984) adaptive, dominant, giant, conglomerate, and niche innovator. As noted in Chapter One, we chose Miles and Snow's typology because of its comprehensiveness and the evolving stream of research it has generated, including research on the hospital industry (Ginn and McDaniel, 1987; Luke and Begun, 1988; Zajac and Shortell, 1989; Keats, Conant, and Mokwa, 1988).

An important issue to consider is the extent to which an organization's *current* strategy facilitates or impedes strategic change. For example, broadly conceived, flexible strategies may reduce the need for significant change. Whatever change is required can be handled within the context of the current strategic orientation. Strategic refinement or modification may be needed, but not marked change. Thus, in the face of increased competition and regulatory pressures, a firm with some experience in diversification may be able to expand its diversification activities with relative ease. In contrast, the more narrow a firm's strategy, the more difficult it will be to initiate change. The perceived need for change may be high, but the perceived feasibility of making the change may be low. In brief, some strategies may be more intransigent than others.

Given the above, organizations will generally tend to make changes closely related to their current strategies. We suggest that each organization has a strategic comfort zone beyond which it does not wish to venture. This zone represents that area where organizational members both desire and feel able to adapt, given current mission and values, distinctive competencies, technology, product and market mix, structure, management procedures and systems, and available human and financial resources. This concept recognizes and reconciles both the structural inertia and the strategic choice schools discussed earlier: changes are made (strategic choice), but within certain boundaries of what the organization and its members feel comfortable with (structural inertia). Thus, an organization is likely to move from its base business to related diversification rather than unrelated diversification (Rumelt, 1974); from a defender strategy (emphasizing current products and services) to an analyzer strategy (representing some experimentation with new products and services but only after others have tried them first) rather than from a defender strategy to a prospector strategy (constantly developing new products and services; Miles and Snow, 1978); and from a cost leadership strategy to a focused differentiation strategy (based on a few products or characteristics) rather than across-the-board differentiation (Porter, 1985).

These changes, while within the organization's strategic comfort zone, may still be pervasive. They may involve the realignment of many structure and process variables, as Miller and Friesen (1984) suggest in their quantum view of organizations. But by selecting new strategies that are more related to current strategies, organizations can minimize the costs of realignment: the disruption of current policies and practices, norms on how things are done, reward systems and career ladders, and investments in new technology and facilities (Quinn, 1980; Cook, Shortell, Conrad, and Morrisey, 1983; Smart and Vertinsky, 1984). At the same time, organizations facing turbulent environments require leadership that continually attempts to expand the comfort zone.

Miles and Cameron (1982) provide some support for the comfort zone idea. They found that acquisitions made by the big six tobacco companies that were closely related to the distinctive competencies of the companies were more successful than those that were not. To go beyond the comfort zone of current capabilities required strong leaders who expanded the competency base through both outside recruitment and internal development.

The strategic comfort zone concept permits making predictions about the direction of strategic change. We believe that strategic changes will be made within categories that are adjacent on the Miles and Snow continuum (see Figure 2.2), with reactors being a special case (see discussion in Chapter One).

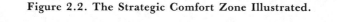

Figure 2.2. The Strategic Comfort Zone Illustrated.

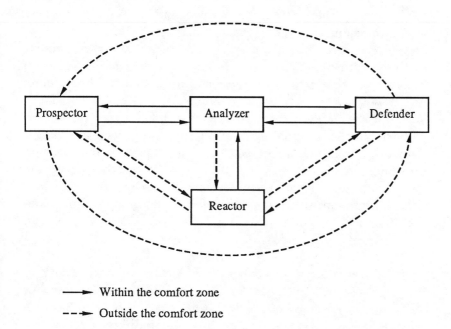

⟶ Within the comfort zone

--⟶ Outside the comfort zone

Thus, to the extent that defenders change at all, they will change to analyzers but not to prospectors, and prospectors will change to analyzers but not to defenders. Reactors, since they sometimes behave as prospectors and sometimes like defenders, could go in either direction but most realistically will become analyzers, since analyzers embody both prospector and defender characteristics but on a more consistent and stable basis than reactors. The strategic comfort zone relationships are summarized in Figure 2.2.

Perceived Feasibility of Strategic Change

Feasibility will be influenced by the characteristics and perceptions of top management and by the content of current strategies. Perceived feasibility, in turn, will influence whether a new strategic orientation is adopted and its content.

Managerial Characteristics. Executives with backgrounds in marketing, sales, research and development, or planning may be more oriented to change than those with production, operations, or finance backgrounds. The former, having dealt more with the external environment, may place greater emphasis on the need to change and give less emphasis to or underestimate the feasibility of making the changes. The latter group, more internally oriented, may exaggerate the difficulties involved and play down the external forces that signal the need to change. Different preferences for risk also play a part in the decision to switch strategies. Also, executives who have been with the organization longer may see less need to change. In fact, a new CEO and management team are often brought in to initiate and implement a major strategic reorientation (Peters and Tseng, 1983; Hambrick, 1985).

Current Strategic Orientation. An organization's current strategy also influences the feasibility of strategic change. For example, if management believes the current strategy has produced a high degree of organizational capability, experience, and resources (that is, slack), then it will be more confident about the organization's ability to implement a new strategy. In contrast, if leaders view the current strategy as somewhat restrictive and the organization's resources and capabilities are very specific to the current strategy, they will be less confident.

An organization's strategic orientation embodies more than the content of the strategy itself. It also contains a set of resources, technologies, skills, norms, behaviors, rewards, and, most significantly, people that have identified with and have lived that strategy. This "strategic web" will influence both the feasibility of strategic change and the content of the new strategic orientation.

New Strategy Selection. Whether a new strategic orientation will be adopted also depends on the characteristics of the available options. Four characteristics are particularly important: (1) complexity, (2) divisibility, (3) reversibility, and (4) diversity. These and related characteristics have been considered in the innovation literature (Pearson, 1988; Walton, 1987; Zaltman, Duncan, and Holbek, 1973) but not by students of strategic adaptation.

Complexity refers to the number and difficulty of the components of the new strategy. For example, a strategy that involves both reducing costs to achieve operating efficiencies and attempting to diversify into new products or markets is difficult to accomplish. *Divisibility* involves the degree to which the new strategy can be subdivided into manageable components. For example, a strategy that can be phased in over time and in incremental steps would be considered divisible. *Reversibility* refers to the extent to which the strategy or its subcomponents can be deleted if they prove problematic without causing the organization much loss in cost, time, or productivity. For example, strategies involving high sunk costs are difficult to reverse and may lead to escalating commitment (Staw, 1976). *Diversity* involves the degree to which the various strategic components are related. For example, an organization involved in many unrelated diversification activities would score high on diversity.

New strategies are less likely to be successful if complexity is high, divisibility and reversibility are low, and diversity is high. Also, the more they depart from current strategies (lie outside the strategic comfort zone), the more likely they will be perceived as complex, indivisible, irreversible, more diverse, and therefore more difficult to implement. These inherent characteristics will interact with the organization's mission, environmental demands, strategic planning and control systems, skills, and related factors as the organization searches for a sustainable competitive advantage.

Management Processes

The change to a new strategy may have a direct effect on an organization's performance, but performance will also be influenced by the management processes associated with strategy implementation, particularly the relationship between the individual business unit and the corporate office and the quality of the strategic planning and control system. The dashed feedback arrow from management processes to new strategic orientation in Figure 2.1 indicates that management processes can also influence choice of strategy by constraining the choices available. From a strategic content perspective, less optimal strategies may be selected because they are more "doable," given the organization's management processes, than one that may be more optimal on paper but has little chance of being implemented.

Corporate Office–Individual Unit Relationship. In organizations with several business units or divisions, the nature of the relationship between them and the company overall becomes a key variable in attempting to explain unit performance. Several observers have suggested that the multidivisional form (M form) of organization offers superior coordinative advantages for pursuing a diversification strategy compared to the functional organizational or unitary form (U form; Williamson, 1975; Williamson and Ouchi, 1981; Armour and Teece, 1978; Rumelt, 1974). Others have questioned the superiority of the M form even for diversified firms, arguing that success depends on the effectiveness of internal coordination and control strategies within a given organization (Hill and Hoskisson, 1987). We consider the issue on a continuum of functional and divisional organization.

The relationship between the corporate office and individual units has received little attention (for exceptions, see Gupta, 1987, and Govindarajan, 1988). For purposes of understanding strategic change, we suggest that the strategic planning and control process is a key barometer for evaluating this relationship. Relevant aspects include the degree of centralization — of the strategic planning process, specific strategic planning functions, and specific content decisions — and the formality of the process. For example, experienced units operating in familiar business lines may be given more autonomy than newer units or units operating in newly diversified businesses. Similarly, a strategy of related diversification may be associated with greater decentralization than a strategy of unrelated diversification.

Strategic Control System. Strategic control systems are the activities established by the organization to oversee strategy formulation and implementation (Camillus, 1986; Lorange, Scott-Morton, and Ghoshal, 1986; Schendel and Hofer, 1979). Strategic control is different from operational control, which involves job scheduling, production scheduling, statistical quality control, budget variance analysis, and related activities. Strategic control involves both feedforward and feedback (Michael, 1980; Veliyath, 1987). Feedforward processes are concerned primarily with strategy formulation and involve environmental scanning, competitive analysis, assessment of strengths and weaknesses, and market research. Feedback processes are concerned primarily with strategy implementation and outcomes and include monitoring reports, activity reports, performance appraisal, consumer satisfaction studies, and the like. While little is known about the influence of strategic control systems, different types of control systems seem to work better with different types of strategies. For example, organizations pursuing diversification strategies in new markets may require a greater emphasis on feedforward control systems than feedback systems, and the opposite may be true for organizations protecting current markets.

In addition, different demands may be placed on the control system by different organizations operating in different environments. These demands will be highest for organizations operating in dynamic, rapidly changing environments pursuing significant strategic change. The ability of the strategic control system to deal with these changes is an important factor for performance.

Among the specific dimensions of interest are the perceived quality of the organization's information systems, imple-

mentation processes, market research, involvement of key stakeholders, and assistance provided by corporate and regional
offices. The perceived quality of market research and the involvement of key stakeholders are important aspects of feedforward control systems, while the perceived quality of information
systems and implementation processes are key aspects of feedback control. Assistance from corporate and regional offices can
contribute to both feedforward and feedback control.

Prospectors may need to give relatively greater emphasis
to feedforward dimensions (market research and key stakeholder
involvement) than defenders, who give relatively more emphasis
to feedback mechanisms, such as information systems that provide tight planning-budgeting linkages and more formal implementation processes. Analyzers will fall in between the two.
This is because the prospector's emphasis on being first in new
product or market development places great reliance on market
research and the involvement of key people to generate creative
ideas and gather support for new initiatives. Defenders have
less need for such activities and, instead, need a control system
that will tightly monitor technical efficiency and consistently let
the organization know where it stands. The analyzer has need
for a relatively tight formal control system in its stable product
and market domain and a more market research–oriented and
stakeholder involvement–oriented approach in its more active
product and market domain. The reactor, reflecting its lack of
a consistent coherent strategy, will reveal a very diffuse control
pattern across the five dimensions.

In sum, the extent to which a prospector, analyzer, defender, or reactor strategy is successful depends not only on the
"correctness" of the strategic choice, given the environment facing
the organization, but also on the ability to manage the strategy
as suggested by these dimensions.

Performance

The relationship between organization strategy and performance has usually been assessed through economic and financial indicators. These indicators have also been used as a general

measure of organization effectiveness (Goodman, Pennings, and Associates, 1977; Kanter and Brinkerhoff, 1981; Cameron and Whetten, 1983)—sometimes with theoretical justification, sometimes merely because they were readily available.

When evaluating the effectiveness of strategic change, it is particularly important to know what the strategy is intended to achieve (Fahey and Christensen, 1986). While it might be argued that in investor-owned organizations all strategies are intended to affect shareholder value (Rappaport, 1986), the linkage may be long-term and indirect. For example, a strategy to enter a new market to preempt a competitor may contribute to the long-run survivability of the firm even though the new venture loses money the first five years. In contrast, a strategy of vertical integration may show short-run profitability because of economies of scope but have little long-run financial value.

Are these strategies successful or unsuccessful? Are they effective or ineffective? It is not clear that simply associating the strategies with return on investment or sales growth answers these questions. We must carefully separate short-run from long-run effects and carefully choose appropriate measurement points. The further away an intended effect of a strategy, the more difficult it becomes to attribute the effect directly and unequivocally to the strategy.

The issue becomes even more challenging in not-for-profit organizations with multiple objectives that extend beyond profitability. As with investor-owned firms, their basic goal is survival. But the range of stakeholders involved is often more diverse, and they have varying expectations (Freeman, 1984). For example, in nonprofit hospitals, physicians want a technologically modern place to practice medicine; consumers want prompt, safe, courteous treatment; employers want the same for their employees but at as low a cost as possible; and the federal government is most interested in purchasing cost-effective care for its beneficiaries. Various community groups and coalitions have their own sets of demands. Because of these varying constituencies, the strategic issue set (see Dutton and Duncan, 1987) is likely to be quite broad, and the performance measures must match specific strategies. Profitability measures are important, of course, but so are other measures: the amount of uncompensated care provided, the ability to diversify services, the quality of services provided, the ability to satisfy professionals and consumers, and the ability to contain costs. The hospital example can be easily extended to other nonprofit community service organizations. Thus, any model of strategic adaptation that hopes to fit a wide variety of organizations must recognize the diversity of stakeholders involved and include nonfinancial as well as financial measures of performance.

Summary

    Significant environmental change poses a distinct threat to organizations, particularly to those not well positioned to deal with the change. Environmental jolts (Meyer, 1982) representing sudden and significant change are likely to affect the performance of all organizations. To achieve high performance levels, organizations must do three things well: (1) they must interpret the significance of the environmental change in terms of the perceived need for strategic change; (2) they must choose a strategy that appears to be well suited to the new environmental state; and (3) they must be able to execute the new strategy successfully.

    Environmental jolts provide unusually good natural experiments for examining strategic adaptation, because they cause an organization to seriously reexamine its strategic orientation and mission — even if the outcome of that process is to stick with the current strategy. More often, jolts result in at least some organizations changing their strategic orientations. The nature of the jolt may favor one strategic orientation over another. For example, the rapid deregulation that occurred in the banking and airline industries would appear to favor a more prospector-oriented strategic orientation, emphasizing diversification and focusing on new-product and new-market development. In contrast, an expansion of antitrust legislation in other industries would tend to favor a more defender-like orientation, emphasizing staying with the current product or market domain. A jolt that is more difficult to assess — such as the ultimate effect of the October 19, 1987, drop in stock market prices — or one that has a succession of aftershocks may favor a more analyzer-like strategy. This strategy involves covering one's bets with some new-product or new-market experimentation but continuing the commitment to existing products and markets. However, this decision will also be influenced by the organization's immediate local task environment, particularly in terms of the intensity of competition and the availability of resources. Thus, the tendency to lean toward one strategic orientation versus another will also be conditioned by local circumstances.

In the working model of strategic adaptation outlined in Figure 2.1, we argue that changes in the organization's environment or performance gaps influence the perceived need for strategic change, which, along with the perceived feasibility of enacting the change, influences the adoption of new strategies. The effect of these strategies on performance will depend largely on the organization's management processes involving both the relationship between corporate office and individual business unit and the nature of the organization's strategic planning and control system. The perceived need for change will also be influenced by characteristics of the top management team as they read the environment, evaluate past performance, and assess the organization's capabilities. The perceived need for change will also be affected in important ways by the organization's mission and current strategies. Given the impetus for change, the type of new strategies adopted will be a function of current strategies and the perceived feasibility of implementing a different strategy. Finally, the model reflects the dynamic process of strategic adaptation; feedback arrows suggest that performance at a given point exerts an impact on the organization's environment, mission, and future strategies.

Changes within an organization's strategic comfort zone are more likely to be adopted and implemented than changes outside the zone. The size and nature of the comfort zone are determined by current mission and strategies, management processes, and top manager's perception of the degree of change required.

3

Strategic Change,
Corporate Goals,
and Management Processes

Profiles of the Eight Systems

American Medical International. American Medical International (AMI) is an investor-owned system founded in the late 1960s. By the early 1980s it had become one of the more aggressive independent-minded investor-owned systems. Its 1984 annual report described the system as "leading the trends." In the early 1980s, it rapidly diversified into urgent care centers, ambulatory surgery centers, substance abuse centers, HMOs, and other activities. When the financial effects of the new competitive and regulatory environment hit the industry, AMI's bottom line, like those of other systems, was deeply affected. The system lost $97 million in 1986.

By 1986, AMI's diversification efforts could no longer be sustained. With the assistance of an outside consulting firm, AMI divested most of its nonhospital activities and recommitted itself to the acute care hospital business. To provide further focus, the system reduced its international operations and sold thirty-six of its hospitals through an employee stock ownership plan. During this period of uncertainty and structural change, AMI also fought off several outside acquisition bids until being acquired by IMA Holdings Corporation in July of 1989.

Among all the systems, AMI experienced the most turnover in the corporate CEO position. At present, it is the only system to be working with its third CEO. The owner-founder CEO relinquished the reins in 1986 to an insider executive who had been groomed for the position for several years. This individual was the major force behind the corporation's strategic reorientation efforts described above. These efforts were, in fact, beginning to pay off, resulting in a $111 million profit in 1987 and faring equally well in 1988. But in mid-1988, a small but influential group of investor board members grew impatient with the pace of change and called for the CEO's resignation. The founder CEO temporarily returned until a permanent successor was found. Meanwhile, AMI is placing more emphasis on local control of hospitals in markets where they have a reasonable chance of enhancing market share. They have also instituted an incentive pay system linked to achieving patient satisfaction and clinical indicator targets. AMI is also giving greater attention to physician participation in management and strategic planning throughout the system.

Hospital Corporation of America. Hospital Corporation of America (HCA) began as a family-owned service business in the late 1960s. It is a second-generation system run by the son of the founding owner; both are physicians. It grew rapidly into a major hospital company projecting a "blue chip, conservative, physician friendly" image. It also recruited an expert influential outside board, many of whose members are from industries outside of health care. It has historically been a highly decentralized organization, and this, combined with its size, has created some challenges in implementing rapid changes.

HCA, too, explored diversification efforts, but more cautiously than AMI. A brief attempt to develop its own insurance company was quickly scuttled after local Blue Cross and Blue Shield plans threatened to drop HCA hospitals from local PPOs. HCA also had a financial interest in twenty-two nursing homes sold to Beverly Enterprises for stock as part of HCA's purchase of Hospital Affiliates. This investment was dropped in 1988. An attempt to merge with American Hospital Supply Corporation in the mid-1980s proved unsuccessful. During the study period (1984–1987), there was a refocusing on acute care hospitals, streamlining of operations, a systemwide emphasis on quality, and an attempt to give local CEOs more responsibility. In the process, HCA spun off 104 of its smaller hospitals through an employee stock ownership plan (ESOP) while retaining most of its urban and suburban hospitals, which serve as market leaders. HCA's president took the company private in a leveraged buyout in March 1989. At that time, HCA owned seventy-nine hospitals with an average bed size of 230, up from an average of 160 beds prior to the ESOP arrangement.

National Medical Enterprises. National Medical Enterprises (NME) is the most diversified of the corporations studied, with major business initiatives in long-term care, rehabilitation, and psychiatric and substance abuse, in addition to its general acute care hospital business. Also started in the late 1960s, the system briefly dabbled in HMO activities but quickly withdrew. In general, it has been somewhat less affected by the financial constraints of the mid-1980s than its counterparts. Nonetheless, the company experienced a $53 million fourth-quarter loss in 1986.

Unlike AMI and HCA, NME's strategic response to the environmental pressures of the mid-1980s called for greater investment in specialty hospitals and long-term care. As a result, it has divested a number of its poorer performing acute care hospitals, consolidated its regional offices, combined its domestic and international hospital operations, and significantly increased its number of psychiatric, substance abuse, and rehabilitation hospitals through both new construction and acquisitions. The system's investment in specialty hospitals has already begun to pay off. Its overall strategy is to focus on markets where it can integrate its diversification efforts to achieve synergy.

It is interesting to note that during this period of significant change, NME has enjoyed stable corporate office leadership from the original owner-founder. In this regard, it remains a first-generation system. There has, however, been considerable turnover at divisional and regional levels and considerable experimentation in structuring the relationship between the corporate office, individual hospitals, and the other divisions.

Evangelical Health System. Evangelical, the smallest and most geographically concentrated of the systems studied, is a second-generation not-for-profit system operating in the metropolitan Chicago market. Founded in the early 1970s, the system has undergone changes in its leadership style and culture. A visionary, entrepreneurially oriented president launched the system and then was followed by a professional leader. The new CEO has introduced considerable management discipline and strategic analysis into the organization to better position the system for growth in the 1990s.

An initial merger attempt with Lutheran General Health System, which would have nearly doubled the size of the corporation's assets, did not occur. Evangelical closed one inner-city hospital to better focus resources on a second inner-city hospital designed to serve the poor. The ability to serve the inner-city poor, which is a part of its corporate mission, is facilitated by a strong network of suburban hospitals and growing diversification efforts in long-term care and retirement centers. Like most other hospitals, its patient days declined in 1986 but have since bottomed out somewhat.

Evangelical perceives the need to become larger to succeed as a major metropolitan system. To do so, the system is building "continuum of care clusters" around its existing hospitals, working more closely and effectively with its physicians, containing its costs, and driving strategic thinking down to the middle-manager level throughout the system. In fact, among the eight systems studied, Evangelical gave the greatest emphasis to the need both to build and maintain inpatient market share and to expand its involvement in managed care activities. It plans to attract major areawide purchasers by emphasizing reasonable costs and accessibility while attracting local market clientele primarily on the basis of quality features.

Health Central (Health One). Health Central is an aggressive, innovative not-for-profit system operating in both a highly competitive metropolitan market and in rural areas. It was formed in the early 1970s as Health Central and recognized the need to grow in order to survive. An initial merger attempt in the 1980s proved unsuccessful, but in 1987 Health Central merged with the Health One Corporation and the combined organization adopted the Health One name. This increased Health Central's ability to link its primary, secondary, and tertiary care capabilities as part of an integrated system.

Health Central has enjoyed stable, innovative leadership since its inception. Like most systems, it overdiversified in the early 1980s and found itself having to retrench by dropping its involvement in consulting activities, dental clinics, and other initiatives. It also assumed greater control over the policymaking activities of its hospital boards, striving to behave more as a system and to respond better to systemwide opportunities.

In recognizing the changing role of physicians, Health Central is actively working to increase physician involvement in management and governance, evidenced by the creation of a senior vice-president for medical affairs. Operating in a highly competitive market, the system had launched a number of joint venture relationships, some of which have included direct contracting with providers. In the process, renewed attention has been given to making strategic planning more of a line management function throughout the organization, with particular attention to marketing.

Interestingly, Health Central gave the least emphasis of all the systems to basic survivability issues such as the ability to contain costs. Given its competitive market, which includes a number of HMOs and managed care providers, the system's managers believe that cost differentiation alone is not sufficient. Market share gains are now sought primarily through selected diversification and quality differentiation strategies.

Intermountain Health Care. Intermountain is a regional, financially conservative not-for-profit system with a strong religious heritage, although it no longer has formal ties to the Mormon church. Founded in the 1970s, the system has enjoyed stable corporate leadership since inception. Operating in a relatively more favorable environment than many of the other systems, it has been better able to withstand the environmental turbulence of the 1980s. Its leaders see Intermountain as a "model health care system" emphasizing learning, excellence, and selective diversification, including an HMO and several surgery centers. Among the eight systems, Intermountain's managers report the highest emphasis on the importance of demonstrating a high-quality image in order to compete successfully. It has also developed a systemwide physician corporation to help strengthen hospital-physician relationships and to explore mutual interests.

Hospital operating margins fell from the 6 to 8 percent range in 1985–86 to approximately 2 percent in 1988. The system currently faces challenges to requirements for defining and documenting its not-for-profit status. Intermountain is attempting to better focus its activities in acute care while continuing to pursue selected diversification initiatives. Profits from the recent sale of a successful software business for $10 million will be used to fund increased charity care and mission-related initiatives.

Sisters of Mercy Health Corporation. Sisters of Mercy Health Corporation (SMHC) is a Catholic not-for-profit system in Farmington Hills, Michigan, sponsored by the Sisters of Mercy, Province of Detroit. The corporation was formed in 1976 by consolidating separate hospital corporations. The system is highly committed to Catholic values, including service to the poor. SMHC has enjoyed stable, visionary leadership by its CEO.

During the study period, a systemwide strategic plan was developed to define the evolution of the Sisters of Mercy ministry in health. As a result, SMHC experienced turnover and reorganization within its divisions and overall corporate structure. Mercy Health Services (MHS) became the parent company of SMHC in 1984, and other subsidiary corporations were developed during the next few years (alternative financing, aging services, home care, fund raising, insurance, information services, and consulting) to address various dimensions of the evolving ministry. SMHC continues to be the major subsidiary, with responsibility for operating the hospital divisions and related community programs. Over the 1980s, it has faced major challenges in developing the system, increasing managerial discipline and financial orientation, and meeting the expectations of the sponsors.

The system's commitment to serve the poor and enhance financial viability placed some inherent limits on its strategic options during the transitional period. To fund selected diversification efforts and to support inner-city and rural hospitals serving the poor, prudent cost-containment activities had to be initiated in other operating areas.

As a result of its strategic plan, MHS is working to develop a Community Health Care System, a focused, integrated system for delivering and financing comprehensive health care organized within a local community. It is also working to strengthen physician partnerships, and toward this end developed a corporate officer for medical affairs in 1981. Project Partnership, an initiative to study and strengthen relationships between hospital chief executive officers and physician leaders, was undertaken with systemwide hospital and physician participation in 1984. The four objectives of the study were to (1) explore alternative financing and delivery systems; (2) facilitate joint ventures between physicians and hospitals; (3) conduct clinical and physician practice analyses; and (4) identify new methods for achieving more effective physician involvement. Some progress in each area was occurring by the end of the study period.

SMHC has targeted the elderly as a main area of growth, developing a range of residential, health, social, and recreational services to meet their needs. In addition, SMHC has become a major national leader facilitating alliances and collaboration with other hospitals and systems of similar philosophy or religious orientation.

Southwest Community Health Services. Southwest is a not-for-profit regional system with large hospitals in Albuquerque and a network of smaller hospitals in rural areas. It owns seven hospitals, leases two, and manages four. It has enjoyed considerable stability in corporate office leadership. The current CEO succeeded the founding CEO shortly after system formation in the early 1970s. Southwest has consistently emphasized controlling costs and recognized early the importance of involving physicians in planning and managerial decision making. Most of its hospitals are low-cost leaders, a strategy that system managers believe is essential for doing well in the tighter financial environment of the late 1980s. Organization leaders anticipate an even more stringent environment in the 1990s, particularly for the system's rural hospitals. At the same time, Southwest managers perceive the need for selective diversification, with a focus on activities compatible with physician interest. Diversification efforts have included sponsorship of an HMO and development of an information systems business and a materials management entity.

Common Threads. Overall, from around 1969 to 1989, the eight systems have passed through three general development stages. The *startup phase* was characterized by rapid growth (particularly for the investor-owned systems) in a relatively benign environment. The systems focused their energies on establishing their mission and identity and pursuing economies of scale that could result from being a system.

The second stage was one of *maturation,* characterized by the development of management infrastructures and a broadening of services. Planning, finance, marketing, human resources, and management information systems were developed as management processes became more formalized and sophisticated. This period was also marked by considerable experimentation regarding the appropriate levels of centralization and decentralization. Overall, the investor-owned systems adopted a more decentralized posture with the exception of overall financial controls. In contrast, the not-for-profit systems were somewhat more centralized. The period was marked by some degree of conflict between corporate offices and local hospitals as the not-for-profit systems sought to gain sufficient authority to behave as a single enterprise.

In recent years, the systems have entered a third phase best described as *refocusing* or *renewal*. Almost every system experienced significant change and reorganization during the study period (1984 to 1987), a trend that has continued. Health Central successfully merged with Health One; HCA's efforts to merge with American Hospital Supply Corporation were scuttled by Baxter Travenol's acquisition of American Hospital Supply. Evangelical's attempt to merge with the Chicago-based Lutheran General Health System eventually proved unsuccessful. AMI has been the object of three takeover bids. Both AMI and HCA have divested large groups of hospitals to their employees through stock ownership plans. HCA has been involved in a leveraged buyout. Most of the other systems have experienced significant reorganizations. Rarely has a week gone by without one or more of the study systems making national health care headlines.

At present, each is trying to figure out how best to run a multidivisional organization in an industry still fragmented and rapidly changing. Each is attempting to integrate primary, secondary, and tertiary levels of care in primarily local and regional markets. Each recognizes the need for strong physician partnerships to achieve these linkages. Each is experimenting with different levels of centralization and decentralization of planning, decision making, and support functions. In the process, most management structures have been streamlined as the corporations try to position themselves to move more quickly to meet the challenges of a demanding environment.

The remaining sections of the chapter highlight selected components of the model of strategic adaptation presented in Chapter Two (see Figure 2.1).

Overview of Findings

Strategic Change. Overall, half of the system hospitals changed their strategic orientations between 1983 and 1987 and half did not. Among the investor-owned, 51 percent switched their strategies versus 47 percent of the not-for-profit hospitals. Among those that switched strategies, 32.8 percent became prospectors, 10.9 percent became defenders, 32.8 percent became analyzers, and 23.5 percent became reactors. Thus, nearly two-thirds of those that switched strategies became prospectors or analyzers, with some flow back and forth between these categories as well as gains from the defender and reactor categories. Among those that did not switch strategies, 14.8 percent were prospectors, 2.2 percent defenders, 77.5 percent analyzers, and 5.5 percent reactors. The popularity of the analyzer strategy will be discussed later.

The most significant predictor of those that switched strategy from 1984 to 1987 versus those that did not was the hospital's strategic orientation in 1984. The importance of prior strategic orientation has been documented in previous analysis (Zajac and Shortell, 1989). Altogether, 83 percent of the hospitals studied either did not switch their strategies or switched within their strategic comfort zone. Only 17 percent, equally divided between investor-owned and not-for-profit systems, shifted outside their comfort zone. Table 3.1 shows the degree and direction of strategic change for each of the eight systems studied.

Perceived Quality of Strategic Planning. Table 3.2 summarizes each system's perceived quality of strategic planning, as rated by the hospital CEOs. It is important to note that the CEOs based their ratings on their own independent perceptions and needs, not in comparison to others. As a group, the not-for-profit system hospitals were perceived to have a higher quality of corporate and regional office assistance in strategic planning, stronger information systems, and slightly better overall quality of strategic planning than the investor-owned system hospitals as a group. These findings may be surprising to some who believe that investor-owned systems are more businesslike and, in particular, have more sophisticated management information systems. There was more variance in the perceived quality of information systems among the not-for-profit system hospitals. On the five-point scale they had both the highest (3.2) and the lowest score (1.9), whereas the investor-owned systems had a much more restricted range (2.1 to 2.4).

Table 3.1. Changes in Strategic Orientation by System.

	Prospector		Defender		Analyzer		Reactor	
	1985	1987	1985	1987	1985	1987	1985	1987
AMI	42.6% (N = 23)	37.0% (20)	0% (0)	9.3% (5)	53.7% (29)	37.0% (20)	3.7% (2)	16.7% (9)
HCA	16.0 (36)	21.3 (48)	4.9 (11)	4.9 (11)	62.2 (140)	59.1 (133)	16.9 (38)	14.7 (33)
NME	6.9 (2)	34.5 (10)	3.4 (1)	6.9 (2)	75.9 (22)	41.4 (12)	13.8 (4)	17.2 (5)
Evangelical	25.0 (1)	0 (0)	0 (0)	0 (0)	50.0 (2)	75.0 (3)	25.0 (1)	25.0 (1)
Health Central (Health One)	0 (0)	16.7 (2)	0 (0)	8.3 (1)	75.0 (9)	75.0 (9)	25.0 (3)	0 (0)
Intermountain	25.0 (4)	18.8 (3)	12.5 (2)	6.3 (1)	56.3 (9)	68.8 (11)	6.3 (1)	6.3 (1)
Sisters of Mercy	10.5 (2)	15.8 (3)	10.5 (2)	10.5 (2)	68.4 (13)	52.6 (10)	10.5 (2)	21.0 (4)
Southwest	0 (0)	14.3 (1)	0 (0)	28.6 (2)	100.0 (7)	57.1 (4)	0 (0)	0 (0)
Total	18.6% (68)	23.8% (87)	4.4% (16)	6.5% (24)	63.1% (231)	55.2% (202)	13.9% (51)	14.5% (53)

Table 3.2. Perceived Quality of Strategic Planning by System.

	Investor-Owned				Not-for-Profit					
	AMI (N = 55)	HCA (N = 227)	NME (N = 30)	Investor-Owned Group Average (N = 312)	Evangelical (N = 4)	Health Central (Health One) (N = 12)	Intermountain (N = 16)	Sisters of Mercy (N = 19)	Southwest (N = 7)	Not-for-Profit Group Average (N = 58)
Corporate and regional office assistance	2.8	2.9	2.7	2.9	4.2	3.6	3.7	3.5	3.6	3.6[a]
Information systems	2.1	2.2	2.4	2.2	2.3	2.5	3.2	1.9	2.9	2.5[b]
Implementation	3.1	3.0	3.1	3.0	3.5	3.0	3.6	2.9	2.9	3.2
Market research	2.6	2.8	2.9	2.8	2.6	2.8	3.3	2.2	3.4	2.8
Board and physician involvement	3.1	3.1	3.2	3.1	3.5	2.7	3.0	2.9	3.5	3.0
Plan innovativeness	3.6	3.6	3.7	3.6	4.1	3.4	3.6	3.8	3.1	3.6
Overall quality of strategic planning	2.9	2.9	2.9	2.9	3.3	3.0	3.4	2.8	3.1	3.1[b]

1 = Low perceived quality.
5 = High perceived quality.

[a] $p \leq .001$ Not-for-profit group significantly different from investor-owned group.
[b] $p \leq .05$ Not-for-profit group significantly different from investor-owned group.

These differences might be due to differences in system size. For example, the investor-owned systems might be perceived by their individual hospitals as offering less assistance because of the larger number of hospitals to which such assistance must be provided; each hospital might feel that it does not receive enough attention. Results, however, indicated that independent of system size, investor-owned hospitals still perceived their corporate and regional office as providing less assistance than did the not-for-profit system hospitals.

A common pattern identified in Table 3.2 is the greater degree of variability among the not-for-profit system hospitals on almost all items. This is partly the result of geographical dispersion and differences in size, mission, and strategies. The Evangelical and Sisters of Mercy systems provide an interesting and contrasting example. While both are religiously affiliated, Evangelical is the smallest system ($N = 4$) among the not-for-profits and Sisters of Mercy is the largest ($N = 19$). Evangelical concentrates its activities in a single metropolitan market; Sisters of Mercy spreads its activities across three states. Evangelical is perceived to have the highest degree of corporate and regional office assistance in strategic planning and is also high on plan implementation, board and physician involvement, plan innovativeness, and overall quality of strategic planning. Sisters of Mercy, in contrast, is relatively low in regard to corporate and regional office assistance, information systems, implementation, market research, board and physician involvement, and overall quality of strategic planning, but is relatively high on plan innovativeness. The management processes behind some of these differences are discussed later in this chapter.

Cost-Containment Strategies. Table 3.3 summarizes the reported use of specific cost-containment strategies for each system. There was not a great deal of variation between systems in the use of staff reduction, program or service consolidation, or efficiency and productivity improvements. Among the investor-owned systems, AMI gave the greatest attention to staff reductions and program or service consolidation. Among the not-for-profit systems, Sisters of Mercy gave the greatest atten-

Table 3.3. Cost-Containment Strategies by System.

	Total Cost-Containment Score	Staff Reduction	Program/Service Consolidation	Efficiency and Productivity Improvements
Investor-Owned				
AMI	3.3	3.6	3.0	3.2
HCA	3.1	3.2	2.5	3.3
NME	3.1	3.2	2.7	3.2
Investor-Owned				
Group Average	3.1	3.3	2.6	3.3
Not-for-Profit				
Evangelical	3.0	2.8	2.4	3.3
Health Central (Health One)	2.8	3.0	2.5	2.9
Intermountain	3.0	3.0	2.7	3.2
Sisters of Mercy	3.1	3.5	2.8	3.1
Southwest	3.1	3.2	3.0	3.0
Not-for-Profit				
Group Average	3.0	3.2	2.7	3.1[a]

1 = We have not implemented this strategy.
3 = We utilize this strategy somewhat.
5 = We utilize this strategy a great deal.

[a]$p \leq .06$ Not-for-profits as a group significantly different from investor-owned.

tion to staff reduction, while Evangelical placed the greatest emphasis on efficiency and productivity improvements.

Factors Influencing Future Viability. Each system hospital CEO was also asked to rate the importance of various factors associated with the hospital's future viability. Table 3.4 provides a summary of the responses. On average, the hospitals rated all the surveyed items as relatively important, somewhere between "important" (rating of 3) to "essential" (rating of 5). There was not much variation between systems, although economic viability concerns were particularly strong for Intermountain and Southwest's hospitals. The importance of having a market orientation was particularly important for Evangelical.

Within the context of this overview, the following sections elaborate on each system's goals and values, perceived strengths and weaknesses, further perceptions of its strategic orientations

Table 3.4. Factors Influencing Future Hospital Viability by System.

	Investor-owned				Not-for-Profit					
	AMI	HCA	NME	Investor-Owned Group Average	Evangelical	Health Central (Health One)	Intermountain	Sisters of Mercy	Southwest	Not-for-Profit Group Average
Economic survivability	4.0	4.2	3.9	4.1	4.4	3.7	4.6	4.3	4.6	4.3
Capital maintenance/ technology enhancement	3.8	3.7	3.6	3.7	3.6	3.4	3.4	3.7	3.7	3.6
Quality and image	4.3	4.1	4.0	4.1	4.1	4.0	4.4	4.1	4.2	4.2
Diversification	3.6	3.7	3.7	3.7	3.8	3.4	3.6	3.8	3.5	3.6
Market orientation	4.5	4.4	4.4	4.4	4.9	4.3	4.5	4.5	4.3	4.4

Note: 1 = less important; 3 = important; 5 = essential.

and planning processes, and corporate leaders' insights into the changes that occurred over the period of the study.

American Medical International (AMI)

Goals and Values, Strengths and Weaknesses. AMI's culture emphasized that "managing is managing" regardless of the industry. When executives were asked to describe strongly held beliefs within their organization, the responses consistently referred to pride in management excellence, entrepreneurial spirit, and reputation as a "high-class" organization with the money available to do things right. Only one out of eight top executives mentioned the organization as a health care provider. The diversity, individualism, and professionalism of the management team were seen as key characteristics that made AMI "unique."

The system's major strengths as perceived by corporate leaders in 1985 were its financial resources and the external perception of its financial influence. Weaknesses identified included the need to be more innovative, to develop better marketing plans, to do more career-path planning, and to improve the cost accounting systems.

Strategic Orientation: The Corporate Perspective. Considering their system as a whole, most of AMI's corporate executives perceived it as an analyzer with an average score of 4.2 on a scale of 1 to 7 (7 = high change). When they were asked to assess the system as it was two years before (1983) and as they predicted it would be two years hence (1987), a consistent pattern of strategic orientation change from analyzer to prospector emerged.

When asked to indicate the strategic orientations for their acute care hospitals, AMI's corporate executives reported 26 percent of their hospitals to be defenders, 13 percent reactors, 25 percent prospectors, and 36 percent analyzers.

Strategic Orientation: The Hospital Perspective. In contrast, when AMI's hospital CEOs assessed their hospitals' strategic orientations in 1985, they overwhelmingly saw themselves as analyzers (53 percent) and prospectors (43 percent). Only 4 percent of the hospitals saw themselves as reactors, and no hospital perceived of itself as a defender. Further, whereas the corporate executives had predicted that the system as a whole would move toward a prospector orientation by 1987, the hospitals assessed themselves in 1987 as retrenching toward a defender orientation (9 percent), moving toward an uncertain reactor orientation (17 percent), and moving away from analyzer (37 percent) or prospector (37 percent) orientations. AMI's hospitals gave considerable emphasis to cost containment (see Table 3.2), which is associated with a defender strategy. At the same time, the data indicate that as they attempted to retrench from some of their overly diversified prospector activities, some hospitals lost their strategic focus.

Strategic Planning Process and Outcomes. To some extent the disparity between corporate and hospital perceptions of strategic orientation is understandable, given the system's involvement in diversified activities. The system is perceived by its executives as a business that extends in vision and scope beyond the "sum of the parts" of its acute care hospitals, even though they are the corporation's primary source of revenue.

The disparity may also be understood by studying the content and process of strategic planning at the corporate level. The top strategic priorities reported by AMI executives in 1985 involved further diversification into nonhospital but health-related lines of business, growth in revenues and prestige, and strengthening the management infrastructure of the corporation. The movement predicted by corporate executives, from analyzer to prospector, was based on diversification, growth, and development *unrelated* to hospital-level operations or strategies. The corporate priorities for AMI's hospital line of business reflected a dominant defender orientation: downsize operations and improve efficiency, marketing, and management information systems. Although there were analyzer and prospector strategies related to acute care hospitals, they involved corporate decision making pertaining to acquisition of and affiliation with major medical centers and acquisition or construction of more international facilities. The justification for the corporate-level priority to diversify was overwhelmingly reported to be the need to "protect the base business" of general acute care, which was perceived as facing current and increasing hostility in the public and private payment environment. The system's strategic response to that hostility was to create new sources of revenue outside this hostile environment and "hunker down" for defense within that environment.

Corporate executives unanimously reported the hospital strategic planning process as "bottom up," that is, it developed its content and form at the hospital level and worked up through the regional level. Corporate marketing, management information systems, and human resources departments provide direct support and education opportunities to the hospitals but not strategic direction. The system's strategic planners were reported to play a minor role in hospital planning, instead focusing their efforts on the system as a whole. There were no systemwide criteria for medical staff credentialing and no standard criteria for service pricing at the hospital level. Hospital CEOs were evaluated on their ability to make their bottom line, achievement of individually determined performance objectives, demonstration of strengthening relationships with their medical staffs, and, more recently, achieving patient satisfaction and clinical standards.

1987 Followup: What Happened? Between 1984 and 1987, AMI underwent a marked metamorphosis similar to most other systems. Losses in diversification efforts, as well as unrealized goals in hospital efficiency, acted as a collective slap in the face to the "managing is managing" and "greater than the sum of the parts" philosophies that had driven AMI's strategies in 1984. Believing that AMI had lost sight of the importance of hospitals, physicians, and local markets to the survival of its base business, the new CEO led his management team back to basics by 1987. It divested all nonhospital subsidiaries except psychiatric facilities, and committed the system to defending and enhancing hospital market share, physician relations, and planning and marketing efforts at the local level. As Chapter

Six highlights, a successful prospector orientation requires an understanding of *what* you are prospecting, *why* you are prospecting, and *who else* is prospecting *where*. AMI learned that it could answer only one of those questions in 1984. Executives knew *why* they were prospecting: to find new sources of revenue to subsidize a base business that was suffering from hostile environmental forces. But instead of choosing to innovate from the base-business level, they chose to seek new ventures in arenas where markets and competitors were not well understood.

This is why the corporate executives' 1985 predictions of AMI's 1987 strategic orientation were not realized. It is also why, by 1987, the cumulative strategic orientations of the system's hospitals more accurately reflected the orientation of the corporation. Now, instead of a diversified system revolving around a technical core, AMI is moving toward a synergy between corporate business expertise and hospital technical expertise to achieve locally relevant and profitable business units. A new CEO, the third in six years, has been recently hired to futher implement the changes initiated by his predecessor. The strategic planning department has changed structure, focusing now on developing strategies with member hospitals. AMI has also begun recruiting physicians to serve on hospital boards of directors and to provide advice on corporate marketing strategies.

The implications of AMI's experience will be discussed in conjunction with the adaptations of all eight systems in the final section of this chapter. In brief, however, AMI's experience is not unique. Similarities in the interactions of internal and external forces were experienced by all systems studied.

Hospital Corporation of America (HCA)

Goals and Values, Strengths and Weaknesses. HCA's top corporate leaders' strongly held beliefs included local autonomy, provision of high-quality care to the community, a belief in long-run performance, and the imperative to hire managers and make operational decisions consistent with those philosophies. They believed these qualities made their system unique. They also frequently referred to the vision of the company's founders and its ability to pursue its philosophies by virtue of its strong financial foundation.

The system's most frequently reported strengths included quality people, financial strength, and high morale, especially among corporate staff. At the same time they also noted weaknesses related to their information systems, career-path planning, and ability of the organization to take risks, to move strategically, and to move quickly.

Strategic Orientation: The Corporate Perspective. Consistent with their hospital operations philosophy and conservative management characteristics, HCA executives assessed their corporation as primarily a defender with an average score of 2.3 on a scale of 1 to 7 (7 = high change). Tracing perception of strategic orientation from 1983 through what it would be in 1987, responses showed a stable defender orientation from 1983 through 1985, with a movement toward an analyzer and prospector orientation predicted for the next two years.

In contrast with AMI, HCA executives assessed their member hospitals as having a greater propensity for change than their system as a whole. On average they assessed 33 percent of their hospitals as prospectors, 31 percent as analyzers, 23 percent as reactors, and only 13 percent as defenders.

Strategic Orientation: The Hospital Perspective. On the whole, individual hospital CEOs agreed with the corporate office perception of their hospital's strategic orientation in 1985, except even higher percentages of them perceived their hospitals as prospectors (16 percent) and analyzers (62 percent). Only 5 percent of the hospitals perceived of themselves as defenders, and the remaining 17 percent as reactors. Responses of the same hospitals in 1987 showed the greatest amount of stability over time of any of the systems. The only change was that 3 percent of 1985's analyzers and 2 percent of 1985's reactors became prospectors by 1987. This movement toward a prospector orientation is generally consistent with the corporate executives' prediction for the system as a whole.

Strategic Planning Process and Outcome. The corporate-level knowledge of and interest in hospital operations carry over into the strategic planning process. Unlike AMI, which left hospital-level planning almost completely to individual hospitals, HCA was more involved in directing or negotiating hospital strategic plans. Corporate executives described a "top down" procedure for setting strategic priorities and guidelines for hospital performance but referred frequently to seeking input from hospitals and regional executives. The divisional vice-presidents were reported as playing key roles in communicating priorities between the field and the corporate office.

Corporate executives' reports of top strategic priorities were consistent with those of a system dedicated to the hospital industry, with one interesting and expensive twist. For the most part, HCA's strategic priorities of 1985 revolved around inpatient care: growth through hospital acquisition and enhanced market share, maintenance and promotion of prestigious image to the hospital industry and the investment community, and strengthening corporate infrastructure (management and information systems capabilities).

The twist is that HCA executives included in their strategic priorities a new diversification effort into alternative delivery systems and health insurance. In 1985 the company had just reorganized, allocating a large sum to a nonhospital development division. After initial attempts to do it themselves failed, the division then formed a joint venture with an insurance company with a goal of implementing a national prepaid plan and several smaller ventures. At this writing, the success and stability of this relationship are uncertain.

1987 Followup: What Happened? As we will see, organizational slack (resources that can be used for future investment and for experimentation) is critical to undertaking new ventures that entail financial risk. But organizational slack alone, no matter how abundant, is not enough to make a new venture succeed. In the 1970s and early into the 1980s, HCA grew rapidly through successful acquisition, management contract expansion, and financial investments. However, because the system saw itself as solely a hospital company, because the national payment and regulatory environment was favorable, and because the company, by its own report, acted from a defender strategic orientation, there seemed little need to diversify into new lines of business.

By 1985, the payment, regulatory, and competitive environments had become increasingly hostile, representing a threat to the company's long-term growth. By that time, however, a considerable amount of organizational slack had been accumulated — perhaps too much. The system, experienced in using organizational slack only for enhancing its image, reinvestment, and upgrading facilities, sailed into uncharted waters when it decided to diversify. The new nonhospital development division was given access to considerable resources and was able to buy actuarial expertise by way of the insurance company joint venture. There was an air of excitement and optimism in which the objectives were "to spend money and have fun." The national growth in prepaid plans and the numerous, widespread system of hospitals that would provide inpatient care discounts to the new network led to the belief that the new venture could not lose. The importance of linking diversification with strong market research was not sufficiently emphasized. The strategy did not take into account the potential alienation of physicians and hospital CEOs at the local level, or the unique management requirements of prepaid plans. (These points will be elaborated in Chapters Six through Nine.)

By 1987, HCA withdrew from the insurance business and greatly reduced the scope of its strategy for prepaid plans, returning its focus to hospital operations, with a new commitment to enhancing physician relations in local markets. In early 1987, the system trimmed its administrative staff at corporate headquarters, and later spun off 104 hospitals through an employee stock ownership plan. Goals focused on improving efficiency and market share at the hospital level, strengthening corporate-hospital relationships, and providing support services (housekeeping, dietary, information systems, consulting) to member and nonmember hospitals. This streamlining left the organization with a similar look and strategy in 1987 to AMI's. However, the process of organizational learning was very different. At AMI, the process was one of understanding the unique requirements of its base business. HCA learned what organizational slack will and will not buy.

National Medical Enterprises (NME)

Goals and Values, Strengths and Weaknesses. NME executives emphasized their system's diversified approach. They viewed their organization as a "total health care company" involved in nursing home care, psychiatric care, and rehabilitation as well as general acute care. They were pleased to see that changes in the hospital environment were beginning to bring their "dark horse" image into the light. Other systems, just beginning to diversify, could now look at their organization as a model. They also reported a strong belief in the important role of physicians, a belief put into action with physician advisory boards more active in decision making than any of the other study systems in 1985.

The diversified approach was felt to be NME's "uniqueness." The system's perceived strengths were diversification, a belief in local autonomy, and entrepreneurship. However, executives also raised concerns that so much autonomy, individualism, entrepreneurship, and divisionalism lead to considerable difficulties in integrating products and services at either the corporate or local level. Indeed, they frequently referred to the different lines of business as different companies, loosely connected by the corporate parent.

Strategic Orientation: The Corporate Perspective. Not surprisingly, the assessments of NME's executives placed this organization closer to the prospector end of the scale, with an average score of 5.2 on the seven-point scale. Asked for their perceptions of the system's strategic orientation from two years prior (1983) to predictions of two years hence (1987), the executives reported a stable analyzer/prospector orientation from the past through the present, and predicted further movement toward a prospector position.

NME's corporate executives also perceived their member hospitals as high on the strategic change continuum, on average ranking 44 percent as prospectors, 28 percent as analyzers, 20 percent as defenders, and 8 percent as reactors.

Strategic Orientation: The Hospital Perspective. NME's hospital CEOs were not as wedded to a prospector orientation as their corporate counterparts in 1985. Only 7 percent of the hospitals considered themselves prospectors, 76 percent analyzers, 3 percent defenders, and 14 percent reactors. By 1987 the analyzers had decreased to 41 percent, changing for the most part to prospectors, who increased to 35 percent. Reactors increased to 17 percent and defenders to 7 percent.

Strategic Planning Process and Outcome. NME executives reported a "top down, bottom up" flow for strategic planning. Although they consider the system informal, the corporate office presents each hospital CEO with a set of assumptions and goals that, along with personally determined objectives, are the basis for performance evaluation. The acute hospital division works in concert with the corporate planning office to prepare the strategic plans for all hospitals. Although this belies NME's otherwise divisionalized and decentralized style, it reveals two important issues. First, although the system prides itself on its diversified portfolio, general acute care is still considered the "base business," and is therefore held under greater corporate control. For example, the acute hospital division was the last to be separated physically from the corporate office. Second, the company's founder and CEO continues to play a strong role in corporate and hospital decision making. During interviews, his name was mentioned three times more often than any other. He not only formed the company but continues to shape it, closely monitoring the direction of the diversified units and particularly the base business.

In 1985, NME planned to continue its growth in the diversified lines of business already established and expand into new areas. Like AMI and HCA, it aspired to become a major player in the health insurance and alternative delivery system market but quickly retrenched to focus on other areas where it had more experience. Unlike the other two investor-owned systems, NME's diversification plans were generally closer to local markets, the technical and medical expertise it already possessed, or both. For example, seeking to adapt to the hostility in the acute care environment, NME planned to convert unused acute care beds into rehabilitation or psychiatric accommodations, contracting with their subsidiaries in those specialties. Also, it planned to expand interests in long-term care, rehabilitation, and home health care, predicting that when the prospective payment system and increased competition provided incentives for early discharge from acute facilities, patients and their families would seek additional services. They also planned more market-area specific research to discover niches for development, such as freestanding treatment centers for Alzheimer's disease and kidney dialysis.

NME also set a strategic priority to link the diversified arms of its system, where possible, at the local level. In some areas the system operates a long-term care or rehabilitation facility as well as an acute hospital and, sometimes, a medical supply company distribution business. Previously these organizations were free to interact with system-owned or other providers, based on each CEO's criteria, such as price and location. In 1985 the system began offering financial incentives for facility executives to form relationships with system-owned providers on a local level.

1987 Followup: What Happened? Like AMI and HCA, NME discovered that diversification into managed care requires intimate knowledge of and strong relationships with physicians and local community networks. As one executive explained NME's deemphasis of managed care, "We didn't understand the business." This statement was also an accurate assessment of the system's efforts in home health care. However, all the other priorities of 1985, including expanded efforts in psychiatric care, long-term care, substance abuse, rehabilitation, development of niches, and integration of system subsidiaries at the local level, were being actively pursued in 1987. NME had built a broad base before the environmental jolts of the 1980s and used that foundation to implement a prospector strategy of diversification at both the system and hospital levels. The system's sensitivity to local market research and the relatedness of its diversification efforts, together with its willingness to take risks, helped it weather the storms of environmental change brought on by PPS and increased competition.

Evangelical Health System

Goals and Values, Strengths and Weaknesses. At the core of Evangelical's belief system and sense of uniqueness was the synthesis of its religious mission and financial viability. As one corporate executive put it, "We must do well to do good, and we are doing both." Another executive phrased this goal a bit less eloquently: "No money, no mission." Executives believed that the system had done well by acquiring a top management team, diversifying on a corporate level, focusing on a geographical area, and operating profitable suburban hospitals. They reported a corporate dedication to use this financial and political security to do good: to serve the inner-city poor, improve societal and individual justice, and be a responsible employer.

A new CEO and newly reorganized corporate structure brought a new challenge to Evangelical in 1983: to bring the church mission that had been embodied in the hospital company into the 1980s — into a hostile payment and regulatory environment where "doing good wouldn't pay the bills." The new corporate parent would oversee subsidiaries responsible for long-term care facilities, subsidized senior housing, and other efforts in harmony with the church's traditional mission. But it would also oversee for-profit subsidiaries, pharmaceutical companies, and joint ventures with insurance companies and investor-owned hospital systems. These latter efforts, while not in concert with a pure religious mission, would allow the company the financial security to pursue its mission in other arenas.

The corporation had bought itself, with this new structure and management, a profitable, influential new image. Even so, by 1985 there was still an uncomfortable and tentative balance between the cautious, mission-driven board and the management team it had hired. Managers referred to "analysis paralysis," and the "need to *move,* not just plan." The greatest example of mixed messages between the board and management of Evangelical comes from the review of an attempted merger with another innovative, influential, locally based religious system, Lutheran General. The merger was an "off the record" topic during 1985 interviews, but we were told by management that discussions were under way and could conclude within a few months. The new titles and positions of the executives from both systems, the arrangements for shared ancillary services and information systems, even the new system name were busily, albeit secretly, being negotiated. The merger did not occur in 1985, and negotiations were placed on hold. But at the time of the 1987 interviews, discussions were again active, and the system's planners predicted no major barriers to the merger, which they felt would occur within several months. In the final analysis, however, Evangelical's board decided against relinquishing full ownership of the system.

Strategic Orientation: The Corporate Perspective. In 1985, Evangelical's corporate executives placed the system slightly on the defender side of an analyzer, with an average score of 3.7. The analyzer strategy represented the common ground between the defender tendencies of the corporate board and the prospector goals of the corporate management. When executives were asked to categorize their organization as it was two years earlier (1983) and predict what it would be two years in the future (1987), they portrayed the system as moving steadily toward the analyzer/prospector end of the continuum.

Evangelical corporate executives perceived their hospitals as having a greater affinity for change than the parent corporation as a whole. In 1985, an average of 34 percent were assessed as prospectors, 41 percent as analyzers, 23 percent as defenders, and 2 percent as reactors.

Strategic Orientation: The Hospital Perspective. The system hospitals in general agreed with the corporate perceptions of their ability to change; 25 percent ranked themselves as prospectors in 1985, 50 percent as analyzers, and 25 percent as reactors. In 1987, the one prospector had converted to analyzer, leaving 75 percent analyzers and 25 percent reactors. No hospital perceived of itself as a defender in either 1985 or 1987.

Strategic Planning Process and Outcome. Evangelical executives unanimously assessed the hospital strategic planning process as "top down" in 1985. This process became even more corporately controlled by 1987, when hospital CEOs were allowed input only into "tactical plans." In both years, hospital and regional executives were under close corporate scrutiny.

The system's strategic priorities of 1985 were those of a prospector: diversification and growth. Executives placed priority at the corporate level on diversification into health care financing and for-profit subsidiaries on the nonprovider side, such as pharmaceutical manufacturing; and at the hospital level into high-technology advances, such as hospital specialty cardiac units. Executives perceived of the system as staying close to home in its hospital operations and branching out in new directions corporately: urgent care centers, alternative delivery systems, and for-profit subsidiaries.

1987 Followup: What Happened? By 1987, Evangelical had learned, like AMI and NME, that urgent care centers were a "strategic flash in the pan," with a high potential to alienate physicians and member hospitals and a low potential for positive returns in the long run. The system, like so many others, had also begun to take an arm's length position with its insurance company joint ventures. However, unlike all the investor-owned study systems, Evangelical enjoyed some measure of success in developing local prepaid plans and was in discussions with other provider-based plans to expand its interest through joint venture partnerships. Its high-technology diversification efforts at the hospital level were beginning to be realized in 1987, and its further acquisition of for-profit nonprovider companies was progressing on schedule. Its long-planned growth through merger encountered a setback when the merger failed in 1987. The system, however, was close to acquiring another facility with which it had been in negotiations for several years.

Evangelical's intimate knowledge of its hospital line of business, gained through a tightly centralized system of decision making, allowed it to diversify appropriately at the hospital level, while its decentralized, looser-reigned approach with its for-profit subsidiaries allowed them to flourish. While the diversification efforts and their outcomes reflected Evangelical's orientation and behavior as a prospector, including the acceptance of failed ventures, the growth through selective acquisition and merger efforts reflected its emphasis on an analyzer strategy.

Health Central (Health One)

Goals and Values, Strengths and Weaknesses. Health Central executives prize an organizational environment that fosters individual achievement, an entrepreneurial spirit, innovation, creativity, and risk taking. At the same time they stressed the importance of being sensitive to local markets, emphasizing the autonomy of local administrators, a belief in a strong community base (including ties with local businesses and local physicians), and "problem solving as close to the problem as possible."

Perceptions of the system's weaknesses, as in most systems, reflected the downside of its strengths. The decentralized decision making so valued by executives came with a perceived price. As one executive said, "Collective decision making is messy." Executives reported that consensus gaining is difficult and time consuming. Further, although they highly valued individual achievement, the 1985 restructuring that promoted individuals into multiple roles left some executives confused. It was unclear to many just exactly how the new system was really different, given that the same executives were at the helm. Although these executives had different titles, some of their functions did not yet have departments to go with them. Executives also stated concerns over more standard organizational weaknesses, as did most systems, such as the quality of their information systems and their ability to do competitor analysis.

Strategic Orientation: The Corporate Perspective. In 1985, Health Central was equivalent to Evangelical in terms of executives' perceptions of its place on the strategic continuum, placing themselves slightly on the defender side of analyzer with a score of 3.7. Executives' perceptions of changes over time, however, were quite different from any other system. Most respondents in other systems, both at the hospital and corporate level, traced a path of change from defender to analyzer to prospector. Health Central's executives, however, perceived a change path from analyzer *to reactor* to prospector, sidestepping the defender orientation altogether. Predicting change from 1983 to 1987, Health Central executives viewed their system as in transition from analyzer to prospector but predicted the route would be through a reactor orientation.

When assessing their hospitals' strategic orientations toward change, Health Central executives saw an average of 25 percent of their hospitals as reactors, the highest percentage of any of the study systems. They categorized 18 percent of their hospitals as prospectors, 36 percent as analyzers, and 17 percent as defenders. The corporate assessment of the system as a whole could be closely related to the structural changes taking place at the corporate level and the environmental changes occurring in the industry. Being headquartered in a competitive and progressive state, Health Central executives had perhaps a more urgent sense of the changing roles of hospitals, physicians, payers, and patients than executives in other systems. The new corporate structure was an attempt to better adapt to that changing environment. But the adaptation itself posed uncertainties, and executives reflected this in their responses. The general impression communicated was that dark days were upon them, but that it is always darkest before the dawn.

Strategic Orientation: The Hospital Perspective. Responses of Health Central's hospital CEOs on orientations toward change were somewhat unusual. In 1985 not one hospital reported itself as either a prospector or a defender. Exactly 25 percent of Health Central's hospitals perceived themselves as reactors, and the remaining 75 percent perceived themselves as analyzers.

By 1987, to a great extent, the predictions of corporate executives were realized. There were changes in every category, resulting in 17 percent of the hospitals reporting themselves as prospectors, 75 percent as analyzers, 8 percent as defenders; no hospital perceived itself as a reactor. Clearly for Health Central, the reactor category was seen as a largely transitory state on the way to refocusing efforts toward a prospector orientation.

Strategic Planning Process and Outcome. The strategic planning process at Health Central was very formal and centrally driven in 1985. Hospital, regional and corporate executives participated in structured management retreats, and the corporate office directed environmental assessments. One executive characterized the system's strategic planning activities as exhibiting the qualities of "participative management in its infancy." He praised the system for attempting to perform sophisticated strategic analysis while simultaneously educating both the corporate board and all levels of management on the importance and process of strategic planning. The system was evolving from a paternalistic to a participative organization. This change was not a revolution — it was not being led by those willing but unable to participate — but rather a guided transformation, brought about through the deliberate design of the top management team.

The system's strategic priorities of 1985, in fact, included the education and development of board and management, to strengthen the system following its recent restructuring, to establish a stronger corporate identity, and to prepare the board and management for the other strategic priorities: growth and diversification. The growth priorities were planned to be realized on three dimensions: (1) the merger and acquisition of general acute care hospitals, (2) expansion of international markets, and (3) economic growth through enhanced ability to raise capital. The third goal was to be achieved through diversification at both the corporate and hospital level. The growth and diversification priorities were part of a larger priority to develop a regional health care system. Unlike the other systems described, however, Health Central had *no* plans to diversify into new lines of business. All its plans, instead, were based on geographical expansion of current diversification efforts, such as long-term care and prepaid plans, or bringing corporate efforts closer to the local hospital level, including linkages with physicians, increasing efficiency, expanding prepaid plans, and promoting consumer satisfaction and marketing research.

1987 Followup: What Happened? The biggest change in Health Central between 1985 and 1987 was its merger with Health One, making it the largest provider in the market. The overall priorities of the system in 1987 reflect the adjustment to the merger. The goal to develop a regional health care system was rethought, as management learned from experience the difficulty and expense of just one merger. The growth imperative was adjusted to target, in order of priority, the Minneapolis–St. Paul metropolitan area, the state of Minnesota, and, finally, the Midwest. As with other systems, Health Central also rethought its plans for HMO development, choosing to retreat from that strategy and instead negotiate with established HMOs as a provider. Other diversification efforts — senior housing, dental centers, and consulting — were also abandoned. These businesses were not new efforts to the system in 1985, but it was decided by 1987 that enough time and effort had been expended to determine their long-run viability — or lack of it. The system also retreated from the international market, discovering that the capital costs related to international competition were best suited to the pocketbook of an investor-owned corporation.

The strategic priorities that remained the same over the two-year period were the overall goal of regional growth, enhanced efficiency and marketing capabilities at the hospital level, and enhanced physician relationships throughout the system, including the creation of a systemwide corporate division of medical affairs. The system's activities in long-term care and behavioral medicine also remained part of the strategic portfolio.

Health Central experienced many of the shocks from the environmental jolt of the 1980s, particularly in the arenas of managed care and unrelated diversification efforts. The strength of the system in 1987 is largely a result of its awareness in 1985 of the uncertainty that hospitals and physicians faced in their local markets, and its understanding of the value of acute inpatient care to long-range viability.

Intermountain Health Care

Goals and Values, Strengths and Weaknesses. Intermountain was similar to Evangelical in its emphasis on both financial strength and a mission to provide high-quality health care. Almost every executive discussed the system's financial strength, the integrity, quality, and progressiveness of the management and board, and the system's commitment to excellence in health care services. Executives reported that the system's high-quality management, "conservative, yet wise" financial decisions, and the geographical concentration of hospitals had been the primary contributors to the system's continued financial stability. Respondents frequently lauded their organization as "the best-run not-for-profit system," a system that "sees itself as a corporation" with a "stable, far-sighted, progressive" management team. They also considered their quality assurance systems to be at the forefront of the field.

Intermountain executives believed that a major challenge lay in balancing their strong financial orientation with their values, emphasizing community responsibility. They also felt that they needed to strengthen their marketing and public relations efforts, and give greater attention to determining their future role in long-term care and related initiatives.

Strategic Orientation: The Corporate Perspective. Executives in 1985 placed Intermountain somewhat on the defender side of the analyzer category, with a mean score of 3.5. This is validated by the discussion above, highlighting the conservative financial practices, limited diversification efforts, and close corporate control over hospital operations. Like Health Central, although not to the same extent, Intermountain executives perceived an increase in a reactor orientation from 1983 to 1987, ultimately resulting in an analyzer/prospector orientation. They were particularly concerned with changes occurring in managed care and long-term care and the need to define a clearer strategy for these areas.

Given the corporate control over many of the hospital activities related to strategic orientation, it is somewhat surprising that Intermountain executives perceived their individual hospitals as more oriented toward change than the system as a whole. Executives on average perceived 33 percent of the system's hospitals as prospectors, 40 percent as analyzers, 22 percent as defenders, and 5 percent as reactors.

Strategic Orientation: The Hospital Perspective. Intermountain's hospital CEOs reflected an even greater orientation toward being prospectors or analyzers. In 1985, 25 percent of the hospitals viewed themselves as prospectors, 57 percent as analyzers, 12 percent as defenders, and 6 percent as reactors. By 1987, 6 percent of 1985's prospectors and 7 percent of 1985's defenders believed that they had become analyzers, resulting in 19 percent prospectors, 69 percent analyzers, 6 percent defenders, and 6 percent reactors.

Strategic Planning Process and Outcome. Intermountain's executives perceived the strategic planning process as primarily "top down" and very formal. Those closer to marketing and environmental assessment saw a greater level of participation by hospital CEOs than did executives at the highest levels in the company. There were no individual hospital representatives on the top-management committee that met monthly to review strategies. However, bimonthly strategic planning sessions are held by the hospital division president and the three regional hospital vice-presidents. Hospital CEOs are evaluated on their ability to meet financial and strategic goals, and subjectively on their teamwork and cooperation with other hospital and corporate executives, but not on their ability to contribute to new strategies.

In 1985 the system's strategic priorities were aimed primarily at corporate level diversification: development of free-standing ambulatory care facilities, prepaid plans, and industrial medicine. Locally, executives stated a priority to integrate the system on a regional level and to build strong relationships with physicians. However, no specific plans for integration or relationship building were described. Again, similar to HCA, Intermountain sailed into relatively uncharted waters in 1985 when it turned the use of its slack resources outward toward diversification efforts in which it had limited previous experience.

1987 Followup: What Happened? Like HCA, most of Intermountain's diversification efforts were unsuccessful. By 1987 diversification into freestanding centers in distant states was terminated, and centers within Intermountain's region were tied more directly to their inpatient facilities. Like AMI, Intermountain renewed its commitment to the viability of its inpatient acute care, and like Health Central it retrenched geographically in its diversification efforts, involving industrial medicine, medical supplies, and ambulatory surgery centers. The exception to geographical restraint was in the area of computer software marketing, which continued to be promoted on a national level until it was sold in late 1988.

Unlike any of the other systems, Intermountain was able to build an evolving HMO managed care network in its home region. In fact, by 1987 the system was the third largest managed care provider in its state, with approximately 100,000 enrollees. The network is expected to break even by 1991.

The strategic priorities of 1985 involving local integration and building relationships with physicians were formalized and implemented by 1987. The system withdrew from long-distance efforts at diversification to devote more attention to integration among the system's individual units. A regional critical emergency network and a regional rehabilitation services network were established. Like many of the systems already described, Intermountain experienced a jump in the organizational learning curve during the study period. By 1987 a more sophisticated organization emerged, aware of the importance and potential of the base hospital business and of the dangers in unrelated or geographically remote diversification efforts.

The system's success in managed care may be closely related to its ability to pursue its other strategic priority: building strong relationships with physicians. From the developmental stages of the system's HMO and PPOs, physician support and participation were crucial ingredients. Informally, the system became increasingly active in bringing physicians into hospital and corporate-level decision making. By 1987, three physician members had been added to the corporate board, and the system had formed a physician corporation to promote partnerships with physicians. Intermountain's knowledge of its local hospital environments, combined with its growing sensitivity to the role of physicians, helped to facilitate development of the managed care network.

Sisters of Mercy Health Corporation

Goals and Values, Strengths and Weaknesses. Sisters of Mercy is a strongly mission-driven system with an emphasis on serving the poor and those in need. The dedication, integrity, and strong values of the corporate board and management were highlighted. The system belief that "health care is a right, not a privilege" drove decisions to diversify into long-term care and inner-city ambulatory care centers. Some felt that the system's relatively large size (nineteen hospitals) was also an asset.

Many of the top executives perceived the system as weak in financial productivity, lacking in capital, and not sufficiently "strategically driven." These characteristics represent, to some degree, the "costs" of being a mission-driven, charitable organization, seeking to "do good" but having to learn to "do well." One of the system's top priorities for 1985 was to increase its provision of charity care as a corporatewide percentage of inpatient revenues from 1.25 to 2 to 4 percent, through better internal management of its resources.

Sisters of Mercy's mission-driven goal to serve the poor, its need for stronger information systems and increased efficiency and productivity, and the relatively hostile external environment in which it operated posed major challenges. Unlike Evangelical or Health One, which began systematic strategic planning for change in the early 1980s (or NME even earlier), or AMI, HCA, and Intermountain, which faced the 1980s with a strong financial foundation from which to experiment, Sisters of Mercy was somewhat less prepared financially and strategically to deal with the rapidly emerging issues.

Strategic Orientation: The Corporate Perspective. Sisters of Mercy executives perceived their organization as very low on the strategic orientation continuum in 1985, with an average score of 2.4, making it clearly a defender — second only to HCA in this respect. Sisters of Mercy executives saw themselves to be moving slowly toward an analyzer orientation, with some prospector orientation predicted by 1987, but not as much as the other study systems.

Sisters of Mercy, like Intermountain, perceived its hospitals in 1985 as having a greater propensity for change than the system as a whole. On average, corporate executives considered 39 percent of their hospitals as prospectors, 30 percent as analyzers, 16 percent as defenders, and 15 percent as reactors. Interview findings did not provide a totally clear picture of the conflict between corporate self-perception and members' perception of the corporation. The positions being filled at the time and the relatively short tenure of most respondents could indicate that respondents were uncertain about their hospitals' orientations. One indication of this "misreading of the system" is that, although the responses on organizational decision making reveal the system as highly centralized, some of the corporate executives reported that they believed their organization was too decentralized.

Strategic Orientation: The Hospital Perspective. Sisters of Mercy hospital CEOs did not agree with the corporate perception of their strategic orientation in 1985, another sign of "corporate confusion." Only 11 percent of the CEOs perceived of their hospitals as prospectors, 67 percent as analyzers, 11 percent as defenders, and 11 percent as reactors. By 1987, 20 percent of 1985's analyzers had changed their orientations to either prospectors or reactors, resulting in 16 percent of the hospitals perceiving of themselves as prospectors, 52 percent as analyzers, 11 percent as defenders, and 21 percent as reactors. The increase in reactors, and perhaps in prospectors as well, reflects the significant organizational structure and decision-making changes experienced during the study period. In addition, by 1987 the hospital division radically changed the role of hospital executives in strategic planning. Those executives willing and able to rise to that challenge became prospectors; others, who may have perceived this new role as one thrust upon them, had not yet developed a consistent strategic orientation.

Strategic Planning Process and Outcome. As of 1985, Sisters of Mercy was the only one of the study systems whose acute care hospital line of business did not have a formalized strategic planning process. The position of assistant vice-president for strategic planning had been created with the newly restructured organization and had been filled for only seven months during 1985. Before that, the corporation had an overall strategic plan — formal, centrally determined, and process oriented — to which the hospital members conformed. However, hospital CEOs were not evaluated on criteria related to the system's strategic planning process or outcome, but on subjective bases.

The primary corporate-level goals of the system in 1985 were to diversify into health care financing and to grow through merger with and acquisition of not-for-profit freestanding hospitals and systems with compatible religious values and interests. The hospital-level priorities were to downsize hospitals through layoffs and bed closure, to create linkages with physicians, and to provide health care services to a greater number of poor and elderly. Sisters of Mercy and Southwest were the only study systems in 1985 that planned diversification efforts outside health care; namely, real estate development and construction. The primary purpose was to generate revenue to subsidize care for the poor and elderly.

1987 Followup: What Happened? In 1987, Sisters of Mercy published an internal document describing its approach to strategic planning. For the first time, hospital CEOs were asked to participate in the process. The document states: "This report differs from its predecessor in that it is less prescriptive and more outcome oriented. It recognizes the increasing sophistication of our management teams. As a result, it places greater emphasis on outcomes rather than process. This document will be considered a success if it leads to strategic plans that are more results oriented than previous plans." In the report, hospital CEOs were provided detailed guidelines on what information to collect, and over what period of time, to do an environmental assessment; the overall goals of the corporation and the role of each subsidiary in achieving each goal; the specific goals of each hospital in the development of managed care products; and the time line for each hospital for completion of strategic planning drafts, reviews and site visits by corporate and regional staff, proposal of plans to the corporate board, and action by the board.

The new strategic planning process, while highly formal and centralized, contained significant new responsibilities for local hospital CEOs. Certain overall corporate plans were the primary responsibility of the acute care hospital subsidiary: development of linkages with other not-for-profit systems of the same religious sect, provision of health care services to the economically disadvantaged, vertical and horizontal integration in current service areas, creation of linkages with physicians to develop alternative delivery and financing options, and enhancement of the financial position of the company to pursue these priorities. This was an ambitious set of goals, especially given the financial and strategic position of the company in 1985. However, they are almost exactly the same as the corporate-level priorities reported in 1985.

In the span of two years, surrounded by a sea of regulatory and competitive forces, Sisters of Mercy came to grips with the many challenges it faced. Some were internally generated, such as having initiated corporate restructuring without securing a sufficient core management team to lead the transition. It also faced challenges in assessing its financial and strategic capabilities to pursue diversification efforts. It pursued many efforts simultaneously, resulting in less progress in any one effort than might have been accomplished otherwise. Sisters of Mercy has been able to maintain its financial viability through its ability to climb a steep organizational learning curve, characterized by stabilizing the organizational structure and developing and decentralizing strategic planning. The current challenge is to secure the financial strength needed to develop community care systems consistent with the corporation's values.

Southwest Community Health Services

Goals and Values, Strengths and Weaknesses. "Doing well and doing good" were strong messages articulated by Southwest's corporate executives, who emphasized attention and responsiveness to patients, the community (including employees), and the external environment as a whole. Executives perceived strength in the system's religious roots (although it is now a secular system), its board and management excellence, and the geographical concentration of its member hospitals.

Attention to the needs of the community comes with a weighty price tag. Executives believed the "white knight" activity of saving rural hospitals, although serving the system's mission and supporting its political strength in the state, had been detrimental to its financial position. They also perceived weaknesses in the system's position on alternative delivery systems and out-of-hospital services.

Strategic Orientation: The Corporate Perspective. In 1985, system executives rated their organization as an analyzer, with an average score of 4.5. They predicted a gentle change from analyzer toward analyzer/prospector in 1987, the most modest trend predicted by any system. The hospital characteristics described above are reflected in corporate executives' perceptions of the abilities of their member hospitals to make strategic change. On average, executives perceived 61 percent of their hospitals as prospectors, 32 percent as analyzers, 5 percent as defenders, and 2 percent as reactors. Like Intermountain, Southwest executives believed their hospitals had a higher propensity toward change than the system as a whole, but for different reasons. Unlike Intermountain, which provided strong central direction for its member hospitals in 1985, Southwest had already "given away" some of its central direction to its urban hospitals, which were more likely to be viewed as prospectors than the rural affiliates.

Strategic Orientation: The Hospital Perspective. In an unprecedented response pattern, 100 percent of Southwest's hospital CEOs rated their hospitals as analyzers in 1985. It appeared that urban hospital CEOs, faced with stiff competition, were seldom first to develop new services across the board but relied more on a market-niche strategy characteristic of analyzers. On the other hand, the system's rural hospitals, by virtue of being part of a strategically sophisticated corporation, also viewed themselves primarily as analyzers, even if, for the most part, they were defending their own turf and struggling to maintain current services and products.

By 1987, hospital CEOs' perceptions had altered but, generally, not in the direction predicted by the corporate staff in 1985. On average, 14 percent now perceived of their hospital as a prospector, 57 percent as analyzers, and two (29 percent) as defenders. The increase in defenders may reflect rural CEOs' greater understanding of their strategic role within the system. In sole-provider rural communities, a hospital that offers a stable set of services and products may serve the community and the system better than a hospital engaged in a great number of high-risk initiatives.

Strategic Planning Process and Outcomes. Southwest's strategic planning process provides a useful example of identifying a strategic focus within an overall service mission. In the early 1980s, seeing competitive changes beginning in their metropolitan area, the board and management of Southwest hired an outside consulting firm to help formulate a strategic plan. The firm, and one consultant in particular, convinced the corporate leaders that the downward trend in admissions was not a temporary "blip" but an indicator of the future. After working together closely for several months, the consultant and the system executives developed a formal strategic plan for both the corporate and hospital levels. The system then wooed the consultant away from the firm to direct a newly created strategic planning department.

Thus, Southwest accepted its lack of expertise in strategic planning and acquired that expertise from outside. As the CEO of the company said in 1985, "I'm just an old-fashioned hospital administrator who believes that operations are the guts of the organization, as opposed to planning. I'm more of a manager than a visionary."

The new vice-president for strategic planning set out to create an ongoing strategic approach for the system, to develop plans with an intent to implement them, and to legitimize the place of strategic planning in the organization. He created a top-down, centralized planning function that by 1985 was still not tied to the system's budget cycle or CEO evaluation criteria, but that moved the system closer to a strategic direction. He developed and implemented plans, some of which succeeded and some not, teaching the system, in increments, how to be an analyzer/prospector.

Southwest's corporate-level plans in 1985 focused on diversification, growth, and linkages with physicians. The primary diversification goal, which also included linking with physicians, was the further development of managed care and alternative delivery options. The system had unsuccessfully attempted an HMO earlier in the decade. Executives reported that they had learned from this experience and were ready to try again. They also planned to expand their successful computer software subsidiary. New areas planned included long-term care and behavioral medicine. Southwest was the only system besides Sisters of Mercy that had plans unrelated to health care—also in real estate ownership and also for revenue generation.

The system's hospital-level plans for 1985 included downsizing current facilities, concentrating on efficiency, especially in rural operations, and expanding, after carefully planned market research, into "high tech and high touch" units in its urban facilities. The goal was to develop a clinically integrated tertiary regional referral system to keep patients within the Southwest umbrella of care.

1987 Followup: What Happened? With few exceptions, the plans and priorities of 1985 were realized by 1987, although progress was slower than some top executives anticipated. Southwest, like Evangelical and Intermountain and unlike the other five study systems, experienced success and growth in its managed care activities. A high degree of sensitivity toward local markets and physician relationships played a key role in this success. To a greater degree than Evangelical and Intermountain, Southwest looked toward future growth and expansion in HMOs, PPOs, and other managed care opportunities. Like all the other study systems, Southwest found urgent care centers a disappointment in their ability to generate revenues or hospital referrals, and decreased involvement in these efforts. Also like the other systems, Southwest strengthened its commitment to "provider activities" and reduced its interest in diversification for its own sake.

Although other systems experienced turnover in hospital CEOs during our study period, Southwest actively encouraged it. Inefficient managers were moved down or out, and new ones were brought in from the outside. This change could explain the change in CEO perceptions from 1985 to 1987 on system centralization and strategic orientation. The new "lean and mean" set of CEOs was perceived as "the strongest administrative team we've ever had" by the vice-president of strategic planning. These executives were placed on an incentive pay schedule relating to their skills as facility managers and to their role in strategic planning and implementation. The imbalance between rural and urban facilities still existed in 1987, but the rural hospitals were no longer considered a "mission-driven writeoff." The system was actively exploring new strategies for some of its rural hospitals, including closing some or converting them to specialty hospitals.

By achieving greater strategic sophistication, however, the executives reflected fewer of the mission-driven priorities in 1987 than they did in 1985. Like all the systems with formal or informal religious ties, Southwest had difficulty doing good and doing well simultaneously.

Conclusion: Pieces of the Model

It is useful to step back from the individual histories of the eight systems. All faced a similar national environment, different state environments, and multiple different local environments. They possessed, in varying degrees, different missions, strategic orientations, and managerial characteristics, and had different levels of past performance. As we will see in later chapters, their strategies had different levels of success. What do these histories have to contribute to an increased understanding of strategic adaptation?

It is clear that no single variable adequately explains an

organization's perceived need for strategic change or its selection of a specific strategy. Considerable trial-and-error learning was involved. However, it is clear that during the study period:

1. All the participating systems perceived the need for some degree of strategic change as a *system*.
2. Before the early 1980s, all but one of the systems (NME) perceived little or no need for strategic change.
3. Approximately half the individual hospitals changed their strategies while half did not.
4. The *systems'* selection of specific strategies, given their different missions and orientations, was strikingly similar in their response to the national competitive environment.
5. Some systems were overly diversified, and some were less prepared for the changes than others.

   Did the larger environment, then, reduce the influence of other organizational characteristics on the perceived need for change and the selection of specific strategies? To some extent, yes. All eight systems, on however unequal strategic footing at the beginning of the decade, benefitted from a leap in organizational learning brought on by the environmental changes of the mid-1980s. Changes in regulation, to some extent, and competition to a great extent, provided opportunities for the organizations predisposed to change, but also forced open the eyes of those less predisposed. Varying levels of difficulty were faced, and will continue to be faced, by systems as they experiment with horizontal and vertical integration, national and local consolidation and affiliation, and the continued imperative of the health care industry to balance the need to do well with the desire to do good. The most lasting impression, however, was the extent and speed of strategic change that occurred in an industry that before had never been required to behave strategically. As noted in Chapter One, the speed of the change was fueled not only by PPS but by the related cost-containment approaches of other payors, by the growing influence of employers, by the increase in competition for patients, and by the continuing decline in inpatient admissions.

4

Structuring the Relationship Between the Corporation and the Hospital

This chapter explores the element of the model of strategic adaptation (Figure 2.1) that is related to management processes, particularly the relationship between the corporate office and the strategic business unit (in this case, the individual hospital). These relationships are little understood in the literature, particularly how they are structured during times of significant environmental change.

Table 4.1 summarizes our findings on three centralization measures; Table 4.2 presents the degree to which each system is organized along functional versus divisional lines. The not-for-profit systems as a group are more centralized than their investor-owned counterparts, but this was primarily because of differences in size rather than ownership form. Being smaller, and relatively more geographically concentrated, the not-for-profit systems found it easier to exert more centralized control over their hospitals.

The advantages and disadvantages of different organization designs are well documented in the literature (Galbraith, 1973; Duncan, 1979; Leatt, Shortell, and Kimberly, 1988). *Functional* designs exist where each individual in the organization

Table 4.1. Centralization of Strategic
Planning and Decision Making by System, 1987.

	Overall Centralization of Strategic Planning[a]	Centralization of Specific Strategic Planning Functions[b]	Centralization of Specific Decisions[c]
Investor-owned			
AMI	30.5	1.5	3.2
HCA	26.8	1.4	3.0
NME	27.1	1.4	3.3
Investor-owned group average	27.5	1.4	3.0
Not-for-profit			
Evangelical	30.0	1.9	4.2
Health Central (Health One)	31.3	1.7	3.2
Intermountain	34.2	1.6	3.7
Sisters of Mercy	28.4	1.4	3.3
Southwest	32.8	2.2	3.5
Not-for-profit group average	31.3[d]	1.6[d]	3.5[d]

[a]See Resource A; 3–42 scale based on weighted responses.
[b]See Resource A; 1 = individual hospital to 3 = corporate office.
[c]See Resource A; 1 = individuals below CEO level to 6 = corporate board.
[d]$p \leq .001$; not-for-profit as a group significantly different from investor-owned as a group.

responsible for a given function (such as finance, marketing, planning, or human resources) reports to the corporate officer responsible for that function. In a hospital system, for example, this would mean that all individual hospital controllers would report to the corporate chief financial officer. Functional designs tend to work best in single-product companies operating in low-complexity environments.

In contrast, *divisional* designs duplicate many functions (finance, marketing, planning, and human resources) within every division. Hospital systems might create divisions based on geography or product lines (for example, acute care hospitals, psychiatric hospitals, or managed care activities). In a divisional organization, each staff support person reports to the head of the division rather than to the corporate officer. Divisional designs tend to have advantages in multiproduct organizations

Table 4.2. Organizational Reporting Structure.

System		Offices Reporting to Hospital COO		Offices Reporting to Corporate CEO		Total Functional/ Divisional Ratio
		Functional	Divisional	Functional	Divisional	
Investor-owned						
AMI	1985	2	3	3	2	5/5
	1987	4	4	8	1	12/5
HCA	1985	2	12	5	5	7/17
	1987	3	6	4	3	7/9
NME	1985	0	10	4	7	4/17
	1987	0	4	1	3	1/7
Investor-owned group average	1985	1.3	8.3	4.0	4.7	5.3/13
	1987	2.3	4.7	4.3	2.3	6.7/7
Not-for-profit						
Evangelical	1985	3	3	8	2	11/5
	1987	3	2	7	4	10/6
Health Central (Health One)	1985	3	2	5	1	8/3
	1987	0	3	2	3	2/6
Intermountain	1985	6	6	7	2	13/8
	1987	2	2	1.5	2.5	3.5/4.5
Sisters of Mercy	1985	5	3	3	3	8/6
	1987	5	3	0	7	5/10
Southwest	1985	7	6	3	4	10/10
	1987	4	6	4	3	8/9
Not-for-profit group average	1985	4.8	4.0	5.2	2.4	10/6.4
	1987	2.8	3.2	2.9	3.9	5.7/7.1

operating in more complex environments. Resources are concentrated to enable each division to respond effectively to its needs. The downside is that it can become difficult to address organizationwide issues that cut across divisions. *Matrix designs,* incorporating both functional and divisional features and involving dual reporting relationships, also exist. Among the systems studied, however, functional and divisional designs dominated.

Using organizational charts for both 1985 and 1987, supplemented by telephone interviews, we were able to calculate the number of activities organized around functions versus divisions for each system. The functional/divisional ratios (Table 4.2) show that the investor-owned systems were more divisional than the not-for-profit systems in 1985, while in 1987 both not-for-profit and investor-owned had an approximately equal ratio of functional to divisional groups. Most of the systems felt that organizing around divisions, with some of the planning, marketing, finance, and human resource support functions located within the divisions, provided greater flexibility for responding to the changing environment. It is interesting to note that AMI was the only system that became *more functionally* oriented between 1985 and 1987.

In the sections that follow, issues involving centralization versus decentralization of decision making, functional versus divisional organization, and the dynamics of the corporate office–hospital interface are highlighted for each system.

American Medical International (AMI)

Centralization/Decentralization. Among all the systems, AMI's corporate executives perceived themselves as the most decentralized in decision making. Its hospital CEOs had a similar view. This was consistent with AMI's philosophy of granting operational autonomy to individual CEOs while still maintaining a fair amount of control over the strategic planning function. In fact, AMI was the most centralized among the investor-owned systems in overall strategic planning control. This helps to explain AMI's emphasis on a greater number of functional reporting lines than the other investor-owned systems.

Functional/Divisional Organization. AMI reflected an even balance of functional and divisional reporting lines in 1985 but more than doubled its functional reporting lines by 1987. The change was entirely accounted for by the addition of functionally responsible executives at the corporate office. In 1985, AMI's functional/divisional profile was more similar to the not-for-profit organizations, which were also smaller and more centralized in their decision making. The addition of more functional reporting lines sent a mixed message to AMI's individual hospital CEOs; on the one hand, they believed they had operational autonomy but, on the other hand, found themselves involved in more and more reporting relationships. Some of the difficulties this caused are elaborated below.

Corporate Office–Hospital Interface. The changes in AMI's structure over the study period had less to do with the system's hospitals than with the balance of power in the executive suites. During the study period, AMI's founding CEO resigned. The chief operating officer (COO) moved into the top position, and an executive from within was promoted to COO. At the time of the 1985 interviews the new "executive team" had not yet been fully determined. Personality and general business acumen were portrayed as more important executive characteristics than industry knowledge or function-specific expertise. In AMI, more than any other system, executives insisted that "managing is managing, whether you run a hospital company or make widgets." Corporate executives were recruited almost exclusively from other industries, deliberately *not* selected from the hospital or regional management levels. Hospital CEOs were portrayed as technicians—experts in the areas of managing nurses and physicians and daily hospital operations, but generally not capable of managing the complexities of the system as a whole.

This accounts for the seemingly contradictory findings of decentralization matched with heavy functional reporting lines noted above. AMI's corporate staff was a business "cabinet" to the CEO, and was recruited based on the CEO's needs and preferences. However, delegating divisional responsibilities to corporate staff would require these executives to have enough industry knowledge to effectively lead regional and hospital managers. Instead, AMI attempted to delegate some of these responsibilities, such as formal strategic planning, to hospital CEOs who were unprepared for them, while at the same time the corporate office staff, lacking industry experience, did not relate well to some of the operating problems faced by local CEOs. This void led to problems in strategy implementation, as we will see in Part Two.

Hospital Corporation of America (HCA)

Centralization/Decentralization. HCA corporate executives also perceived decision making to be relatively decentralized. HCA's individual hospital executives felt decision making was even more decentralized. Decentralized decision making is one of HCA's most strongly held corporate values. Although there were many advantages to such decentralization, it sometimes created problems for reactor- and defender-oriented hospitals, which required more centralized control and guidance.

Functional/Divisional Organization. HCA, more in keeping with its decentralized operational decision making than AMI, was organized largely along divisional lines in 1985. A few functionally responsible executives operated at the corporate level, but for the most part the organization was divided into geographical divisions. Between 1985 and 1987 HCA streamlined its structure dramatically, resulting in eight fewer divisions. Unlike AMI, HCA fills many of its regional and corporate staff positions with individuals who have had some hospital operational experience. This helped to facilitate relationships between the corporate office and individual hospitals.

Corporate Office–Hospital Interface. HCA provides a fascinating contrast to AMI on many dimensions. Unlike the "managing is managing" hallmark of AMI, HCA perceived itself as hospital oriented. A number of corporate executives had an orientation toward hospital activities, and many of those responsible for owned and managed facilities had firsthand knowledge of hospital operations. In fact, in 1985 corporate executives voiced concern that the rapid growth of the company had created a large pool of hospital CEOs aiming for the corporate office. Advancement from the field, high job satisfaction, and long tenure of corporate office staff had already resulted in a large support staff at corporate headquarters. In 1985 the corporate office conducted a job satisfaction campaign for hospital CEOs, including a new bonus program, to convince executives in the field of the prestige and monetary benefits of their current positions.

HCA prided itself on the autonomy it allowed local hospital CEOs but, unlike AMI, not because they were perceived as technical experts. Most of the corporate office staff was intimately aware of the local forces with which a CEO must deal, and to which even a knowledgeable corporate office might not respond quickly enough or appropriately. Corporate executives did not perceive the system as an entity that revolved around the technical core of individual hospital operations, as did AMI executives. On the contrary, executives frequently referred to the system as a loosely tied federation of hospitals, and hoped that the members of the federation might be drawn together into a tighter network with one another and with the corporate office.

An important dimension of HCA's activities is its relationship with its managed hospitals. These hospitals provide the system important distribution channels for achieving local market continuums of care; career-path opportunities for young administrators; opportunities to spread the name and influence of the system across a wider geographical base; and, to a lesser extent, a "trial marriage" for potential acquisition candidates. Systems, particularly investor-owned systems, tend to avoid hospital ownership in heavily regulated states (those with restrictive rate regulation, certificate of need, or all-payor programs), for example the New England states. Contract management of facilities in these states allows systems access to the provider and political networks without the financial risks of ownership, although executives report that lobbying efforts are lower in states with only managed facilities.

In HCA, managed hospitals report through a different line of regional and corporate executives than do owned hospitals, but are considered full members of the system in terms of access to corporate resources. Unlike some of the other systems to be described below, HCA believes the decision to initiate and terminate a management contract should be solely in the hands of the hospital board, not in the hands of the system. In 1985, the managed hospitals were considered a more highly valued resource than they had been before because of the broader geographical base they provided for a planned managed care network.

National Medical Enterprises (NME)

Centralization/Decentralization. Similar to AMI and HCA, NME corporate executives saw decision making as relatively decentralized. This was generally supported by the individual hospital CEOs, although they perceived NME as even more decentralized than did the corporate executives. Decentralization was facilitated by having a very lean corporate staff with relatively few functional responsibilities.

Functional/Divisional Organization. In 1985, NME, along with HCA, was the most divisionalized of all the systems. By 1987, the number of divisions had been reduced by more than half, and only one function remained (governmental and external relations). Some corporate office staff wore two hats, being responsible, for example, for planning and an operating division. NME strongly felt that this organization structure best suited its diversification philosophy.

Corporate Office–Hospital Interface. Like HCA, decentralization was part of NME's culture and operating philosophy, but for different reasons. NME's divisional and decentralized structure stems from the diversified nature of the company. No one executive or department could efficiently balance the demands of acute care hospitals, psychiatric and long-term care facilities, and medical equipment companies. Different client types, regulation, competition, payment sources, and technical expertise in each area would make integration of budgeting, management information systems, marketing, and strategic planning inappropriate. Further, NME expanded into new lines of business primarily by acquiring entire companies and has attempted to retain their management teams when possible. These acquisitions had already developed functions suited to their needs; creating corporate functions to support them would have been redundant. But the primary reason for the system's divisional structure was a matter of design rather than convenience. The original vision of the company's founder and CEO was a diversified, decentralized, divisionalized health care organization. Even though the system's structure is closer to HCA's, the philosophy behind that structure—holding operations expertise at arm's length from corporate office—is more similar to AMI's.

Like HCA, NME also pursues management contracts to gain a foothold in a geographical area, to enhance its image, or to court a potential acquisition candidate. NME, however, differs from HCA in that it will not renew the contract if the hospital is not meeting the system's expectations. Also unlike HCA, managed and owned facility CEOs report through the same regional and corporate managers. Managed hospitals do not receive the management information services of the corporate office that owned hospitals receive, but in other respects the facilities are considered full system members. Although a few hospitals terminated their management contracts during the study period, there was far less turnover in NME than in HCA.

Evangelical Health System

Centralization/Decentralization. In 1985, Evangelical's corporate executives perceived their organization as one of the most centralized among those studied. Marketing, strategic planning, and management information support functions were all highly centralized at the corporate office. While hospital CEOs did not perceive this degree of centralization in 1985, they clearly did by 1987, when they showed the highest centralization score among all the systems. This centralized structure was largely a reflection of the new corporate CEO who was brought in to provide a professional management focus to guide the corporation toward further growth.

Functional/Divisional Organization. In keeping with its centralized decision making and with the close geographical proximity of its hospitals, Evangelical was primarily organized along functional lines, especially at the corporate level. All divisional heads, at both the acute care hospital and corporate level, were housed in the corporate headquarters building.

There was little change in the organizational structure from 1985 to 1987. New lines of business brought in as subsidiaries required divisions of their own, and the closure of one hospital eliminated the need for one of the hospital-level divisions. However, the corporation remains predominantly functionally organized.

Corporate Office–Hospital Interface. Evangelical executives emphasized the efficiencies of a centralized, functionally organized company, given the concentration of business units in one metropolitan area. They also expressed some of the "managing is managing" philosophies of AMI, particularly in the area of finance. The corporate chief financial officer (CFO) had been wooed into the system from private industry and knew very little about the health care industry. His job was to manage debt, investments, financing of the corporate subsidiaries, and employee pension funds. Unlike AMI, Evangelical did not pursue corporate management as a separate goal, leaving hospital operations to "the experts." Rather, it extended its "managing is managing" philosophy, at least in terms of finance, to the hospital level. All member hospitals' controllers reported directly to the corporate CFO.

The value placed on management sophistication in 1985 was a side effect of the transition the company was then making to a new structure and a new CEO. The new CEO had been recruited from outside, although from within the health care industry, five years earlier. Two years before the study, the company was restructured into a parent corporation with a hospital company and nonhospital subsidiaries. The former company president became chair of the new corporate board and entered semiretirement. The company was in transition throughout the study period. Issues involved in balancing the religious mission and professional management were highlighted in Chapter

Three. Basically, Evangelical executives felt that a more centralized structure helped to manage this balance.

By 1987, management of the nonhospital subsidiaries had become, as one executive said, "too damn complex" to maintain centralized decision making. The system then released its centralized grasp on some of its subsidiaries but simultaneously tightened that grasp on its hospitals. As the CEOs' responses reflected, the system executives reported that by 1987, hospital CEOs had little input to the *system's* strategic plan, which was primarily developed at the corporate level. The hospital division, however, developed its own plan with input from individual CEOs. These plans were more tactically and operationally oriented. Each hospital, in turn, had its own plan within the context of the hospital division and overall system plan. Because Evangelical is a small system, this approach has worked well to date. The quality of strategic planning is well respected internally, and individual hospital CEOs seem to have bought into the process.

Health Central (Health One)

Centralization/Decentralization. In 1985, Health Central's executives perceived their system to be highly decentralized in decision making, looking much more like the investor-owned systems than other not-for-profit systems. These perceptions were largely shared by individual hospital CEOs in both 1985 and 1987.

By 1987, the relationship took on a different tone as Health Central engaged in merger discussions with Health One. Decentralization of operating responsibilities continued, but greater emphasis was placed on establishing more direct accountability between the local hospital governing boards and the corporate office. To better compete as a system and work through the merger details, Health Central executives felt the need for greater policymaking authority at the corporate level.

Functional/Divisional Organization. In 1985, Health Central had just undergone corporate restructuring. The acute care hospital line of business had become a subsidiary of a new parent organization. New subsidiaries had been developed for long-term care and consulting. The hospital system's president had become president of the corporate parent, and a chief operating officer had been promoted from within to lead the hospital subsidiary. The new structure had many more functional than divisional lines of reporting, but relatively few individuals filled those positions. That is, the executives from the "old" hospital system had been promoted into at least one position in the new structure. Many individuals held dual roles, even though each slot in the new structure was intended to be a full-time position. The corporate restructuring had taken place without a great influx of executives, from either within or outside.

By 1987, the system had adjusted to the new structure and had divisionalized almost completely, both at the hospital and at the corporate level, while reducing the number of functional reporting lines from eight to two. Fewer individuals wore two hats by 1987, mostly because positions and reporting lines were reduced and responsibilities were pushed down to the regional and hospital level.

Corporate Office–Hospital Interface. Although in 1985 the functional organizational structure of Health Central appeared to counteract its decentralized decision-making style, the structure itself was somewhat artificial. Having just undergone a corporate restructuring, the system was, as executives reported, "just settling in." Some individuals who had been valued executives in the hospital system were promoted into new positions to "fill in the blanks" in the new organizational chart. In 1985 their positions were less meaningful as functions than as representations of continuity of management. Health Central, like NME, placed a high value on the individual and on entrepreneurship, although Health Central consistently reflected a closer bond to the acute care hospital industry. Also like NME, Health Central executives referred frequently and with pride to the presence and guidance of their CEO, which had resulted in a centralized, formal, but supportive strategic planning function. But this example of centralization was the exception rather than the rule. For as much as the system was similar to NME in the executives' frequent references to individualism, it also resembled HCA in their frequent mention of local autonomy and in their reports of support and communication with hospital-level executives.

As a result of its proposed merger with Health One, Health Central's organization structure in 1987 was again in flux. As one executive reported, "The current structure won't last. It's designed around people. Ninety percent of the people will still have jobs, but they will be different. Most of the changes will be made at the corporate level, not the hospital level." This comment reflects the continued balance between a support of individual excellence at the corporate level and respect for the knowledge and authority of the local hospital CEO.

The system divisionalized by 1987, and did so dramatically. Management retreats were taken off the agenda after the merger, and the corporate office ceased performing environmental assessments for local hospitals. Hospital CEOs and physicians were now responsible for developing the hospitals' strategic plans. Hospital CEOs gained authority to change product lines. The corporate office–hospital relationship became what one executive described as similar to the relationship between General Motors and its auto dealers.

Health Central also operated a few hospitals under management contract. These were generally requested by local hospital boards and involved a longstanding relationship. These hospitals had access to the same management expertise and corporate resources as did their owned counterparts. In terms of marketing support, however, corporate staff focused more attention on the owned than the managed hospitals.

Intermountain Health Care

Centralization/Decentralization. Intermountain executives saw themselves as a highly centralized system in 1985, a view essentially shared by hospital CEOs in both 1985 and 1987. They were the most centralized of all systems in overall strategic planning. Of all the systems, Intermountain gave particular emphasis to monitoring physician performance. HMO/PPO contract negotiations were also centralized. In fact, the managed care contracting was so tightly centralized that information on HMO discounts had to be obtained from the corporate office; individual hospitals were unaware of their percentage discount.

Functional/Divisional Organization. In 1985, Intermountain had an even number of functional and divisional reporting lines within the acute care hospital line of business, but was heavily weighted toward a functional structure at the corporate level. This functional-divisional blend places the system somewhere at the midpoint of organizational structure in comparison to the other study systems, similar to its position on the centralization continuum.

By 1987, Intermountain consolidated the three hospital divisions under a single individual who, in turn, reported to an overall hospital division head. This resulted in two divisions and two functional areas reporting to the hospital head. At the corporate level, a number of functional lines were reduced while the number of divisional lines remained essentially the same. One individual held both functional responsibility as vice-president for finance and divisional responsibility as head of the health plans division. Overall, Intermountain executives felt the new structure made them more responsive to their regional marketplace.

Corporate Office–Hospital Interface. Intermountain was similar to HCA in its industry reputation for profitability, after accounting for differences in ownership status. The two systems also shared a tradition of internally directed use of slack resources. Both had also directed resources toward upgrading physical plant, investment, and image enhancement. Intermountain also focused much of its organizational slack on quality enhancement in the areas of patient outcomes, patient satisfaction, staff development, utilization review, and physician relations.

The system's religious heritage sheds light on its centralized decision making and organizational structure. Decisions about the purpose and future of the group as a whole were made centrally, as were a general set of values that guided members' behavior. Intermountain's centrally controlled pursuit of quality enhancement reflected the system's values. While the system members were allowed some flexibility in adapting to their immediate environments (percentage of charity care offered, pricing of specific services), they were similar enough to one another (in corporatewide medical staff policies, staff development programs, marketing, information systems, managed care negotiation) to be easily identifiable as members of the same group. Thus, some of the decentralization implied by greater divisionalization occurred within a strong commonly held value system involving clear understanding of "how things are and should be done." This philosophy generally extended to Intermountain's managed hospitals, which reported to the same management structure as the owned hospitals and generally received the same level of support and resources.

Sisters of Mercy Health Corporation

Centralization/Decentralization. Mercy Health Services executives saw themselves as a centralized system in 1985 — the most centralized of the eight systems. Services such as purchasing, personnel benefits, and insurance had been coordinated since the early 1970s. Many of the hospital CEOs essentially concurred with this perception in 1985 when major steps were taken to refine line management relationships between the CEOs and the regional executive vice-presidents. By 1987, they saw the system's decision making as somewhat less centralized. Changes in strategic and financial planning responsibilities, system performance, and organization structure were responsible for this shift.

Functional/Divisional Organization. Reflecting the direction of their strategic plan and similar to Health Central and Intermountain, Sisters of Mercy Health Corporation (SMHC) experienced significant organizational change during the study period. In 1985, at both the corporate and acute care hospital levels, the system was nearly evenly balanced in functional and divisional reporting lines, although the hospital level was slightly heavier on the functional side. By 1987, the structure had evolved. Four more divisional (subsidiary) reporting lines had been created, reflecting the corporation's evolution into managed care, elderly services, home care, and related initiatives. The hospital-level reporting lines remained stable during the study period.

Corporate Office–Hospital Interface. Just prior to the study, SMHC corporately restructured. The hospital corporation's president became the CEO of the new parent company and retained responsibility for the hospital subsidiary until a new president was appointed in 1986. The vacancies in the hospital subsidiary were mirrored in other divisions (subsidiaries) as they were being established by the restructuring. The leadership in corporate-level function positions was evolving as well. Many interviews conducted in 1985 were with "interim" and "acting" division heads or corporate staff as the permanent leadership team was in the process of being recruited.

Mercy Health Services' 1985 structure was a reflection of its recent ministry evolution, strategic planning, and organizational restructuring. By 1987, the leadership team was in place and the strategic plan was being implemented. The president of the hospital subsidiary had designed a matrix reporting structure that was implemented at the end of the study period. The evolution of the system's strategic plan and the associated changes partly explain the number of SMHC hospitals that became reactors during the study period.

SMHC and its divisions operate a number of hospitals under management contract. The system uses formal criteria for the contracts, based primarily on compatibility with philosophy and mission, what makes sense in the local service area, and compatibility with the hospital's management staff. The managed hospitals report to the same management structure through the owned hospitals, based on their geographic location.

Southwest Community Health Services

Centralization/Decentralization. Southwest's corporate executives perceived themselves in 1985 as a moderately centralized system, similar to Intermountain. Like Intermountain, however, Southwest's hospital CEOs considered the system highly centralized, particularly in 1985 and somewhat less so in 1987. Part of the overall perceived centralization can be attributed to strong centralized strategic planning initiated in the early 1980s, which held implications for many operating decisions as well.

Functional/Divisional Organization. Similarities to Intermountain also exist in the area of organizational structure. In both 1985 and 1987, Southwest had a fairly large number of total reporting lines evenly balanced between functional and divisional. Only Evangelical shared such stability in organizational structure. Southwest's stability in structure was matched by a stability in corporate staff unequaled by any other system during the study period. No new executives were brought in to the top corporate staff and none left from 1985 to 1987. Also, other than minor title and position changes, the executives did not change roles during this time. No other system experienced such consistency.

Corporate Office–Hospital Interface. Southwest's unique combination of centralization and organizational structure has a great deal to do with the location and characteristics of its member hospitals. The urban hospitals represent the "best and the brightest" jewels in the system's corporate crown, while the rural facilities are, for the most part, recipients of a mission-driven orientation. In many cases, if the system had not acquired a rural hospital, it would have closed, leaving a large geographical area without an acute care facility. All the rural facilities are small with relatively low occupancy rates. Patients requiring sophisticated technology or intensive services are transported to urban facilities, some into Southwest's Albuquerque hospitals but others to urban tertiary care centers outside the system. The state as a whole has a lower than average physician to population ratio, but the state ratio masks a large imbalance between rural and urban areas. Southwest executives report serious physician shortages in the outlying areas and a "physician glut" in the metropolises.

More than other systems, Southwest for all practical purposes operates two systems: one metropolitan-based, successful, divisionalized organization with participative management, and one that is more centrally directed, designed to keep rural hospitals viable. The urban hospital group enhances its efficiency by using centrally available functions, such as marketing, human resources, and finance, although CEOs participate in marketing and planning groups for hospital and areawide services. The rural hospitals are corporately supported to varying but higher degrees in all functions. Understanding this bifurcation between urban and rural environments sheds light on the balance of functional and divisional reporting lines and the differences in the perception of centralization by the hospital CEOs and corporate executives.

Southwest also has a small number of hospitals with management contracts or leases. They report through the same management structure as the owned hospitals, have access to similar levels of corporate resources, and most have been relatively long-term members of the system.

Summary

In general, we found the not-for-profit systems more centralized in their decision making than the investor-owned. For the most part, individual hospital executives agreed with their corporate office counterparts. Organizational structure (functional versus divisional) was an open target for change from 1985 to 1987 and, in turn, influenced centralization and the nature of strategic planning. Contract management of hospitals was pursued for slightly different reasons by systems of different ownership status. For investor-owned systems, the contract was a potential source of market integration, revenue generation, and image building, and was a way to secure a fit with a hospital for later acquisition. For most not-for-profit systems, management contracts were primarily a reflection of the mission to serve a given community. For the most part, the reporting lines and services offered were similar to those experienced by the owned hospitals.

By far the most salient feature of the corporate office–hospital interface was the marked changes in the structures of these relationships over a relatively brief time period. With the exception of Southwest, every system corporately reorganized or restructured at least once; some went through several reorganizations. The changes were perhaps most dramatic for AMI, HCA, Health Central, and Sisters of Mercy. For the not-for-profits, there was a general trend toward creating more divisions and reducing the number of functional lines reporting to the corporate office. This was congruent with a greater emphasis on diversification and the need to respond more rapidly and flexibly to the dynamic changes in the environment. For the investor-owned, particularly HCA and NME, a reduction in the number of divisions reflected their need to streamline and consolidate some of their diversification activities.

The major lesson derived from this experience was the need to match corporate structure and decision-making levels not only with the demands of the larger environment but also with the specific strategic orientations of local hospitals and the demand, needs, and skills of local hospital CEOs. Different mechanisms are required, depending on the needs of different units (Govindarajan, 1988). In a more stable environment, functionally organized companies with relatively centralized decision making had cost and efficiency advantages. But in more rapidly changing environments, more divisionalized structures and decentralized decision making had effectiveness advantages associated with getting things done more quickly and letting those closest to the decision with the requisite expertise take action. Some systems, such as AMI and Sisters of Mercy, got caught in the transition of making these matches and, consequently, experienced some difficulties. Others, such as Evangelical, found they could stick with a functional centralized organization despite the changes in the environment because of their small size and geographically concentrated facilities. Thus, there are no universal guidelines or blueprints to be offered. In turbulent environments, the corporate office–strategic business unit relationship is likely to be in continual flux.

A corollary to the issues of functional versus divisional organization and centralization versus decentralization of decision making is the degree to which these attributes are related to the system's ability to behave as a system rather than as a loose collection of hospitals. (In Chapter Eleven, we suggest seven criteria of "systemness.") The trend, seen in almost all the systems, to move toward greater divisionalization created some problems in their ability to behave as a system. While all systems instituted various systemwide financial planning and management control mechanisms, they varied widely in the other "system" attributes. Each system was strong on one or more dimensions but none was strong across all dimensions. As we will see in Chapter Eleven, the ability to develop systemwide capabilities on all dimensions is likely to be a key factor in systems achieving their goals and objectives.

Part One has used a broad brush to paint the picture of strategic adaptation within the hospital industry. We have focused on the degree and direction of change, system goals and values, strengths and weaknesses, overall structure and decision making, and the nature of the interface between the corporate office and individual hospitals. In Part Two we turn to a more fine-grained analysis of hospital-specific strategic orientations— prospector, defender, analyzer, and reactor—and their performance consequences. The focus is on the requirements for successfully managing these strategic approaches within the context of the overall corporate office–hospital relationship just described.

Part Two

Managing Change
and Adaptation:
Four Strategic Orientations

5

The Four Orientations:
Their Environments, Performance,
and Management Processes

In this section we look in detail at the four strategic orientations. The focus is on three aspects of the model of strategic adaptation outlined in Figure 2.1 — environment, managerial processes, and performance. We consider these in relation to the four orientations and assess the extent to which ownership (investor-owned versus not-for-profit) makes a difference. Chapters Six through Nine then provide detailed examples and guidelines for managing each of the strategic archetypes.

General Background Characteristics

In 1987, 87 of the study hospitals — nearly one-fourth — were prospectors, 24 were defenders, 210 analyzers, and 57 reactors. Of the 87 prospectors, 27 were prospectors two years earlier, 46 were previously analyzers, and the remaining 14 were previously reactors. No defenders attempted to make the jump to the prospector strategy. Of the 24 defenders, 4 were defenders two years previously, 15 were previously analyzers, 4 were previously prospectors, and 1 was a reactor. Of the 202 analyzers, 145 were analyzers two years previously, 23 were previously prospectors, 25 were previously reactors, and 9 were previously defenders. Among the 53 reactors, 9 were previously reactors, 29 were analyzers, 12 were prospectors, and 3 were defenders. Overall, prospectors showed a net gain of 19 hospitals, defenders 8, and reactors 2; analyzers showed a net loss of 29 hospitals. But of the 90 analyzer hospitals that switched strategies, 46 became prospectors, while 29 fell into the reactor category, while only 15 became defenders. Overall, however, the analyzer and prospector are the most prevalent strategic orientations, a finding consistent with other recent studies of health care organizations (Keats, Conant, and Mokwa, 1988; Ginn and McDaniel, 1987).

Table 5.1 summarizes some background characteristics of the prospector, defender, analyzer, and reactor. On many characteristics, defenders are different from the other three. They tend to be smaller, are more likely to be the only hospital in their community, and have CEOs with the shortest job tenure. As expected, they give less emphasis to developing new services or new markets and are less likely to be involved in economic joint ventures with their physicians. They are also less likely to differentiate their services based on technical quality and are more likely to emphasize access and convenience features. They appear to have less slack (they had a lower percentage of profitable services in 1984 and a somewhat lower operating margin in 1983). In contrast, prospectors and reactors are generally larger, more diversified organizations with somewhat higher operating margins in 1983. Prospectors are much less likely to be the only hospital in their community and are the least likely of the four to differentiate their services based on the technical quality of care provided. How these background characteristics affect the hospital's ability to implement the various changes is discussed in Chapters Six through Nine.

Environment

Table 5.2 summarizes three key environmental characteristics — community wealth and resource availability, competition, and regulation — for each strategic orientation.

Table 5.1. Background Characteristics of the Strategic Archetypes.

Characteristic	Prospector	Defender	Analyzer	Reactor	Total Sample Average
Bed size	160	96	147	172	150
Years as a system member	10.1	7.8	8.2	8.5	8.7
Sole provider[a]	9.1%	40.0%	33.3%	24.1%	26.6%
Average years CEO in position[a]	4.2	2.2	3.1	3.4	3.4
Average years CEO with system	7.6	5.7	7.0	7.3	7.1
Number of diversified services offered (bed size adjusted)	10.0	7.3	9.5	9.5	9.5
New service or new market development score[a,b]	79.3	60.2	72.0	67.8	72.4
Own or sponsor an HMO	10.4%	4.0%	8.0%	4.0%	7.7%
Have economic joint venture with their physicians[a]	43.4%	12.0%	20.6%	38.5%	27.9%
Emphasize low-cost provider strategy	17.0%	20.0%	12.4%	13.0%	14.1%

Table 5.1. Background Characteristics of the Strategic Archetypes, Cont'd.

Characteristic	Prospector	Defender	Analyzer	Reactor	Total Sample Average
Differentiate services based on superior technical quality[a]	28.4%	16.0%	22.9%	24.1%	23.9%
Differentiate services based on superior access or convenience	38.6%	60.0%	50.2%	40.7%	46.7%
Differentiate services based on how well they are managed	35.2%	24.0%	28.4%	31.5%	30.2%
Diversified services profitable in 1984[a]	40.0%	29.7%	34.3%	35.4%	33.5%
Fifteen services profitable in 1984[a]	81.4%	66.3%	82.5%	77.4%	76.0%
Operating margin as a percent of net revenue, 1983 ($N = 195$)	8.6%	6.7%	6.9%	8.2%	7.6%

[a]$p \leq .01$; one way analysis of variance
[b]On a scale of 0–200.

Table 5.2. Environmental Characteristics and the Strategic Archetypes.

Environmental Characteristic	Prospector	Defender	Analyzer	Reactor	Total Sample Average
Community Wealth and Resource Availability					
Population below the poverty line	13.3%	15.9%	13.9%	13.9%	13.9%
Median family income adjusted for manufacturing wage index[a]	$18,753	$16,494	$17,367	$18,093	$17,743
Median home value	$47,007	$43,044	$43,810	$45,327	$44,741
Median years of education	11.9	11.8	11.7	11.8	11.7
White-collar and health care professionals in labor force[a]	58.5%	54.6%	54.1%	55.6%	55.4%
Number of active physicians per 1,000 population[a]	1.83	1.47	1.42	1.59	1.55
Population growth 1975–1982	64.8%	49.6%	61.2%	59.1%	60.9%
Competition					
Two or more competing hospitals[a]	67.0%	56.0%	45.3%	50.0%	51.9%

Table 5.2. Environmental Characteristics and the Strategic Archetypes, Cont'd.

Environmental Characteristic	Prospector	Defender	Analyzer	Reactor	Total Sample Average
One or more ambulatory surgery or urgent care center[a]	19.3%	12.0%	5.0%	14.8%	10.3%
Number of HMOs in the market	4.7	2.5	3.3	3.9	3.7
Perceived intensity of market area competition[a] (1 = least intense to 5 = most intense)	4.4	3.8	3.7	3.9	3.9
Regulation					
Stringency of certificate-of-need legislation (0 = least stringent to 22 = most stringent)	9.0	10.6	9.4	9.6	9.5
Stringency of rate-review legislation (0 = least stringent to 14 = most stringent)	4.1	4.0	4.6	5.1	4.3

[a]$p \leq .01$; one way analysis of variance

Source: The primary data source for most measures is the 1980 Area Resource File and updates; secondary data source is the strategic planning questionnaire.

Community Wealth and Resource Availability. Defenders stand out as operating in the least munificent environments. A higher percentage of their population is below the poverty level, with lower median family income and median home values; they have fewer physicians per capita and, perhaps most significant, the lowest population growth of the four groups between 1975 and 1982. Defenders were more frequently found in collar counties and rural areas surrounding metropolitan areas. Given the constrained local environment, they had a particularly difficult time responding to the extensive changes associated with PPS and related developments. Their experience is highlighted in Chapter Seven.

In contrast, prospectors operated in generally the most favorable environments, particularly in regard to the availability of physicians and population growth. As we will see in Chapter Six, both were important ingredients in successfully executing a prospector strategy. Analyzers' environmental characteristics were generally closer to defenders (with the exception of population growth); reactors were generally closer to prospectors.

Competition and Regulation. The favorable environments occupied by prospectors also attracted competition. Prospectors experienced the greatest degree of competition in their local markets, as indicated by the number of competing hospitals, competing ambulatory or urgent care centers, the number of HMOs in the market, and the perceived intensity of competition. At the same time, prospectors operated in relatively less regulated states. As discussed further in Chapter Six, competition gave prospectors the incentive to diversify into new markets with new services, while the relative lack of regulation, the availability of resources, and population growth helped them do so.

Defenders faced the most regulated environment in regard to the stringency of certificate of need, suggesting that they may have had problems maintaining facilities and technology. Decisions about new facilities and technology often favored the larger suburban and urban hospitals, where a greater volume of patients could be used to justify expansion. This placed the smaller defender hospitals at a competitive disadvantage, making it more difficult for them to attract and retain physicians, nurses, and other health professionals. As a result, defenders had problems in further penetrating their markets.

Interestingly, analyzers did not have particularly competitive environments. As we will see in Chapter Eight, this gave them time to "straddle the fence" and observe what was going on, rather than being pulled toward either a prospector or defender strategy.

Reactors found the most stringent regulatory environments, particularly in rate review. Interviews with reactors suggested that stronger regulation may have been a factor in their lack of a consistent strategy. Several reported the futility of trying to "outguess" the regulators. Others believed they were being "jerked around" by the regulatory process. Reactors also faced relatively stiff competition from HMOs and other managed care providers. Overall, the combination of stringent regulation and heavy competition made it difficult for reactors to develop a stable approach to the environmental forces. Others have also found a greater number of reactors present in "hostile and complex" environments (Zahra, 1989).

Performance

The performance of most corporations can be measured by financial and accounting indicators such as operating margins, return on investment, return on equity, earnings per share, and market share. These financial measures tell us whether any business organization is "doing well." But hospitals occupy a special role in society; their fundamental purpose is to care for the sick and injured. Their performance cannot be judged by financial indicators alone but, rather, must be judged by their ability to fulfill their healing and social missions. In brief, hospitals must also be evaluated on their ability to "do good." Tables 5.3 and 5.4 summarize the ability of the study hospitals to both "do good" and "do well," broken out by strategic orientation.

Doing Good. For the most part the four archetypes had a similar ability to "do good." One pattern evident from the data

Table 5.3. "Doing Good" Performance Measures.

Performance Measure	Prospector	Defender	Analyzer	Reactor	Total Sample Average
Bad debt and charity care as percentage of outpatient revenue	8.3%	9.2%	10.3%	9.3%	9.6%
Medicaid revenue as percentage of total outpatient revenue	7.7%	10.3%	8.3%	7.4%	8.2%
Uncompensated care (bad debt plus charity care) as percentage of total revenue	3.4%	4.9%	3.9%	3.3%	3.7%
Diversified services for which no charity care provided	11.7%	10.3%	12.8%	15.1%	12.7%
Number of unprofitable services offered	7.2	7.8	7.1	7.0	7.2
Have organized quality assurance department[a]	43.2%	20.0%	35.8%	42.6%	37.5%
Severity-adjusted Medicare patient death rate for 16 selected conditions	11.3%	9.7%	10.8%	10.8%	10.8%
Number of Joint Commission contingencies	.56	1.0	.80	.60	.72

[a] $p \leq .05$; one way analysis of variance

Table 5.4. "Doing Well" Performance Measures.

Performance Measure	Prospector	Defender	Analyzer	Reactor	Total Sample Average
Operating margin as percentage of net revenue	9.4%	3.7%	7.9%	10.3%	8.5%
After-tax net income as percentage of total income	6.8%	2.4%	6.5%	7.6%	6.5%
Diversified services profitable[a]	38.5%	21.7%	36.4%	38.5%	36.2%
Fifteen services profitable[b]	82.5%	68.3%	79.6%	82.2%	79.9%
Adjusted market share score[b,c]	3.84	1.84	2.53	2.50	2.79
High share and high-growth services	22.8%	10.2%	19.2%	18.6%	19.4%
Cost per adjusted admission	$2,771	$2,650	$2,884	$2,863	$2,838
Admissions per full-time-equivalent employee	18.5	18.7	18.2	18.0	18.3

[a] $p = \leq .01$; one way analysis of variance
[b] $p = \leq .05$.
[c] On a scale from 1 to 5 where 5 = 1.5 times or greater market share than any other providers and 1 = at least one other provider with 1.5 times or greater market share; adjusted for number of competitors.

in Table 5.3 is that defenders provided more charity care and uncompensated care than the others. That is consistent with their location in less favorable environments. Defenders are also less likely to have an organized quality assurance department and more likely to have a Joint Commission contingency (that is, less than full compliance on specific quality indicators). This may, in part, be explained by their smaller size. None of the differences among prospectors, analyzers, and reactors is remarkable except for the tendency of reactors to be less likely to provide charity care.

Doing Well. Table 5.4 reveals more marked differences in the ability to "do well." Prospectors and reactors are generally more profitable than analyzers, and the analyzers, in turn, do better than defenders. Regression analysis (see Tables E.1 and E.2, Resource E), which controlled for environmental variables, regulation, competition, ownership, and bed size, also indicated that those with a strategic orientation closer to the prospector end of the scale were significantly more profitable and enjoyed greater market share. Thus, contrary to existing literature (Miles and Snow, 1978; Hambrick, 1981) suggesting that the strategic archetypes can be equally effective in a given environment, it may be that in a rapidly changing environment such as health care, a more active prospector-oriented strategy may be more successful. Others have also recently found prospector-oriented strategies to be positively associated with performance in hostile, turbulent environments (Covin and Slevin, 1989). This is discussed further in Chapter Twelve.

Strategic Comfort Zones and Performance. We expected hospitals that switched outside their strategic comfort zones to do more poorly than those that stayed within their comfort zones. However, there were no statistically significant differences on any of the performance measures. There was some suggestion that those operating outside their comfort zone had somewhat less market share but not significantly less. One explanation may be the short time frame of the study; the performance effects of switching outside one's comfort zone may not be felt for several years. In contrast, the more immediate disruptive effects were process oriented, involving conflict, role ambiguity, and turnover. The qualitative material presented in Chapters Six through Nine highlights some of these effects.

Management Planning and Control

Table 5.5 summarizes the average scores for each strategic archetype in three areas of planning and control — centralization and standardization, perceived quality of strategic planning and control processes, and cost-containment strategies.

Centralization and Decentralization. Somewhat surprisingly, there were relatively few differences by strategic orientation in centralization of decision making. As discussed in Chapter Four, centralization appears to be most closely associated with ownership (investor-owned are less centralized than not-for-profit) and system size (larger systems are more decentralized). The major exceptions are that defenders and reactors tend to be somewhat less centralized in specific strategic planning functions and tend to use less standardized strategic planning reporting formats. The overall lack of differences, however, does not mean that these issues were unimportant to the adaptation process. As suggested in Chapter Four, almost all hospitals and their corporate parents struggled with the issue of what should be centralized and what should be decentralized. These struggles and the lessons learned from them are highlighted in Chapters Six through Nine.

Perceived Quality of Strategic Planning and Control. Table 5.5 indicates a number of differences in this area. On almost all items — overall quality of the process, implementation, plan innovativeness, market research, and board and physician involvement — prospectors were most satisfied and defenders least satisfied. As we will see in later chapters, prospectors' ability to implement strategies through their strategic planning and control system and the relative inability of defenders to do so may partly account for the differences in their performance.

Table 5.5. Management Planning and Control.

Planning and Control	Prospector	Defender	Analyzer	Reactor	Total Sample Average
Centralization and standardization					
Overall centralization of strategic planning[a]	27.7	26.1	28.7	27.4	28.1
Centralization of specific strategic planning functions[a,d]	1.49	1.42	1.50	1.36	1.47
Centralization of decision making	3.12	3.23	3.09	3.18	3.12
Centralization of strategic content decisions	3.69	3.76	3.68	3.78	3.71
Centralization of strategic implementation decisions	2.83	2.96	2.80	2.88	2.83
Standardization of forms[b,d]	1.2	.83	1.05	.87	1.0
Perceived quality of strategic planning and control					
Overall quality of strategic planning and control process[c]	3.07	2.65	2.92	2.91	2.94
Corporate and regional office assistance	3.01	2.86	3.06	2.89	3.01
Information systems	2.36	2.24	2.26	2.14	2.27

Table 5.5. Management Planning and Control, Cont'd.

Planning and Control	Prospector	Defender	Analyzer	Reactor	Total Sample Average
Implementation[c]	3.22	2.70	3.04	3.10	3.07
Innovativeness of plans[c]	3.91	2.86	3.47	3.86	3.59
Market research[c]	3.04	2.44	2.73	2.68	2.77
Board member and physician involvement	3.17	2.80	3.14	3.07	3.12
Cost-Containment Strategies					
Overall cost containment[c]	3.10	2.80	3.10	3.10	3.10
Staff reduction	3.27	3.08	3.34	3.20	3.29
Program or service consolidation	2.60	2.37	2.60	2.58	2.59
Efficiency and productivity improvements[c]	3.27	2.84	3.26	3.25	3.24

Note: Unless otherwise noted, all scales are 1 to 5 (1 = low; 5 = high). See Resource A for further details.

[a]See Table 4.1 for explanation of scale.

[b]On a scale of 0 to 2 (0 = no standardization; 2 = high standardization).

[c]$p = \leq .01$; one way analysis of variance

[d]$p = \leq .05$.

Interestingly, reactors were similar to prospectors on many of the planning and control dimensions but scored the lowest of the four groups in information systems and were also relatively low in assistance received from the corporate or regional office. As we will see in Chapter Nine, lack of strong information systems and lack of direction from the corporate office were factors in the reactor hospitals' inability to achieve a more coherent strategic orientation.

Cost Containment. Table 5.5 indicates that defenders were less engaged in cost-containment activities than any of the others. This was particularly true for efficiency and productivity improvements such as methods engineering, zero-based budgeting, inventory control practices, preadmission screening, cost-containment education programs, and incentives to reduce length of stay. As we will see in Chapter Seven, these findings shed considerable light on the relatively poorer performance of defender hospitals. They showed significant structural inertia as the result of having lived in a relatively benign environment before the early 1980s, and were slow to recognize the need to adopt tough cost-cutting approaches. As one defender executive noted, "We thought we just needed to do more of what we were doing. We didn't perceive the significance of the [prospective payment] change."

In efficiency and productivity improvements, prospectors were particularly active in reducing length of stay by emphasizing strong discharge planning and utilization review. Some of the diversified activities that prospectors engaged in (for example, home care) facilitated earlier hospital discharge, thus representing a "two-for-one" solution.

Does Ownership Matter?

We examined differences in ownership across the strategic archetypes for forty-six measures, including all the performance measures, centralization of decision making and strategic planning, the perceived quality of the strategic planning process, cost-containment strategies, and factors felt to influence the continued viability of the organization. Not-for-profit hospitals were somewhat more likely to be analyzers than investor-owned hospitals (62.1 versus 53.2 percent) and also somewhat more likely to be defenders (10.3 versus 6.1 percent). Not-for-profit hospitals were somewhat less likely to be prospectors (15.6 versus 25.5 percent). There was little difference in the percentage who were reactors: 15.2 percent for the investor-owned versus 12.2 percent for the not-for-profit. Despite the percentage differences, the rank order of strategic orientations was the same for both ownership types: the analyzer strategy was by far the most popular, followed in order by the prospector, reactor, and defender. Slightly more of the investor-owned hospitals (51 percent) changed their strategic orientations than of the not-for-profit (47 percent).

Controlling for strategic orientation, we examined whether there were any significant differences between investor-owned and not-for-profit hospitals on each of forty-six measures. We found significant differences ($p \leq .05$) in only 18 percent of the relevant comparisons (33 out of 184), suggesting that ownership differences are not prevalent. Other studies also suggest few differences by ownership form (Kralewski, Gifford, and Porter, 1988).

The most consistent statistically significant differences were in hospital-specific diversification, overall profitability, centralization of strategic planning functions, and perceived quality of strategic planning assistance provided by the corporate office. Investor-owned hospitals were less diversified but had higher levels of profitability; their strategic planning process was more decentralized; but they also reported less satisfaction with the perceived quality of strategic planning assistance provided by the corporate office. Analysis indicated that while system size largely accounted for the greater decentralization of investor-owned hospitals, size did *not* account for the lower perceived quality of strategic planning assistance. Interview data and related information suggested that too much "strategic" autonomy may have been delegated to some investor-owned hospitals without sufficient corporate office backup.

Among defenders, investor-owned hospitals appeared to recognize more quickly and give greater emphasis to cost-containment strategies. They scored significantly higher on the overall cost containment scale (3.0 versus 2.2) and the overall efficiency scale (3.1 versus 2.1). They also scored significantly higher in plan implementation (2.8 versus 2.2).

Analyzer investor-owned hospitals had significantly greater perceived appropriate involvement of physicians in the strategic planning process than not-for-profit analyzers (.09 versus − .36 factor analysis score). This largely reflects the fact that most investor-owned hospital boards are composed of from one-third to two-thirds physicians. During the study, the not-for-profit hospitals, recognizing the need for greater physician involvement, significantly increased the number of physicians serving on boards and key committees.

Among reactors, not-for-profit hospitals gave greater emphasis to survivability issues (4.6 versus 4.2). This reflects, in part, the generally much poorer financial condition of not-for-profit reactor hospitals.

Interestingly, among prospectors, investor-owned hospitals were significantly more likely to reduce staff (.00 versus − .65, factor analysis score) as a way of containing costs. Interview data suggested that this was done in part to streamline inpatient care in order to focus greater attention on diversification. Overall, however, not-for-profit hospitals were significantly more diversified (at the hospital level) than investor-owned hospitals.

Finally, while there was relatively little overall difference in the total amount of reported uncompensated care provided, not-for-profit analyzers provided somewhat more uncompensated care than investor-owned analyzers (4.9% of net revenues versus 3.6%) and not-for-profit defenders provided more than twice as much uncompensated care as investor-owned defenders (9.3% versus 3.9%). The uncompensated care burden of not-for-profit defenders, combined with their relative lack of emphasis on aggressive cost containment, readily explains the concern for their continued viability.

Overall, most of the findings are not strongly influenced by ownership form. Nonetheless, the differences that emerged are important. For example, regardless of strategic orientation, investor-owned hospitals were more profitable. The differences in profitability, however, began to narrow between 1983 and 1985. For example, while after-tax income margins as a percentage of total income were 7.6 percent for investor-owned hospitals in 1983 versus 5.6 percent for not-for-profit hospitals, by 1985 the respective figures were 8.4 percent versus 7.5 percent (Friedman and Shortell, 1988, p. 254). In more recent years, hospital profit margins have declined for all hospitals as payment rates have tightened.

Regardless of type, the perceived quality of strategic planning assistance from the corporate office is perceived to be higher among not-for-profit hospitals. This could not be explained by their smaller size. While the poorer perceived quality of assistance did not appear to greatly affect investor-owned hospital profit margins, it did appear to hamper some of their attempted diversification efforts.

In general, decision making and strategic planning were more centralized among the not-for-profit hospitals, largely because their smaller size makes it easier to centralize functions. As not-for-profit systems grow in size and become more geographically dispersed, they may face some of the same decentralization issues as their investor-owned counterparts.

Thus, ownership does make some difference but the differences are not pervasive. All hospitals, regardless of ownership, faced significant challenges in the mid-1980s, causing them to reexamine their basic strategic directions. Whether, how, and how much they changed direction were largely independent of their form of ownership.

A View to the Future

In addition to the differences described in previous sections, we examined each hospital's future intentions. We found a continuing shift toward analyzer and prospector orientations and away from the defender. Prospectors and analyzers were expected to increase from 78.7 percent to 82.5 percent, with most of the growth coming in the prospector category, which was expected to increase from 23.8 percent to 38 percent. The overall percentage of analyzers was expected to decrease from

54.9 percent to 44.5 percent, primarily due to most analyzers evolving toward the prospector orientation. Interestingly, the percentage of reactors was expected to remain stable at around 15 percent.

Thus, while a continuing shift toward the prospector strategy is expected, the evidence also suggests that diversification activities associated with this strategy will be highly focused and that prospectors cannot ignore their commitment to their acute inpatient care business lines. For example, prospectors received the highest mean score (4.4 on a five-point scale) on a cluster of items involving a focus on inpatient market share (gaining greater inpatient market share, recruiting and retaining physicians, enhancing revenues, and increasing marketing activities). Relatively high mean scores (4.2) were also given to basic survivability issues (for example, controlling costs, maintaining multi-institutional system affiliation, and gaining political influence) and to developing a perceived high-quality image (for example, ensuring quality of care, improving community relations, attracting and retaining effective administrators, and improving physician/administrative relations). In contrast, diversification activities (for example, diversifying into related health care activities and developing joint ventures with physicians) were awarded an overall average importance score of only 3.6. In brief, the trend toward the prospector orientation is accompanied by a continuing focus on cost containment, maintaining and building inpatient market share, and improving quality of services.

Summary

There are both similarities and differences in the background characteristics, environments, performance, and management processes of prospectors, defenders, analyzers, and reactors. Defenders are smaller, operate in generally less favorable environments, and generally have less slack. Prospectors are larger, have generally more slack, and operate in more competitive environments. There are virtually no significant differences by archetype in the provision of charity care or in selected process and outcome measures of quality of care. But prospectors and, to a lesser degree, reactors do better financially. While there are few differences in the centralization and standardization of the strategic planning process by archetype, the perceived quality of various elements of the process is generally highest for prospectors and lowest for defenders. Prospectors were also more likely to be engaged in various cost-containment strategies than defenders.

There were relatively few differences by ownership. Investor-owned hospitals were somewhat more profitable (although the difference was narrowing), more decentralized, and less satisfied with the quality of strategic planning assistance provided by the corporate office. Most hospitals intend to become more analyzer- and prospector-oriented in the future.

6

Managing the Prospector Orientation

"You throw a lot of mud against the wall and see what sticks."

The Prospector: A Mini-Case

"We want to be first and do a lot. We want to deal with the changing role of the doctor." So spoke the CEO of Wells Fargo Memorial Hospital, a classic prospector. Operating in a highly competitive market, Wells Fargo developed a cardiac and pulmonary rehabilitation program, an acute dialysis program, laser surgery, a hospice, and a fertility center. The hospital has a strong array of outpatient services across the board, most of them organized along product lines. The emphasis is on increasing market share. The cornerstone of its approach is to begin by analyzing the market for its physician practices and then developing programs that will benefit both the hospital and its physicians. Wells Fargo has developed a list of approximately thirty physicians it would like to attract to the staff. If successful, this will enable it to increase market share by 5 percent.

Well Fargo's efforts are supported by a corporate office that shares a strong prospector culture. The corporate office removed one popular hospital CEO because, in the words of a corporate staff member, he was "a caretaker and not a risk taker." The corporate office backs up member hospitals with a strong capability in market research and new-program development, including a "model hospital program" designed to rethink the nature of a hospital from scratch. The emphasis is on organizing technology, work design, and people in the most cost-effective way possible. Experiments are being conducted in a few test hospitals, and successful practices will be transferred to other hospitals in the system.

The system also places considerable emphasis on environmental assessment and competitor analysis while acknowledging the need to do a much better job in both. System leaders talk about "anticipating change and opportunity." They recognize the need to remain flexible in structure. As the system president and CEO put it, "We shed our skin about every two years." Leaders also recognize the importance of collaborative strategies, and the system has entered into joint ventures with other organizations to provide nursing home care. The corporate identity, which was described as being "hid under a bushel basket" in the past, is being actively promoted.

The system and its hospitals are not without problems. Foremost among them are the need to create greater local market integration and synergies among operating units and the need to develop new managerial mind sets to stay with the prospector strategy. As one division CEO said, "Administrators [in the past] were simply technicians carrying out corporate policy. They have to be more freewheeling and have the ability to identify business opportunities, analyze them, determine the level of risk, and decide whether they want to pursue them. This requires a different type of hospital administrator with a different orientation."

The Prospector's Performance

As indicated in Figures 6.1 and 6.2, and by the Wells Fargo case above, prospectors generally did very well on most

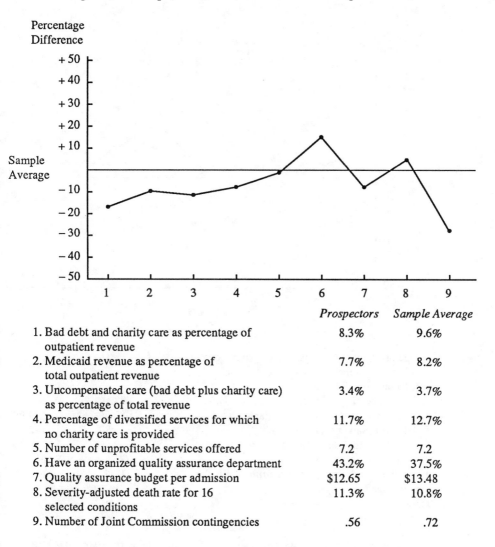

Figure 6.1. Prospector Performance Profile — "Doing Good."

	Prospectors	Sample Average
1. Bad debt and charity care as percentage of outpatient revenue	8.3%	9.6%
2. Medicaid revenue as percentage of total outpatient revenue	7.7%	8.2%
3. Uncompensated care (bad debt plus charity care) as percentage of total revenue	3.4%	3.7%
4. Percentage of diversified services for which no charity care is provided	11.7%	12.7%
5. Number of unprofitable services offered	7.2	7.2
6. Have an organized quality assurance department	43.2%	37.5%
7. Quality assurance budget per admission	$12.65	$13.48
8. Severity-adjusted death rate for 16 selected conditions	11.3%	10.8%
9. Number of Joint Commission contingencies	.56	.72

performance measures. Although they did not provide quite as much charity care as the overall sample, they were more likely to have an organized quality assurance department and have somewhat fewer Joint Commission contingencies. They were generally above the sample average in profitability and market share measures.

Figure 6.2. Prospector Performance Profile—"Doing Well."

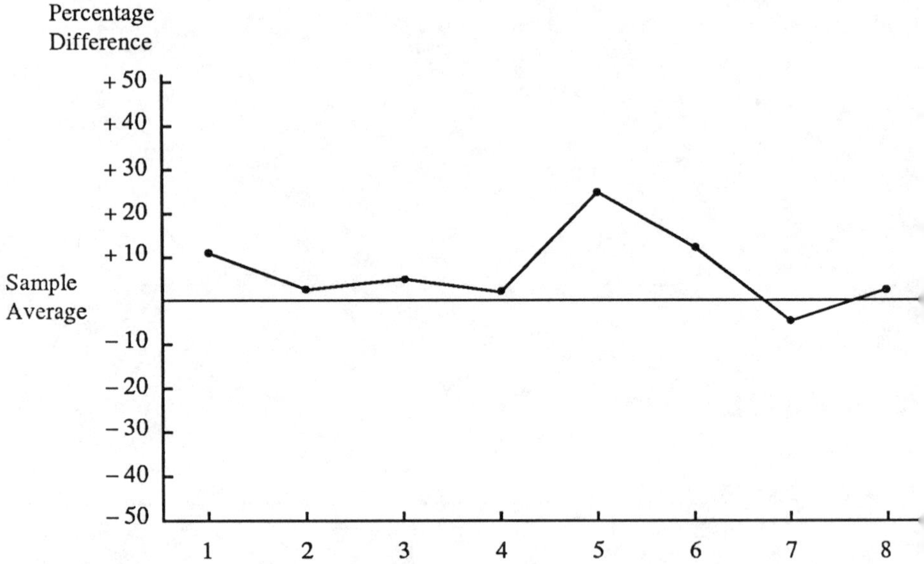

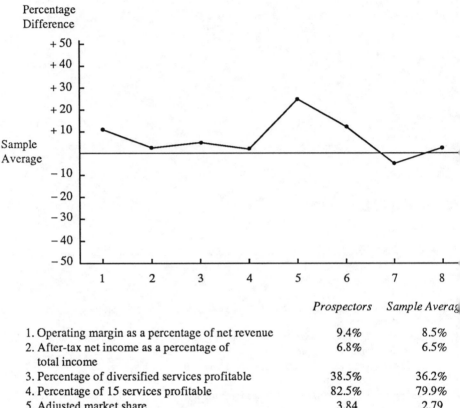

	Prospectors	Sample Averag
1. Operating margin as a percentage of net revenue	9.4%	8.5%
2. After-tax net income as a percentage of total income	6.8%	6.5%
3. Percentage of diversified services profitable	38.5%	36.2%
4. Percentage of 15 services profitable	82.5%	79.9%
5. Adjusted market share	3.84	2.79
6. Percentage high-share and high-growth services	22.8%	19.4%
7. Cost per adjusted admission	$2,771	$2,838
8. Number of admissions per full-time-equivalent employee	18.5	18.3

Part of the prospectors' success can be attributed to the quality of their strategic planning and control system. As shown in Figure 6.3, prospectors score higher than the sample average on almost all dimensions and particularly in regard to market research.

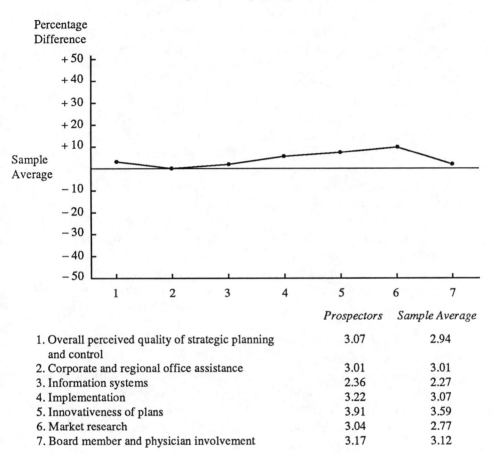

Figure 6.3. Prospector's Perceived Quality
of Strategic Planning and Control.

	Prospectors	Sample Average
1. Overall perceived quality of strategic planning and control	3.07	2.94
2. Corporate and regional office assistance	3.01	3.01
3. Information systems	2.36	2.27
4. Implementation	3.22	3.07
5. Innovativeness of plans	3.91	3.59
6. Market research	3.04	2.77
7. Board member and physician involvement	3.17	3.12

The Prospector's Challenge

The central challenge facing the prospector is successfully managing diversification. By definition, prospectors are involved in the frequent development of new products and services for new markets and are almost always first to initiate such efforts. They must guard against expanding too rapidly, spreading themselves too thin, diversifying into areas where they have little knowledge, and ending up with such a wide array of products, services, and markets that it becomes difficult to achieve any financial or functional synergies. A prospector strategy is facilitated by a favorable environment — some degree of competition, little regulation, and strong resources and population growth. Financial and organizational slack generated from positive performance in the past is also needed, to experiment, innovate, and take calculated risks — not all of which will succeed (Cheng and Kesner, 1988). In highly professionalized organizations such as hospitals, a prospector strategy requires that the professionals understand and support the organization's diversification activities. There must be sufficient commonality of interests between the organization and the professional group.

There are also specific implications that derive from an environmental jolt. In the case of the health care industry, prospective payment meant fewer resources available for inpatient care, greater competition for these resources, and greater competition for the provision of alternative services. Prospectors who had been prospectors and, to a lesser extent, analyzers who became prospectors had already gained some experience in providing out-of-hospital services. The implementation of PPS was largely interpreted by prospector CEOs as a need to accelerate their diversification activities with perhaps fewer resources available from their inpatient activities to support such diversification. Most of these CEOs and their organizations responded very quickly to the change. As one CEO commented, "We have been watching carefully what was going on in New Jersey [which had a PPS-like system several years before the national program was implemented], and we were preparing for something like this." These organizations, in effect, have been creating a strategic comfort zone for themselves.

For defenders who switched to prospectors and, to a lesser extent, reactors who switched to prospectors, the challenge was more difficult. For not only did PPS mean fewer resources, it also meant developing diversification strategies with which they had little experience. Defenders who switched to prospectors generally did less well than prospectors who remained prospectors or analyzers who became prospectors. As a CEO of one defender hospital noted, "We were doing a little bit too much. We sorta got beyond ourselves. We need to get back to some of the basics." In brief, they were operating outside their strategic comfort zone.

Being a prospector in the changing health care environment involves six primary managerial tasks:

1. Understanding the difference between related, partially related, and unrelated diversification and how best to approach each.
2. Learning how to constantly differentiate services.
3. Recognizing the limitations of the experience curve associated with being a "first mover."
4. Understanding how to create local market synergies.
5. Understanding the need to switch back and forth between cost leadership strategies and quality differentiation strategies.
6. Learning to work with physicians in support of the organization's mission.

Diversification. One prospector hospital decided to diversify into home health care services. The nursing department was given responsibility for developing the program. After several months it became obvious the program was having difficulty. Hospital rules, policies, and practices were used that had little relevance to home health care. The program was subsequently split off as a separate entity and charged with developing its own mission, policies, and practices.

A second prospector hospital developed several ambulatory care centers in an effort to attract physicians to outlying areas. The intent was to preempt competing hospitals and physicians from entering these markets and thereby gain a market toehold. The ambulatory care centers were organized as a subunit of the hospital's ambulatory care division. Many of the hospital's personnel, purchasing, and budgeting policies and its information and reporting systems were used. After six months, several physicians resigned from the centers, citing frustration with the "hospital's bureaucratic approach to managing the practice."

In both cases the hospitals misjudged the extent to which the new activities were related to the hospitals' acute inpatient care business. Attempts to manage these new services like inpatient services spelled failure.

For prospectors, two major dimensions of relatedness are important: technical and managerial. Technical dimensions include (1) compatibility with existing technology, (2) consistency with existing technical skills and knowledge, (3) ability to build synergies with existing programs and services (such as an outpatient cardiac rehab program to complement a strong inpatient cardiology service), and (4) compatibility with existing professional interests and values. Managerial relatedness criteria include (1) consistency with mission and philosophy, (2) consistency with existing managerial skills, knowledge, and resources, (3) compatibility with existing management systems, and (4) the ability to serve relevant markets.

Technical and managerial relatedness are part of the overall question of whether diversification activities are related. We found it best to view relatedness on a continuum, from related to partially related to unrelated. The closer the service was to acute inpatient care and its technical and managerial requirements, the more related it was. Ambulatory surgery, outpatient chemotherapy and radiation therapy, nuclear medicine, ultrasound, and cardiovascular and pulmonary diagnostic services are examples of related services. Examples of unrelated services include real estate development, book publishing, and management consulting. In between the two extremes are a large number of partially related services: home health care, adult day health centers, geriatric care, health promotion, sports medicine, occupational health, ambulatory care centers, and HMO ownership or sponsorship.

These partially related services proved to be the most problematic for prospectors because many executives considered them related and believed that technical and managerial resources gained from acute inpatient care could be transferred. Time and again members of the hospital management team were charged with responsibility for developing and managing these new services. Usually, but not always, they failed to recognize that the technical and managerial requirements of delivering home health care service, for example, were different from providing care to inpatients. One manager commented: "You cannot manage this kind of activity [primary care center] as you do the radiology department. They [the physicians] won't stand for it. The needs are different, the markets are different, the kinds of staffing are different, and so are the technologies. We found they didn't even want to use our purchasing system because they [the primary care center] felt they could build good will by purchasing from a local vendor. We learned quickly."

In general, we found that the more related the diversification activity, the more likely it was to be profitable. While this is at odds with an earlier industry study (Clement, 1987), it is consistent with most of the diversification literature (Rumelt, 1974; Montgomery, 1982). We also found, however, that partially related diversification efforts, such as home health care, long-term care, and ambulatory care centers, were successful if (1) the different technical, managerial, and cultural requirements of the services were recognized, (2) resources and attention were concentrated in a few well-selected areas, and (3) market-entry strategies were appropriately matched to the specific activity.

Prospectors with better market research (Walker and Ruekert, 1987) and management information systems generally did a better job of recognizing the different technical and managerial requirements of their diversified services. As in the tobacco industry (Miles and Cameron, 1982), hospital executives both developed talent internally and recruited it from outside. Experience and knowledge were developed internally by seeding startup projects for several years and then carefully monitoring to select the winners. This "greenhouse effect," as one prospector called it, helped the organization accelerate its learning. One system assisted its member hospitals by pilot testing new programs and services in areas geographically removed from local markets. As one executive explained, "We want to make our mistakes in someone else's back yard, not our own. What works, we transport. What doesn't, we don't have any lingering negative effects." Other prospectors went outside to recruit executives with background and experience in long-term care, home health, medical group management, and the like.

A common mistake made by some prospectors, particularly those working outside their strategic comfort zone, was to diversify too quickly. To some extent this was caused by the tension between short-run needs and long-run objectives. In the short run, there was great need to maintain profit margins (particularly for the investor-owned hospitals) and to develop aftercare services to facilitate quicker patient discharge. But often these decisions were made at the expense of longer-run growth objectives, the creation of synergies among services, and competitive positioning. Overexpansion from 1983 through 1985 brought significant losses for both investor-owned and not-for-profit systems, causing major retrenchments in 1986–1987. This included divestment of HMOs, freestanding surgery centers, pharmacies, dental clinics, management consulting services, urgent care centers, home health care services, and the like. A marketing staff member of one system described the frenetic pace of early diversification activity in his organization by noting that "working at [his system] is a lot like changing a tire on a moving vehicle."

In addition to learning how to better focus their diversification activities, the more successful prospectors learned how to match market-entry approaches with specific diversification activities. The guiding rule of thumb appeared to be that the more related the diversification activity, the more amenable it was to being provided by the organization itself (Roberts and Berry, 1985). The major advantage of providing a service oneself is greater control over the activity. Examples included ambulatory surgery centers, outpatient diagnostic centers, and cardiac rehabilitation programs. In these areas, hospitals had the necessary resources to run the service.

In partially related diversification, where one does not possess all the resources to develop this service, a joint venture or network relationship with others has advantages: the opportunity to share costs and risks and the opportunity to learn from each other. Ideally, the joint venture partners complement each other. Major disadvantages are some loss of control and the coordination costs (Williamson, 1975) of maintaining smoothly working relationships. The joint venture approach was used successfully by many prospectors in responding to HMO activity, often after having failed at owning or directly sponsoring HMOs themselves.

Intermediate entry strategies, halfway between doing it oneself and entering into a joint venture with an outside party, were also used. Primarily they involved internal corporate joint ventures, often with members of one's medical staff (Shortell and Zajac, 1988). In an internal joint venture, a separate organization is established to provide a service (for example, a primary care group practice or an outpatient diagnostic center), but it is ultimately responsible to the parent company board, in this case the hospital. This approach has the advantages of promoting innovation while still enabling the hospital to maintain more control than it would have in a joint venture with an outside party. The major challenge lies in balancing the autonomy needs of the professionals working in the new unit with the control needs of the hospital. Hospitals that use this approach successfully let the requirements of the market largely dictate the degree of control. As one physician working in a hospital-sponsored practice said, "We were no different from any other physician in private practice, except we have the financial resources and backup of the hospital. For the most part they [the hospital] left us alone. We did what we felt was needed to to attract patients and build our practice."

A few hospitals used these entry strategies in combination. In one case, a hospital entered into a joint venture with the local visiting nurses association (VNA) to develop a home health care agency. After two years of gaining experience in delivering home health care, the hospital (with the VNA's agreement) took over 100 percent control of the agency, providing greater strategic direction for future growth.

Thus, prospectors met the challenges of managing diversity by assessing the relatedness of the proposed activity in both technical and managerial criteria. Where the proposed activities were different from the technical and managerial requirements of the core business, these differences were recognized and planned for. This was done by developing internal capabilities and recruiting outside expertise, by considering joint ventures, networks, and internal corporate joint ventures to share startup costs and increase learning, and by focusing on a few well-selected activities rather than spreading the organization too thin across too many projects. Strong market research capabilities and management information systems were also important. Perhaps most important of all was the need for patience and determination in "staying the course." As we have noted, a prospector strategy cannot easily be reversed without raising the danger of experiencing the negative consequences of becoming a reactor.

Constant Differentiation. There are few barriers to entry for many of the new services and so they can easily be imitated by others. Thus a second requirement for successful prospectors was the constant need to differentiate their services in order to sustain competitive advantage.

Two examples, one successful and the other unsuccessful, illustrate the importance of continual differentiation. In the first case, two hospitals in a very competitive market had both identified cardiology as an area of distinctive competence. Hospital A felt it could outdistance its competitors by recruiting an outstanding angioplasty specialist from a prominent West Coast medical school who would develop a wide array of diverse cardiology programs, both inpatient and outpatient. Hospital A successfully recruited the physician and began to launch its plans. But, much to its dismay, six months later hospital B (the major competitor) recruited its own specialist from a prominent East Coast medical school to effectively neutralize hospital A's strategy. Within a short period, what little market share had been gained by hospital A was wiped out. The result was a "cardiology standoff," with both hospitals continuing to split the market approximately fifty-fifty.

Hospital A, the first mover, failed to understand the need for an overall strategy of cardiac care differentiation based on many interrelated areas of distinctive competence beyond a single physician. For example, it might have developed a package of cardiac services for a fixed price, followup cardiology rehabilitation services provided at home and in the office, specially trained cardiac counselors, and prevention programs emphasizing nutrition, exercise, and stress management. Ideally, the data to make these decisions would come from market research where the targeted populations expressed their need for the services.

In the second case, an investor-owned prospector hospital operating in a competitive market developed a package of maternity care services (from prenatal care through delivery and after care) for a fixed price of $850. The package became popular and for about a year OB admissions significantly increased. It didn't take long, however, for competing hospitals to put together similar packages at equivalent prices. The original hospital recognized the need to further differentiate its service, so it added a program of two visits to the family's home by nurses from the hospital's home health care agency, three days after and seven days after delivery. The visiting nurse answered questions, provided psychological support, and rendered any care needed. This strategy could not be easily imitated by competing hospitals because they did not have a home health care agency, and the original hospital continues to be the market leader in OB care.

Constant differentiation requires a culture that stresses innovation, a commitment to continual new-product and new-market development, a disciplined strategic planning process, and a strong market research capability. A major problem faced by defenders and reactors attempting to become prospectors was that they did not have a culture of innovation. And such a culture does not occur overnight; the process often takes five to seven years (Bice, 1984; Kanter, 1984).

Successful prospectors continually experiment with new products and services. As noted, one prospector believes strongly in the "greenhouse effect" of developing several programs simultaneously and then seeing what emerges as a winner. This, of course, requires some amount of slack resources. Another hospital provides incentive pay to executives and managers for developing ideas that lead to new programs and services. A not-for-profit system with a prospector culture challenges and stretches its people by creating job descriptions with responsibilities significantly beyond what people in those positions can realistically achieve.

Constant differentiation requires a strategic planning process based on knowledge of the market and knowledge of the organization's capabilities. To recognize the need to differentiate and to select specific points of differentiation that cannot be easily imitated by others, an organization needs reliable sources of information and a process for analyzing that information. For hospitals this meant collecting ideas from physicians, nurses, and other health professionals familiar with the technical requirements of the service, in addition to the financial and managerial requirements. It also meant rigorously evaluating their strengths and weaknesses in relation to major competitors. In general, successful prospectors had a more disciplined planning process, which enabled them to generate an idea and data base for constantly differentiating their services.

For service industries such as hospitals, strong market research is particularly important. All systems recognized this, but some gave more attention to it than others. Also, some were better at executing their marketing strategies than others. Experiences varied; one system characterized its hospital CEOs as "marketing virgins" while another doubled its marketing budget, including specific components for marketing education of its CEOs.

A central issue in differentiation was the ability to determine whether a service was driven by consumers or professionals. For consumer-driven services such as health promotion, sports medicine, and occupational health services, hospitals must focus on identifying specific dimensions of the services most desired by consumers, then package and promote them in a way that meets these needs. For professionally driven services such as cardiology, oncology, and renal dialysis, physicians are the primary target audience. Programs, services, and marketing strategies must be designed to meet their expressed needs. If successful, the physicians will bring their patients to the institution for these services.

Other services, such as obstetrical care, are both consumer driven and professionally driven. Consumers have definite ideas of what they want but physicians act as gatekeepers, channeling patients from one hospital to another. In these cases, the physician *and* the hospital need to be marketed to the consumer.

The more successful prospectors were more adept at assessing whether a given service was consumer driven, professionally driven, or a combination of the two. They committed more resources to upgrading the marketing capability of their organizations and generally supported the philosophy. As one corporate staff member put it, "Those that educate the market will own it." This philosophy, along with a culture supportive of innovation, new-product and new-service development, and a disciplined strategic planning process, helped prospectors constantly differentiate their services.

The Experience Curve. Successful diversification often requires being the first to offer the product or service. By being the "first mover," prospectors can gain a toehold in the market and erect barriers to keep competitors out (Lieberman and Montgomery, 1988). They can also gain experience and learn to improve the method of delivering the service, thereby lowering costs and providing a further entry barrier for competitors. Successful prospectors realized when a first-mover strategy was advantageous and when it was not. Most importantly, they learned to recognize for what specific diversified services a prospector strategy made sense. Three examples illustrate the issues involved.

In the first case, the hospital failed to recognize the first-mover advantage enjoyed by an HMO that had already enrolled more than 100,000 subscribers. The hospital decided to develop its own HMO to protect its existing patient base from further erosion. As the vice-president for strategic planning noted, "We were late into the HMO market. Our enrollment is less than one-third of our major competitor. We lost a million dollars our first year. But 90 percent of employers in the area offer the HMO option. So we feel we have to be involved to prevent further erosion and to be a full-service provider." The question here is whether the revenues used for what is essentially a rearguard defensive strategy could be better deployed in other areas. This example also raises another question: whether the hospital would have been better off entering into a joint venture with one of the existing HMOs or a stronger third party and, thereby, sharing the cost, risks, and learning associated with the HMO business.

In the second case, the hospital needed to expand its primary care base and generate more inpatient referrals. In response, it developed a network of urgent care centers designed to provide low-cost convenient care for minor illnesses and injuries on weekday evenings and weekends. The hospital was the first to develop such centers and hoped to reap the benefits of being the first mover. After eighteen months, the centers were losing money and referrals to the hospital were not being generated, and the hospital dropped three of the four centers. What went wrong?

Basically, the first-mover advantage did not exist. The hospital failed to recognize how easily the urgent care center concept could be imitated by competitors. Not only did physicians expand their office hours to compete, but the hospital's own emergency room developed similar services — a severe case of "service cannibalism" and shooting oneself in one's foot. The urgent care centers actually represented a late entrant into a very crowded market of competitors, who emphasized quality features that could not be duplicated by the urgent care centers. The one urgent care center that enjoyed some degree of success relied on an explicit differentiation strategy, focusing on a carefully targeted market not occupied by current physicians or other treatment centers.

By contrast, the hospital in the third example followed a first-mover strategy in starting the first ambulatory surgery center in its area. The hospital was able to capture learning curve effects by increasing volume over time, gaining experience, and lowering unit costs. It was also able to take advantage of a changing reimbursement climate favoring outpatient surgery. By the time competing hospitals were able to start their own centers, the first-mover hospital had established a stronghold as the market leader, a position it has been able to maintain.

These three cases illustrate the need to consider first-mover and experience-curve advantages on an individual basis, considering the market and the competitors. In the process, answers to six questions need to be found (Ghemawat, 1985):

1. How rapidly will the service become technologically obsolete?
2. How predictable is demand for the service?

3. Will the volume of output increase fast enough for the experience curve to provide sufficient leverage?
4. Is demand sufficiently price sensitive?
5. Can the cost-reduction approach be easily imitated by others?
6. Are there strong competitors who are already following an experience curve strategy?

It may be difficult to gain first-mover advantages where the technology underlying the service is rapidly replaced by more advanced technology. Some hospitals found this to be true with second- and third-generation nuclear magnetic resonance imaging technology. Whether new technology negates first-mover advantages depends largely on the market share captured by the existing technology and the extent to which skills and experience can be transferred. Where a toehold has already been gained and skills and knowledge are transferable, then the hospital's chances for remaining the market leader in that service line are high.

Where demand is unpredictable or volume does not increase fast enough, then first-mover advantages may not materialize. These characteristics are most frequently associated with out-of-hospital services, which tend to be low volume: health promotion services and low back pain clinics, for example. Also, when the demand for service is not price sensitive, attempting to build volume based on low price is not an effective strategy. Thus, some services that are well insured may not be good candidates for an experience-curve strategy — at least not one based on a lower-cost, lower-price strategy.

Problems also arise when the cost-reduction approach can be easily imitated by others and when others are already following an experience-curve strategy. The hospital that found its low-cost maternity package matched by competing hospitals was forced to further differentiate its services through the home visits by nurses. Also, the hospital that started its own HMO was bucking two competitors who had already gained considerable experience-curve advantages.

Hospital executives frequently mentioned the importance of being the first or at least an early entrant into the market.

One system in particular placed great emphasis on adding new services to maximize experience-curve advantages. The personal nature of health services makes it very difficult to recapture market share after it is lost. Most people do not switch physicians or hospitals as quickly as they switch brands of toothpaste. But at the same time, clear thinking and careful planning are needed. Hospitals that used the six screening questions for each service being considered generally did better than those that did not.

Local Market Synergies. Among the challenges most often mentioned by prospector hospital executives was the need to develop an integrated continuum of care in local hospital markets. It was the prospector's way of responding to the diversity of product and service offerings and an attempt to create financial and service synergies. The continuum involved an integrated, coordinated network of primary care, acute care, and post–acute care services. If this could be established, hospitals felt they would have a competitive advantage in marketing their services to local employers, third-party payors, and the public. Comprehensiveness, continuity, and quality were the main attributes of the services continuum. The objective was to "regenerate patients" by offering services that ranged from health promotion and disease prevention, to acute hospital care, to post-acute home health care and long-term care. Using this approach, patients and revenues could be kept under the hospital's umbrella rather than going to competing organizations. As one nonstudy prospector system CEO said, the trick is "to become an effective system integrator without losing the excitement associated with prior initiatives."

Two major problems prospectors faced were a slowness in recognizing the need for local market integration and problems in working with physicians to bring it about.

One investor-owned corporation was a successfully diversified health care company long before the introduction of PPS. It offered general acute hospital care, specialty hospital care, and long-term care in various markets throughout the United States. The problem was that, with a few exceptions, its service lines did not coexist in the same markets. Thus, it was unable to attain the operational and financial synergy demanded by the new environment. Once the need for such synergy in local markets was recognized, the corporation evolved the strategy of a "health campus," centered on carefully targeted markets. The health campus concept essentially defined an integrated, geographically concentrated configuration of facilities and services ranging from multispecialty clinics, to a hospital, to a rehabilitation center, to nursing homes and retirement centers. The services were marketed both individually and as a group and linked where possible to HMOs, PPOs, and related finance and delivery arrangements.

A second system failed to create synergies with an initial wave of diversification that included investment in freestanding surgery centers, pharmacies, HMOs, and the like, mostly because the new services were not located in markets where the system had leading hospitals. In cases where the services were located in the same markets, they often competed with each other. The system eventually divested many of these services and refocused its efforts on building an integrated continuum of care around local hospitals that would serve as beachheads for an array of pre-acute and post-acute services.

Underlying many of the above problems was the relationship between the corporate office and the individual hospital unit. The dilemma involved integrating local planning with corporatewide strategic planning. Some systems made the mistake of granting too much autonomy to local CEOs who did not know how to assess the market or take advantage of corporate resources. At least two not-for-profit systems responded by becoming more centralized and directive in their strategic planning and control; less emphasis was given to consensus building at the local level.

Other systems made the mistake of overly centralizing the strategic planning and control function and granting too little autonomy to local units. These systems were out of touch with local markets and so could not plan effectively for local services integration. Services developed at the corporate office often did not play well in Peoria.

Most systems came to realize the need for a middle ground, decentralizing responsibility for building market share and negotiating joint ventures with physicians (with corporate assistance as needed) while centralizing financial control and final accountability. One system executive called this the "guided autonomy" approach.

Prospectors were not different from the others in overall degree of centralization. However, they did tend to flourish more under "guided autonomy." This approach took the form of well-specified corporate office guidelines and overall strategic directions coupled with the freedom of the individual hospitals and CEOs to make local market choices within these guidelines. In some cases they had the flexibility to set aside corporate guidelines if a persuasive case could be made for doing so. Thus, one hospital formed a joint venture outpatient radiology center with one of its radiologists even though such activities were generally not encouraged by the system.

In a second case, market analysis was done by the local management team with backup support from regional and corporate office staff. The implementation process was dictated by the local market. "Test programs" were developed for targeted programs such as low back pain clinics. Successful programs were made available to other interested hospitals, typically operating in markets similar to the test site. The net result for the system was a process of "transfer learning." This process was further facilitated by a bottom-up planning approach where each hospital's strategic plans were developed and forwarded up the corporate chain for review and comment. Several local hospital executives serve on the review groups and also participate in regional and corporatewide planning task forces.

In some systems, the principle of guided autonomy was also greatly facilitated by the exchange of executives between hospitals and corporate and regional offices. This cross fertilization helped to enhance corporate executives' understanding of local market dynamics while bringing their experience to bear on local issues.

Successful prospectors took advantage of the combined centralized-decentralized approach to strategic planning and control. Overall direction and some market analysis were conducted centrally, but each hospital was left free to determine the mix and amount of services required to meet local needs. Once the broad guidelines were set, serving the local market well became the basis for strategic integration. A hospital located in a young, growing community emphasized services for women and children, health promotion, health education, sports medicine, and fitness centers. A hospital located in a community with a growing elderly population emphasized a continuum of long-term care services including adult day care, hospice care, nursing home care, and continuing care retirement centers.

Managing Functional Strategies. Successful prospectors also recognized the need for a combination of cost-containment strategies and service differentiation strategies. Given the environmental jolt represented by PPS, all hospitals faced the need to lower their costs. In fact, prospectors placed somewhat more emphasis on this than defenders, particularly in staff reductions and productivity improvements. Prospectors made these cuts and improvements to generate additional resources to support diversification efforts. This incentive did not exist for most defenders, who were concentrating only on streamlining current operations.

But, in addition to using both approaches, prospectors also saw the need to switch from one approach to another to sustain competitive advantage as a particular service evolved (Gilbert and Strebel, 1987). For example, one hospital's joint sponsorship of an HMO gained early market share because it was first in the community to offer the service. This source of differentiation, however, was quickly eroded by a second HMO, which undercut the hospital-sponsored HMO in price. To counter this threat, the hospital-sponsored HMO lowered its premiums and adopted an "efficient, accessible, no-nonsense" marketing strategy. This strategy helped the hospital-sponsored HMO regain a major employer that had been lost to the new HMO the preceding year.

In the future, however, there may be limits to the low-cost strategy as employers and other purchasers begin to make choices based on quality, convenience, and related characteristics in addition to price. Thus, to sustain its competitive advantage, the first HMO will need to consider switching back again to a differentiation strategy, perhaps based on superior technical quality of care, expanded benefits, or greater personal attention, which might come from a policy of assigning specific physicians to specific patients.

Switching between a cost-leader approach and a differentiation approach is not easy. It requires slack resources, patience, discipline, a sense of timing, and a flexible skill base. Some of the surplus generated from a differentiation strategy must be invested in productivity and process improvements that will enable the organization to compete on a low-cost basis when it needs to switch to such a strategy. Similarly, surpluses generated from sustaining competitive advantage under a low-cost approach need to be invested in new products and new services that will enable the organization to switch back to a differentiation strategy when required. Because the skills and resources required for a low-cost strategy are often different from those required for a differentiation strategy, few organizations are equally well equipped to do both. Most of the prospectors studied were just beginning to understand what is involved in developing the flexibility and resources to execute the switching strategy.

The Physician Factor. If a single factor influenced the ability to adapt to the changes in the industry, it was the ability to work effectively with physicians (Shortell, Morrison, and Hughes, 1989). This was true for all four strategic archetypes, although each faced particular physician challenges associated with the specific nature of its strategic orientation. For prospectors, the major challenge was involving physicians in a meaningful way in the diversification process.

There were four major sources of physician opposition to prospectors' diversification plans: (1) perceived competition with their own practices, (2) perceptions that one group of physicians would be favored over another, (3) lack of involvement in the decision-making process surrounding diversification plans, and (4) philosophical opposition to what was perceived as the "corporate practice of medicine." These four were often interrelated in complex ways, and it was difficult for hospital executives to diagnose the specific source of the opposition and develop remedial strategies. The situation was further complicated by the lack of a common physician viewpoint or voice on the issue. Specialists such as surgeons and cardiologists generally favored diversification activities that would expand the hospital's ability to generate referrals to themselves. Primary care physicians such as family practitioners and general internists, in contrast, were understandably generally opposed to these efforts, fearing hospital encroachment on their private practices. Some hospital-based specialists such as radiologists, pathologists, and anesthesiologists favored selective joint venture involvement with the hospital. Other physicians opposed such efforts on the basis of favoritism. Hospital executives in prospector organizations quickly learned that in undertaking such diversification activities as ambulatory surgery, outpatient diagnostic centers, primary care clinics, and outpatient cardiac rehabilitation, one does not deal with a "medical staff" but with individual physicians and groups of physicians.

We also identified three facilitating factors: (1) a tradition of a close partnership between the hospital and its physicians, (2) a high percentage of loyal medical staff members with admitting privileges only at the hospital of interest, and (3) a common enemy against which to unite, such as a major competing hospital, HMO, or related managed care plan. The first two facilitators usually went hand in hand and reinforced each other. The third usually provided the immediate trigger for activating specific diversification initiatives, some of which involved joint ventures between the hospital and its physicians.

Two general approaches were used to improve working relationships with physicians: across-the-board strategies on the one hand, and specifically targeted strategies on the other. Among the most prevalent across-the-board strategies were increasing physician involvement in the management and governance of the organization at all levels, developing programs to help physicians maintain and expand their practices, and recruiting CEOs with experience and reputation for working well with physicians.

Greater physician involvement in management and governance included expanding voting physician membership on the hospital's governing board, increasing physician involvement in the strategic planning process of the institution, appointing full-time or part-time medical directors or executive vice-presidents for medical affairs, extending the term of office for elected presidents of the medical staff (for example, to two years instead of one year) to ensure greater continuity, and appointing full-time or part-time section chiefs to give more management and quality assurance focus to individual clinical departments. In addition, many systems created regional and corporate physician planning advisory councils, and a few created divisions of medical affairs at the corporate office level.

For example, at one prospector hospital, three out of five board members are physicians, and a fourth member is a respected, retired outside physician. Three physicians serve on the hospital strategic planning committee, which is headed by one of them. The hospital also has a full-time executive vice-president for medical affairs (a physician, whose main responsibility is to oversee the hospital's quality assurance activities and to ensure integration between the hospital strategic plan and physician interests). Most recently, part-time chiefs for medicine and surgery have been established to provide greater administrative guidance to these areas. The objectives are to: (1) get *early* physician input into the hospital's strategic thinking so that programs can be developed that are largely compatible with physician interests, (2) identify early warning signals and trouble spots where selected initiatives may have implementation problems, (3) educate physicians about the environmental changes taking place within the industry and the specific implications for the hospital and its medical staff, and (4) create a climate of open, honest communication that furthers the development of a more trusting relationship between the hospital and its physicians.

While almost all hospitals were pursuing greater physician involvement in management and governance, most investor-owned hospitals had more active physician involvement, particularly at the board level, than not-for-profit hospitals. For example, two-thirds of the board members of one investor-owned hospital system, and one-third of the two other investor-owned systems, are required to be physicians. This physician orientation comes partly from the fact that one of the investor-owned systems was founded by a physician and is largely driven by his value orientations, and partly from the fact that many of the early hospitals acquired by investor-owned companies were "doctors' hospitals" owned by physicians. But it also reflects the investor-owned companies' early realization that their economic success depended on physicians filling beds and that strong physician involvement would pay dividends.

A second across-the-board strategy has been "practice enhancement" programs. System hospitals, particularly prospectors, recognized the need to assess and then meet physician needs to gain their support for the hospital's strategic plan. Physicians want to know what the hospital and the system can do to help them compete in their own market. Among the programs developed have been patient referral systems, practice-management assistance, including marketing of physician practices, management information systems that link the physician's practice to the hospital and vice versa through computer networks, subsidization of younger physicians' practices, subsidized malpractice insurance coverage, assistance in negotiating managed care contracts, continuing medical education support, quality assurance systems, and personal financial counseling. The more successful efforts have been those that have identified different "market segments" of physicians with different needs and then created services specifically for them.

A third, somewhat more intangible factor involves appointing CEOs with reputations of being "good at working with physicians." They gained their reputations by successfully putting together joint ventures with physicians at other institutions and by effectively integrating physicians into hospital management and governance. They are described by one system executive as "individuals with a genuine respect for physicians without kowtowing to them or feeling the need for one-upmanship." They approached problem solving from the perspective of both physician and hospital and looked for areas of overlap. They were also adept at using the outside environment and physician peer pressure to facilitate change.

In addition to the across-the-board approaches, targeted strategies were needed to meet specific professional and economic needs of physicians. This involved identifying those physicians most likely to be interested in specific diversification efforts, those likely to be neutral, and those likely to be opposed. These lessons were learned:

1. A clear statement of mission and purpose for each *specific* diversification activity is needed.
2. It is important to identify physicians who understand and are willing to take some financial risk. In the words of one executive, "Some physicians' idea of a joint venture is that they get all of the *adventure* and stick us with the *joint.*"
3. A clear specification at the outset of each party's roles and responsibilities is needed. Physicians often operate on short time frames and thus expect financial rewards sooner than can realistically be achieved. Executives must carefully explain the short-run and long-run risks and communicate realistic expectations. Criteria should be developed by which each party may dissolve its interests in the joint venture.
4. A detailed business plan should be developed for each specific program, including target market characteristics, market size, projected market share by segment, projected revenues and expenses (both fixed and variable), and contingency plans.
5. There should be shared (hospital and physician) governance in management of the joint venture consistent with the nature of the risk/reward relationship. Fifty-fifty financial arrangements should be matched with approximately fifty-fifty decision-making authority and influence. If one party bears more of the risk/reward relationship, governance and managerial decision making should be matched accordingly. Several systems, both investor-owned and not-for-profit, established venture development corporations.
6. Appropriate mechanisms must be established for managing conflict. Where the activity level is small, this can be done through close daily interaction between the CEO and key physician leaders. In larger organizations, however, task forces are needed to oversee troublesome areas. It is par-

ticularly important that interested individuals with the appropriate expertise be involved.

7. Sufficient autonomy must be given to the diversification or joint venture unit. Attempts to impose the hospital's cultural rules and decision-making paradigms will fail. A joint venture must be free to experiment and to learn what best serves the intended purpose.

8. It is particularly important that information systems be developed to match the needs of the joint venture activity so that corrective action may be taken in a timely fashion. For example, many HMO and PPO activities have failed partly because of insufficient data on projected enrollment.

Guidelines for Managing the Prospector

Based on the analysis and examples discussed in this chapter, we offer the following guidelines for successfully managing a prospector strategy.

- Diversification activities must be carefully examined for their technological and managerial relatedness to existing businesses. The more unrelated a proposed new venture, the greater the need to develop new technological and managerial resources, the costs of which must be carefully examined against potential benefits and against the opportunity costs involved.

- There is a need to create "greenhouses" to maximize the learning that comes from inevitable failures. This requires the existence of slack resources. Organizations and managers without slack resources should not go prospecting.

- Entry strategies must be matched with the specific requirements of the diversification effort. The more related the diversification, the greater the benefits of doing it oneself. The more unrelated the diversification, the greater the benefits of joint ventures, networks, and related interorganizational arrangements.

- One must recognize the need to constantly differentiate products and services based on criteria that are least likely to be imitated by competitors, now or in the future.

- Strong market research capability is absolutely essential.
- Each product or service must be screened carefully to determine whether the experience-curve effects of a first-mover strategy can, in fact, be achieved.
- In a highly fragmented industry (such as health care), the diversification strategy should create local market synergies. Prospecting has to be localized, with many related "diggings" in the same area.
- Elements of both centralization and decentralization in strategic planning and control are needed in guiding the relationship between corporate office and strategic business unit. This is best expressed by the principle of "guided autonomy."
- There is a need to switch back and forth between cost-leadership and quality-differentiation strategies, depending on the stage of the product life cycle and the degree of market competitiveness. To execute such switching strategies successfully requires slack. Remember, if you do not have slack resources, do not go prospecting.
- There is a need to involve key professional groups in the development of diversification plans early in the process. Professionals' needs must be identified and linked to organizational needs and objectives. The goal is to create "common comfort zones" through exploring joint venture and related opportunities with key professionals.
- Know your strategic comfort zone! Think three times before venturing outside of your comfort zone. If you do not have slack resources, don't think about it at all.

There is more to being a prospector than throwing mud against the wall and seeing what sticks.

7

Managing the Defender Orientation

"It's hard for us to come to grips with change."

The Defender: Two Mini-Cases

"Diversification is not a major part of our strategy. Our focus is on acute inpatient care." These are the comments of the CEO of Community Memorial Hospital, a fairly typical defender. Community Memorial is a member of a very decentralized system that emphasizes local autonomy in decision making. It offers a fairly stable set of services to the community and has been known for strong medical staff relationships. As a result, it has been reluctant to initiate cost-containment strategies and has refused to consider joint venture opportunities because it does not believe in interfering with how physicians practice medicine. As the CEO noted, "We don't compete with our doctors."

At the same time, it has recognized the need to bond its physicians more closely to the hospital. As a result, it has recently established a number of physician services, including a 50 percent reduction in malpractice insurance, data processing support, purchasing assistance, and practice-management support.

Despite these initiatives, the hospital has lost market share in a moderately competitive community.

The system recognizes the challenges Community Memorial and similar defenders face. The corporate office believes it has been "too provincial, too narrow, and too self-satisfied in the past." It had difficulty "coming to grips with change." While still believing in decentralization as an operating philosophy, it now recognizes the need to "centralize things a bit" in terms of planning and control to help Community Memorial reduce its costs. It also plans to "standardize" key hospital departments so they can work with a common data and information base. The primary goal is to increase hospital productivity. Among other things, this will involve downsizing or deleting individual hospital labs and substituting regional labs that can serve several hospitals in a given area. This will require more centralization and less autonomy than Community Memorial (and other hospitals) are used to, but this is the price of remaining competitive.

In a second case, the system's goal is to keep cost increases below the industry average. Toward this end, it has formed a local industry advisory board to examine ways of lowering health care costs. This system currently has the lowest-cost hospitals in its market, but it is working to develop a more accurate cost accounting system. Its defender strategy is best expressed by the system CEO's comment that "responding to current affiliates and patients is a higher priority than system growth."

A major part of the cost-containment effort is focused on small defender hospitals in mostly rural areas. These specific steps were taken: (1) cross-training professional personnel so that fewer people are needed to do the work, (2) developing more efficient elective surgery schedules, (3) reducing the volume of laboratory tests, (4) reducing swing-bed staffing, (5) sending staff home if there's not enough work to do, and (6) instituting a value improvement program designed to eliminate certain procedures while maintaining care and service standards.

The system is also working actively with its physicians on both cost containment and improving quality of care. For example, at Norton Hospital joint hospital/physician committees explore changes needed in the hospital/physician relationship to enhance the competitive position of both parties. They emphasize selective diversification based on compatibility with physician interests. One task force is devoted to streamlining decision making so it is easier for physicians to participate. In addition, program coordinators are used to assess and where possible meet the needs of key physicians in each specialty. At the same time, these coordinators are responsible for monitoring physician activities in their area against cost and quality standards. Project teams, composed of physicians, nurses, and marketing and planning staff, are used to develop new programs and services as needed. Finally, Norton has also developed an array of physician appreciation programs, including recognition dinners, "clinician of the month" awards, and a fund for continuing medical education programs.

The Defender's Performance

As Figure 7.1 shows, defenders are somewhat more likely than the sample average to serve Medicaid patients and to provide a greater percentage of uncompensated care. At the same time, they are somewhat less likely to have an organized quality assurance department, and they experience a greater number of Joint Commission contingencies. This is consistent with the findings in Chapter Five, which indicate that defender hospitals give more emphasis to differentiating their services based on access and convenience and less emphasis on differentiating their services on technical quality of care.

Figure 7.2 shows that on almost every financial dimension, defenders did more poorly than the sample average, particularly in operating margin as a percent of net revenue (130 percent lower) and after-tax net income as a percent of total income (171 percent lower). Part of the reason for the relatively poor financial performance is the perceived weaknesses in their strategic planning and control systems, as shown in Figure 7.3. On every dimension, defenders score lower than the sample average, particularly in implementation, plan innovativeness, and market research.

Figure 7.1. Defender's Performance Profile—"Doing Good."

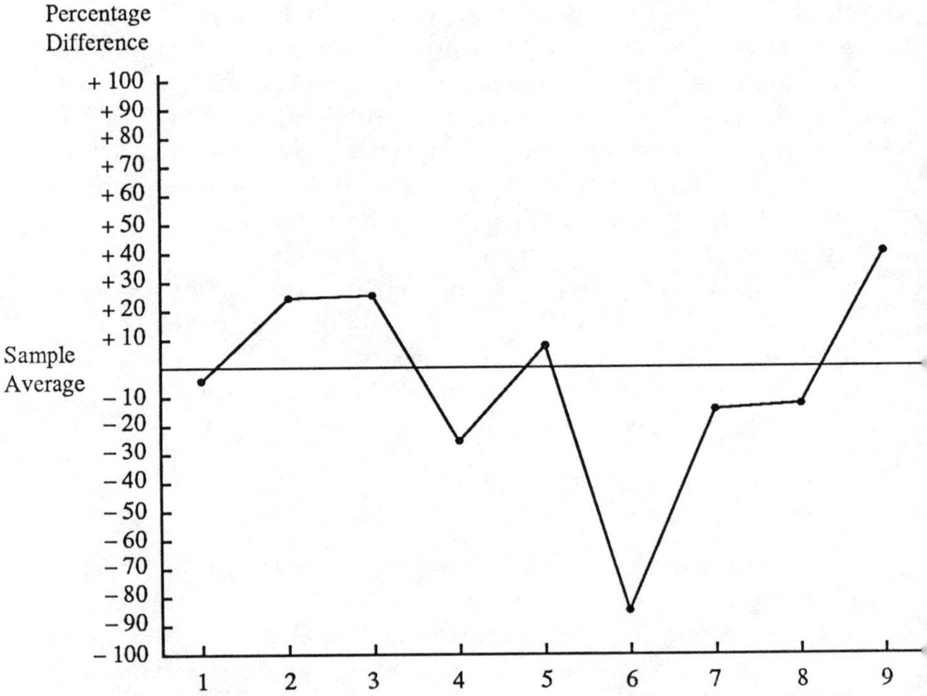

Percentage
Difference

	Defenders	Sample Average
1. Bad debt and charity care as a percentage of outpatient revenue	9.2%	9.6%
2. Medicaid revenue as a percentage of total outpatient revenue	10.3%	8.2%
3. Uncompensated care (bad debt and charity care) as a percentage of total revenue	4.9%	3.7%
4. Percentage of diversified services for which no charity care is provided	10.3%	12.7%
5. Number of unprofitable services offered	7.8	7.2
6. Have an organized quality assurance department	20%	37.5%
7. Quality assurance budget per admission	$11.82	$13.48
8. Severity-adjusted death rate for 16 selected conditions	9.7%	10.8%
9. Number of Joint Commission contingencies	1.0	.72

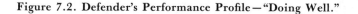
Figure 7.2. Defender's Performance Profile—"Doing Well."

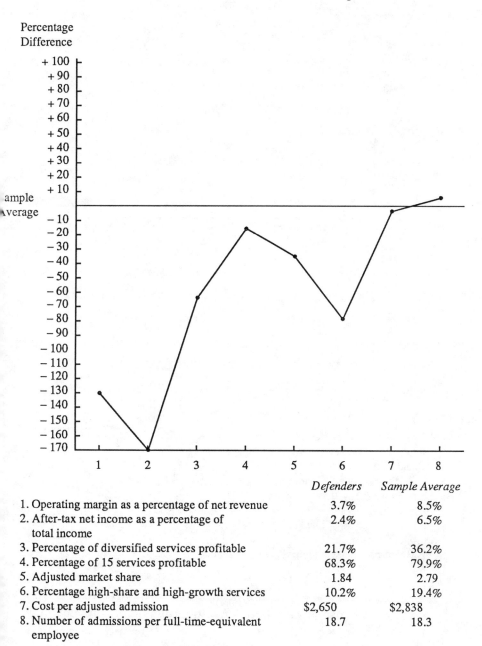

Percentage
Difference

ample
Average

	Defenders	Sample Average
1. Operating margin as a percentage of net revenue	3.7%	8.5%
2. After-tax net income as a percentage of total income	2.4%	6.5%
3. Percentage of diversified services profitable	21.7%	36.2%
4. Percentage of 15 services profitable	68.3%	79.9%
5. Adjusted market share	1.84	2.79
6. Percentage high-share and high-growth services	10.2%	19.4%
7. Cost per adjusted admission	$2,650	$2,838
8. Number of admissions per full-time-equivalent employee	18.7	18.3

Figure 7.3. Defender's Perceived
Quality of Strategic Planning and Control.

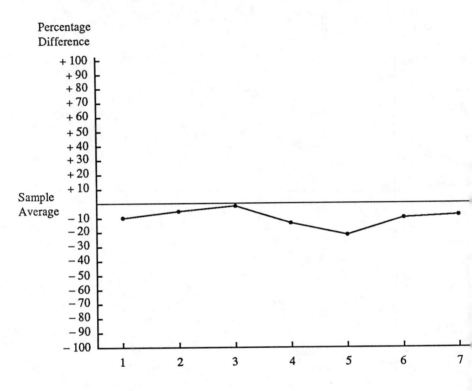

	Defenders	Sample Aver.
1. Overall perceived quality of strategic planning and control	2.65	2.94
2. Regional office assistance	2.86	3.01
3. Information systems	2.24	2.27
4. Implementation	2.70	3.07
5. Innovativeness of plans	2.86	3.59
6. Market research	2.44	2.77
7. Board member and physician involvement	2.80	3.12

Contrary to expectations, defender hospitals also gave less emphasis to cost-containment strategies than others (see Chapter Five). They were slower to recognize the need to take tough cost-cutting measures. As one defender executive commented,

"We thought we just needed to do more of what we were doing. We didn't recognize the significance of the change [prospective payment]." The challenges associated in implementing a defender strategy in a turbulent environment are the central focus of this chapter.

The Defender's Challenge

The primary challenge facing the defender is to protect and, if possible, increase current product or market share. This can be done by emphasizing technical efficiency and cost improvements that facilitate a cost-leadership strategy, or through various strategies designed to differentiate products or services from others in the market. Differentiation may be based on customer access or convenience, customer service, superior technical quality, or other features. Most of the existing literature (see, for example, Miles and Snow, 1978) associates the defender with strategies of cost containment and price leadership. But we suggest that existing product and market domains can also be defended, even extended, through well-selected differentiation strategies. This second way of successfully being a defender was particularly important for hospitals because under prospective payment there was a common incentive for *all* hospitals to contain costs. Thus the opportunity for defenders to maintain market share through cost containment alone was diminished as competitors engaged in cost-cutting activities. It was necesary for defenders to seek additional ways of protecting their domains.

Overall, the relatively poorer performance of defenders, particularly in "doing well" measures, came from two weaknesses: a slowness in recognizing the need to cost costs and the failure to recognize the need for some differentiation on quality dimensions. An important related factor was that defenders operate in less supportive environments that constrain their ability to implement their strategy.

We found that being a successful defender in the changing health care environment involved six requirements:

1. The need to manage costs.
2. The need for focused differentiation of services.

3. The need for selected diversification.
4. The need for slack resources.
5. The need for more centralized strategic planning and control.
6. The need to appropriately involve physicians in the above activities.

While many of these are also requirements for the other strategic archetypes, they take on a particular significance for defenders.

Managing Costs. One way for defenders to protect current product and market domains is to become the low-cost provider of services. Then they can potentially undercut the market and retain market share against possibly larger, more diversified, and more differentiated providers. This strategy requires that demand be price sensitive and that market segments exist for a "no-frills" product or service at a satisfactory level of quality. In the health care industry, these assumptions were essentially met as prospective payment provided incentives for being a low-cost provider, and many employers and third-party payers were interested in aligning with hospitals and physicians who delivered a basic set of health care services at a reasonable price. Technical quality was basically assumed and felt not to vary to a significant degree from one provider to another. Thus, the macro changes in the environment meant that a well-executed defender could potentially succeed.

The major problem, however, was that defenders were slow to recognize the need to actively manage their costs and, once they did, slow to take concerted action. There were three major reasons for this slowness: (1) the relatively benign environment enjoyed by defenders in previous years; (2) the fact that twenty of the twenty-five defender hospitals studied were not previously defenders and therefore did not have a strong cost-containment orientation; and (3) entrenched interests in current products and services, which made it difficult for defenders to divest services, coupled with strong community ties that made it difficult to lay off employees.

Before 1983, defender hospitals, like most hospitals, existed in a relatively benign environment. Third parties paid hospitals their costs plus a markup for capital replacement and expansion. In such an environment, defenders focused on a basic array of acute inpatient services with costs only slightly below their competitors. Competition involved not cost but service amenities for patients and physicians. The primary difference between defenders and the other archetypes was that defenders focused almost exclusively on acute inpatient care services (medicine, surgery, obstetrics, and pediatrics) while the others were significantly more diversified into outpatient srvices. Before 1983, defenders did not give particular emphasis to cost containment. They were not well prepared to deal with the change. In the words of one system executive, "I was as surprised as anyone when the prospective payment system flowed through Congress early last year [1983]. We clearly believed that such a change would not be enacted before 1985." A financial officer in one of the systems that contained a number of defender hospitals commented, "We were one of the least prepared organizations to meet the DRGs (diagnosis related groups). We did not anticipate the depths of the utilization declines."

Defenders' slowness to respond to the change can be partly explained by the phased-in implementation of the prospective payment program. Initial price limits were based on each hospital's historical cost for treating patients in each category in a given geographical area and thus were not particularly stringent at first. In fact, many hospitals found themselves making *higher* profits under the first year of prospective payment. Prospectors and analyzers were better than defenders in recognizing that this was a short-run phenomenon and took action to cut their costs so as to generate resources to support their outpatient diversification activities. Defenders were still focusing on inpatient and market domains and were slower to react. It was only as the DRG limits became more stringent and were blended into one national rate that defenders saw the need to, in the words of one hospital executive, "accelerate our cost-containment strategies."

The general lack of preparedness of defenders was compounded by the fact that many of them (twenty out of twenty-five) had previously been either prospectors, analyzers, or reactors. Many of them were trying to consolidate their programs and services to focus on a narrower product/market domain, but these activities did not involve process cost reductions. In some cases, costs actually increased as off-campus programs established in separate subsidiary corporations were brought back under the hospital corporate umbrella, with associated overhead and operating costs.

Underlying much of the slowness of defenders' responses was the reluctance to divest services and downsize the labor force. The defender strategy is one of the most difficult to reverse because of the interests involved in maintaining the status quo. Commitments and loyalties to existing programs and services had been established over many years. One vice-president of medical affairs noted, "We have always had a pediatric service here. The idea of dropping it, even though we have taken a beating financially, is devastating to some of our people. It's almost like we're not a hospital without it [the pediatrics department]." In almost every defender hospital, at least one program or service was being continued because of the interests of certain physicians or other health professionals. In addition, some defenders, particularly those in rural areas, feared that eliminating a service might result in a permanent loss of patients.

Many defender hospitals, particularly those associated with religiously affiliated systems, also found it difficult to delete programs and services because of their commitment to provide a full range of services to the community, particularly the poor. As one CEO commented, "Our decisions here are based on our mission and secondarily on the economics." A problem arose, however, when the economics failed to support the mission, and the viability of the hospital as an organization was threatened. Some defenders had to make difficult tradeoff decisions.

In considering such dilemmas, defenders had to take into account the attractiveness of programs and services to various groups (the community as well as physicians), the hospital's competitive position in regard to the service (for example, current and projected market share and profitability), and the degree to which the service could be provided by others in the area. A number of strategic alternatives arose from these considerations (MacMillan, 1983). For example, programs with low attractiveness and a weak competitive position and that can be provided by others suggest an aggressive divestment strategy. For one defender, prenatal care for unwed mothers was an example. Programs with a high degree of attractiveness but a weak competitive position and with a large number of other providers available may call for an orderly divestment strategy.

Defenders need to focus on those product and market domains that are most profitable. Therefore, if the organization's competitive position is weak, even though the program may be attractive on other grounds, it may be better to consider deleting the program, particularly since others may have a comparative advantage in offering it. For one hospital, this was the case for its occupational medicine program.

In a situation where few others can provide the service, then the defender strategy might be to build strength or delete it altogether. For another defender hospital, its outpatient behavioral medicine program was an example. The hospital needed to decide how important the service was in its overall strategic portfolio and, if important enough, commit the financial and human resources necessary to make it a success.

In other cases, defenders had strong competitive positions but with programs that were no longer particularly attractive to them. Where other providers were available, a useful strategy might be to support the best competitor, either through a joint venture arrangement or outright sale. In one case, the hospital sold its interest in a durable medical equipment company to use the resources for other purposes.

In other areas, hospitals had a strong competitive position (for example, a mobile diagnostic screening program in rural areas), but the program was unattractive because it was a financial loser and failed to generate sufficient inpatient demand. Yet no one else in the area could or would provide the service. In such a situation, a "bite the bullet" strategy may be the only alternative. The hospital needs to weigh the negative community reaction to eliminating the service against the ongoing losses of continuing the service.

A final situation was represented by a defender hospital that saw an opportunity to provide health promotion services to a growing elderly population. The program initially was not seen as particularly attractive, the hospital was not particularly competitive in providing the service (not having done it before), and yet only one other organization was providing such care. Thus, an opportunity existed that was best captured through a joint venture strategy that enabled the hospital to share in the risks, the startup costs (which in this case were small), and the learning involved.

All these represent divestment or reorientation strategies that the less successful defenders were less willing to consider. These decisions are even more difficult than they appear at first glance because they cannot be considered in isolation from one another. The decision to eliminate a pediatric service, for example, has an obvious effect on obstetrics. The decision to eliminate an outpatient behavioral medicine service will affect the inpatient psychiatric service. Thus, in refocusing the product and market domains as part of their cost-containment strategies, defenders needed to consider the interdependence and potential synergies among their programs and services.

All hospitals in the systems we studied engaged in some downsizing activity, but defenders had a particularly difficult time laying off employees. Partly this was because of the stable mix of basic services defenders offered to their communities. When demand for these services began to slacken, defenders were slow to recognize the overstaffing that resulted. As one chief financial officer put it, "We felt that the decline in utilization was only temporary. We kept thinking it would bottom out, but it never did. We probably reacted too late."

A second reason for slowness to lay off employees was strong ties to the local community. This involved both economic and social/psychological dimensions. Some defenders were the largest employers in their communities and were reluctant to downsize too swiftly or too greatly. In addition, in smaller communities and ethnic areas of larger cities (where some defenders were located), strong friendship and kinship ties exist. In these situations, layoffs can have a devastating effect on community morale. In the words of one CEO, "It is very difficult to downsize employees in an organization that is very people oriented and community minded."

Finally, because defenders engaged in few, if any, diversification efforts, they did not have alternative avenues of employment available for those who were no longer needed to provide acute inpatient services. Prospectors and analyzers, on the other hand, would often transfer employees from the hospital unit to various other units.

For all these reasons, defenders gave less attention to cost containment than might have been expected, particularly in productivity and efficiency improvements and program and staff deletions. But many also failed to take certain positive actions that would have helped them further penetrate current markets. Among these was the need to differentiate their current acute care services.

Focused Differentiation. In addition to the need to be cost efficient, the more successful defenders engaged in focused differentiation of their inpatient services (for example, general and medical surgical care, obstetrics, pediatrics, and psychiatry). The less successful defenders failed to recognize the need for such differentiation and tried to get by with what they had.

Most defenders recognized they could not compete with the generally larger prospectors, analyzers, and reactors on technical quality of care. Instead, much of the service refinement took the form of trying to provide convenient and accessible services: more convenient scheduling of surgical patients, introduction of guest relations programs, reorganization of the emergency room to serve as a convenience clinic, and introduction of "gourmet meal services." One system with a number of defender hospitals encouraged differentiation along a number of lines: (1) providing practice support to encourage physicians to admit patients to the hospital, (2) providing training programs to help physicians communicate more effectively with patients, (3) providing leadership development and continuing education programs for key employees, (4) providing research support to identify the quality of care components of most interest to consumers, (5) developing information systems to monitor quality, (6) developing advocacy programs for quality of care with legislators and policymakers, and (7) including patient comfort and convenience criteria in considering new technology purchases.

A key to successful differentiation was investment in market research and promotion. While prospectors and analyzers focused more of their marketing activities on their diversified services, defenders focused on their stable core of acute inpatient services. One defender emphasized its "family-oriented" care. The hospital was promoted as a family hospital, with an active department of family medicine and an emphasis on obstetrics and pediatrics care. The hospital was actively involved in the community in serving as a sponsor and cosponsor of a number of community events including health fairs, 10K runs, "school adoptions," and homecoming floats.

Another defender placed its primary emphasis on obstetrics care. Working cooperatively with its obstetricians, the hospital provided a nurse to each prospective mother early in her pregnancy. To the extent possible, this nurse carried through with the mother's care in the hospital during labor and delivery and at home for postpartum care. Fathers were encouraged to participate actively in childbirth. The hospital delivered flowers daily to each mother's room, and each baby received a gift. A small gift was sent to the child's home on each birthday for five years. The hospital saw its emphasis on outstanding maternity care as a way of reaching women, who make most of the family's medical decisions. The hospital believed this strategy helped them maintain their occupancy rate while competitors were losing admissions.

Thus, the need for good market research and promotion is not a characteristic of prospectors alone. Defenders with good market research capabilities tended to outperform defenders without such capabilities, particularly in profitability of basic acute care services. Good market research enabled these defenders to tailor their services to fit niches in new and existing markets. It also helped when some defenders undertook selective diversification activities.

Selective Diversification. Just as prospectors need to engage in some cost-containment strategy, so do defenders need to engage in some diversification activities. The problem many defenders had in trying to penetrate current markets with current inpatient services is that these services and markets typically had low-growth or even no-growth potential. In a word, they were "mature." This is typically true of most general medical and surgical services, pediatrics care, and often obstetrics care as well. Even if additional market share could be attained, the profit margins on the "gained shares" were rapidly declining as DRG rates became more stringent over time. Defenders needed some degree of diversification to expand their revenue base.

At the same time, defenders needed diversification activities that would contribute to reducing the cost of inpatient care so that they could better compete under the prospective payment system. Such diversified services as outpatient diagnostic testing facilitated efficient use of inpatient resources once patients were admitted to the hospital. Other diversified services such as home health care helped to facilitate early hospital discharge. In addition, such diversification represented alternative sources of employment for laid-off hospital personnel.

Many defenders failed to recognize the need for diversification. For some, this was due to the inbreeding of senior managers. "We were slow to get into the market," observed one manager. "Diversification requires new forms of compensation, job descriptions, and performance appraisal. Even when we recognized this, I'm not sure we wanted to make the changes." The lessons of successful diversification learned by prospectors apply as well to defenders; the major difference is that defenders had much less experience at diversification and a fundamentally different culture, making the diversification process particularly difficult.

It was also important that defenders' diversification activities be highly related to their inpatient business. Since most defenders did not have an abundance of slack resources to experiment with, it was important that they stay within their strategic comfort zone and build on their current case of knowledge and expertise. Examples included outpatient diagnostic services and ambulatory surgery services, which build on the expertise of internists and surgeons on the staff, and outpatient behavioral medicine (that is, alcoholism and drug addiction programs), which builds on the strength of staff psychiatrists. These services seldom had the volume or profitability on their own to dominate their market; they were needed to serve as feeders to basic acute inpatient services.

Slack Resources. To state the obvious, if an organization is going to pursue a defender strategy, it should first make sure there is something worth defending. If a defender strategy is to be reasonably successful, the organization has to be sufficiently financially viable. Failing this, it may need to merge with other providers in the area or in other ways rethink its strategic role in the system's overall plan. One alternative, of course, is closure. Another is a significant infusion of capital.

Some of the hospitals that maintained or adopted the defender strategy were not financially viable. In normal times, these organizations might have succeeded with a defender strategy. But the period from 1983 to 1988 was not normal. In addition to the macro environmental changes, most defenders faced local environments lacking in resources and support. The lack of population growth meant that market penetration was a zero-sum game. Defenders could gain market share only by taking it away from someone else. Defenders also had problems competing for a more limited supply of physicians, nurses, and other health professionals. Some were located in collar-county semi-rural areas but still had competitors thirty to fifty miles away. These defenders needed to become more technically sophisticated and differentiate themselves more on technical quality to keep local residents but were largely unable to do so. Being a cost or price leader alone would not hold local residents when they perceived themselves to be really sick. Also, being more frequently located in highly regulated certificate-of-need states made it doubly difficult for defender hospitals to upgrade plant and equipment needed to attract both physicians and patients.

Even those defenders that were moderately healthy financially did not have sufficient slack to differentiate their services on quality grounds, to market their services aggressively, or to engage in selected diversification. In a sense, defenders were one cycle too late. The savings that might have accrued from earlier cost improvements could have been used to market services to expand market share. But because they operated in a relatively benign environment before the 1980s, most defenders had not stockpiled the resources to deal with the turbulence created by the shift in the environment. One executive aptly describes the situation: "We were not as rigorous in our cost control as other organizations." This was particularly true in methods engineering, inventory control, and related efficiency and productivity measures.

Centralized Direction. Effective implementation of cost-containment and market-penetration strategies in multidivisional organizations requires centralized strategic planning and control. Implementation itself may be decentralized to the local units, with strong centralized controls necessary to instill the discipline required to make the defender strategy viable. This is particularly true if significant environmental change has occurred. In such situations, defenders may have a tendency to deviate from the course and begin to behave as reactors. A strong, centralized strategic planning and control system can help safeguard against this.

The defender hospitals confirmed the importance of strong centralized direction and control. Defenders if anything were *less likely* to adopt cost-containment strategies than other groups, particularly in efficiency and productivity improvements. They also did less well financially. We believe that both findings were in large part a result of the relative lack of centralized strategic planning and control. Defenders, which we expected to be the most centralized, were actually no different from the other three strategic archetypes in strategic planning and control.

Many defenders were part of hospital systems that emphasized decentralization as part of their culture. These systems saw decentralization, emphasizing local autonomy, as their key value and strength. Because health care is delivered locally, it was important that local hospitals have control over their own destiny. Part of the success of the systems was their ability to provide overall financial and management assistance while granting local hospitals as much autonomy as possible. In a benign environment, this relatively loose philosophy worked well. But with the changes wrought by prospective payment and its associated effects, a decentralized approach was inadequate because the local hospitals could not cope with the changes required. In addition, the systems needed to begin thinking about the local hospitals as a *group* and consider how each fit into the larger hospital system as part of its overall strategy for responding to the environment. Thus, both local and systemwide incentives existed for providing more centralized strategic direction and control.

Understandably, these incentives were fought by many of the local hospitals, which desired to retain their autonomy. Some were simply slow to recognize the need for the change, others denied it altogether. Those who recognized the need for change wanted to play a larger role than the system deemed appropriate. The situation was best captured in the words of one system executive, "We finally pulled it off [centralization of strategic planning and control], but it wasn't without considerable blood-letting. There are still some pretty bruised feelings."

Part of the problem came from the confusion between strategic control and operational control. Some system executives, particularly those who had risen through the managerial ranks, were themselves reluctant to centralize greater authority at the corporate office. They feared that such control would be viewed negatively by the local hospital constituents and would also result in poorer program planning because the corporate office would be too far removed from the local market. They failed to recognize that it was possible to set overall strategic direction and accountability for the system and for each hospital's role within the system, and still delegate operational responsibility to the local hospital management team. As a result of this confusion, system executives were not as rigorous in initiating the cost-control and market-positioning strategies required to execute a successful defender strategy in the new environment.

A related reason for the relatively poor performance of defenders was their lack of adequate management information systems. They were often late in linking financial and budget information with clinical data to track physician performance under the DRGs. For some defenders, such monitoring ran counter to their culture, which emphasized catering to physicians and being as unobtrusive as possible in the practice of medicine. For the same reason, they were slow to recognize market protection and market penetration strategies that could be pursued through physician joint ventures.

Overall, the lack of adequate information systems meant that defenders did not have the data to examine their position relative to the market. Thus, even defenders that recognized the need for cost control, for product and service differentiation, and for selected diversification did not have adequate information upon which to build their plans. This hampered their efforts to convince their physicians of the need to change behavior and to involve physicians in executing a successful defender strategy.

The Physician Factor. While for prospectors a major challenge was involving physicians in a meaningful way in the diversification process, for defenders the major challenge was involving them in a meaningful way in cost containment and in market defense and penetration. A major source of physician opposition was their fear of having their clinical and professional autonomy curtailed. As one hospital executive noted, "Our cost-containment strategy [that is, its effectiveness] will depend in large part on physician support."

Prospective payment put many hospitals and physicians at odds with each other; while there were incentives for hospitals to contain costs, there were no such incentives for physicians. Because physicians are directly or indirectly responsible for approximately 70 to 80 percent of hospital costs, hospitals needed to persuade physicians of the importance of cost containment: discharge patients earlier, reduce treatment inputs such as tests and procedures, and scale down requests for new technologies and equipment. All these go against the physicians' professional culture, which argues for doing everything possible for the patient. Defenders operating in competitive environments faced a particularly difficult task in implementing changes because physicians could threaten to take their patients to competing hospitals. For defenders operating as sole providers in the community, the task was easier because physicians' own professional and economic success was more directly linked to the success of the local hospital.

Thus the ability of defenders to adopt cost-containment strategies was limited by physicians' professional opposition. This is unlike the situation faced by firms in most other industries, where employees generally work to bring about the strategic intent of the business, but is similar to other highly professional organizations such as high-technology research firms, symphonies, and universities where the aspirations of the professionals may differ from those of the organization. More successful defenders had executives who understood physician needs and expectations. They worked patiently with physicians, adopting an educational approach to making physicians more aware of the long-run implications of prospective payment and what it meant for both physicians and hospitals. These executives were also effective in identifying a few key physician leaders who understood the importance of what the hospital had to do to contain its costs. These physician leaders, in turn, helped to educate and influence their peers.

Some defender executives were also good at using the outside environment and circumstances to persuade physicians of the need for change. In one case the threat of an outside organization coming into the community was used to get physicians to adopt stricter utilization review requirements. In another case, an executive used the threat of a merger between two hospitals to persuade his medical staff of the need for change.

These executives were also skillful symbolic leaders of the need for change. They modeled the desired behavior by first initiating budget cuts in administration and support areas. Physicians could see what the hospital was doing to cut its costs, and recognized that the hospital was not simply using them as a scapegoat for cost containment. These executives were careful to make sure that the initial cuts were not made in direct patient care areas (such as nursing), which would be most noticeable to physicians and which would be perceived as a direct threat to quality of care.

While the main physician issue defenders had to deal with was cost cutting, they also faced some problems with their limited diversification activities. In the case of prospectors, physicians feared competition for patients from the diversified activities. But the main problem for defenders was that physicians could not understand why the hospital needed to engage in such activities when hospital occupancy was low, running between 40 and 50 percent. They felt that more attention should be paid to the basic hospital services. The more successful defenders continued to educate their physicians and use outside events and circumstances to encourage prudent use of resources.

Above all, defenders, with their focus on basic acute care inpatient services, needed to recognize the physician as their primary customer in differentiation strategies designed to protect and enhance current market share. For prospectors, diversification activities often involved customers and market segments different than physicians (for example, employers, schools, and women). But for defenders the primary focus had to be on the physicians who brought patients into the hospital. Defenders were largely unprepared for the new and more aggressive approaches to courting physicians required by the more competitive environment. In competitive markets, the annual physician recognition dinner would no longer suffice. Successful defenders had to learn to identify each physician's needs through market research and then design services to meet those needs: office management, assistance with medical records, billing, practice promotion, more convenient patient scheduling, and assistance with malpractice insurance.

Guidelines for Managing the Defender

Summarizing the issues discussed in this chapter, we offer the following guidelines for successfully executing a defender strategy.

- If you are going to be a defender, you have to have something to defend. Some existing programs and services must be doing well.

- Costs must be actively managed on an ongoing basis.
- Selected programs and services must be consolidated or divested. Being a strong defender is like growing a strong tree. It is necessary to prune the dead wood to give light and air so that the healthy branches may grow stronger.
- Program and service interdependency and synergies must be considered in deciding what services to divest. Some unprofitable services should be retained because they are necessary to support or complement a profitable service. Other profitable services might be deleted because they add little value to the overall portfolio of services and consume resources that can be better used for other purposes.
- Managing costs and divesting services are not enough. Defenders must also differentiate their services to hold or gain market share. Sources of differentiation include quality, access, comfort, convenience, and service.
- Defenders must invest in market research and promotion to effectively differentiate their services. Marketing is not the sole province of prospectors.
- Successful defenders must engage in a limited degree of diversification activities highly related to the core business. This is particularly true in competitive markets.
- Being a defender in a resource-constrained environment requires slack resources to selectively differentiate and diversify the existing service mix.
- Being a defender requires discipline. In multidivisional organizations some degree of centralization of strategic planning and control is required.
- Key professionals must be involved in cost containment, differentiation, and limited diversification. Continued education, modeling of appropriate behavior, and judicious use of external events and circumstances and incentives are needed to effectively involve professionals in executing a successful defender strategy.

8

Managing the Analyzer Orientation

"We want to take advantage of opportunities but not create them. We want to be flexible."

The Analyzer: Two Mini-Cases

One analyzer-oriented system was in the midst of a transition from a very entrepreneurial strategy, associated with the system's first executive, to a more professionally managed analyzer strategy represented by the successor. The system grew initially through horizontal integration of several hospitals in a given area. When prospective payment was introduced in 1983, the system saw the need to grow vertically as well, and began to diversify into residential retirement centers, ambulatory surgery centers, physician office buildings, and sports medicine programs, among others. At the same time, it saw the need to significantly upgrade its strategic planning, human resource planning, marketing, and information systems. The system did not attempt to have the lowest (or highest) cost hospitals in its markets but rather to emphasize *cost-effective* care. While launching several successful diversification efforts, it also initiated several cost-containment programs, including centralized purchasing, laundry, data processing, laboratory, and pharmacy, resulting in cost savings of $4.5 million. An additional $2.5 million was saved through joining a nationwide purchasing alliance. Automated cost accounting and inventory control systems were also introduced. Systemwide productivity and monitoring standards were established. Some hospitals established joint hospital-physician cost-containment committees that explored ways of containing costs while maintaining quality. These and other initiatives helped the system hospitals reduce their operating costs 5 percent while most competitors' costs continued to increase.

At the same time, incentives were established to develop new businesses. As one executive noted, "We don't crucify people anymore for making mistakes. We don't rush into things, but we want to promote entrepreneurial risk taking behavior. We use incentive compensation to do this in a culture which says it's OK to fail sometimes. In the past, failure was never forgotten." Among the new initiatives started by member hospitals were alternative birthing centers, industrial health physicals, and HMOs. The overall goal is to build "continuum of care clusters" around the base hospitals. These clusters will contain a variety of pre- and posthospital services, ranging from health promotion to home care. At the same time, the system continues to be committed to core inpatient services. For example, some hospitals have developed centers of excellence in arthritis, cardiology, emergency medicine, open heart surgery, and sports medicine.

Within the system, strong management is viewed as the key to holding diversified subsidiaries together. System leaders feel that too many of their executives still think like defenders, particularly at the middle management level where they have had problems implementing their strategic goals. To continue to walk the analyzer tightrope, they perceive the need for an additional $8 million in cost reductions. At the same time, they recognize the need to give physicians greater involvement in the managerial and governance processes of the system and its member hospitals.

A second system dominated by analyzer hospitals also places primary emphasis on cost effectiveness but is more regionally based. The system also has considerable resources, faces only moderate competition, and has been able to diversify without spreading itself too thin. Among its new activities, usually developed only after careful study and analysis of others, are freestanding ambulatory surgery centers, occupational medicine programs, and practice management. At the same time that it was diversifying, it made considerable financial investment in ongoing inpatient services through capital replacements involving upgrading all its acute hospital facilities.

The system is strongly committed to managing "off its strategic plan." The top management group meets once a month for two days for in-depth review of both short-term and long-term plans. There is a computerized cash projection model that goes fifteen years into the future. The system places high emphasis on developing market niches, such as among self-insured and smaller employers, and believes in trying things on a small scale first, finding out what works before proceeding. As the system CEO noted, "We want to go slow and not stub our toe. We prefer to be small and strong rather than large and weak." At the same time, system leaders are trying to educate a conservative board that they will need to make some mistakes and are trying to install a management culture that says "first mistakes are OK."

To execute its strategy, the central office retains fairly centralized direction and control, including appointing the individual hospital governing boards, which are advisory only. While this makes it easier to coordinate systemwide policies among the hospitals, the system has recognized the need for greater hospital management involvement in strategic planning. It has also recognized the need for stronger marketing support and for developing, in the words of one planner, "a truly integrated regional plan rather than stapled-together individual hospital plans." It has made significant progress in working with physicians through a systemwide physician corporation and appointments of two physician executives at the corporate office, but recognizes the need for continuous cultivation of these relationships. It is unusually well positioned and has considerable capital but "we also need to keep a conservative board comfortable with our plans," at a time when hospitals' operating margins have shrunk from the 6 to 8 percent range to the 1.5 to 2 percent range.

The Analyzer's Performance

Figures 8.1 and 8.2 indicate that the analyzer's performance profile is generally similar to the sample at large. For the most part analyzers do better than defenders but not quite as well as prospectors or, in some cases, reactors. Figure 8.3 indicates that they also resemble the sample average in perceived quality of strategic planning and control systems. Like prospectors, however, they make greater use of standardized forms and formats in their strategic planning process than either defenders or reactors.

The challenge of being an analyzer lies in balancing the competing demands of both a prospector and defender strategy. The lessons learned about this process are the focus of this chapter.

The Analyzer's Challenge

The primary challenge facing the analyzer is to manage the complexity inherent in attempting to pursue new services and new markets and at the same time protect current services in existing markets from erosion. Analyzers have both a stable domain and an innovative domain, which produces a dynamic tension in its planning and management systems, with the need for control on the one hand and flexibility on the other (Shank, Niblock, and Sandall, 1973). Falling in between the prospector and defender categories does not simply mean that analyzers are watered-down prospectors or glorified defenders. Rather, it means that analyzers must be true prospectors in some of their activities and true defenders in other activities. They must know when to use each strategy and how to execute both appropriately. In brief, they must be ambidextrous in their approaches and in their implementation.

Figure 8.1. Analyzer's Performance Profile—"Doing Good."

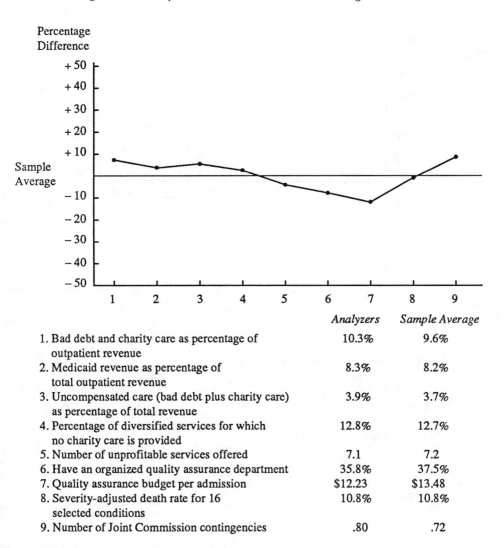

	Analyzers	Sample Average
1. Bad debt and charity care as percentage of outpatient revenue	10.3%	9.6%
2. Medicaid revenue as percentage of total outpatient revenue	8.3%	8.2%
3. Uncompensated care (bad debt plus charity care) as percentage of total revenue	3.9%	3.7%
4. Percentage of diversified services for which no charity care is provided	12.8%	12.7%
5. Number of unprofitable services offered	7.1	7.2
6. Have an organized quality assurance department	35.8%	37.5%
7. Quality assurance budget per admission	$12.23	$13.48
8. Severity-adjusted death rate for 16 selected conditions	10.8%	10.8%
9. Number of Joint Commission contingencies	.80	.72

Because analyzers contain components of both the prospector and defender orientations, many of the requirements for successful execution of prospector and defender strategies apply to analyzers as well. On the prospector's side, these include the need to understand related diversification, to constantly differen-

Figure 8.2. Analyzer's Performance Profile — "Doing Well."

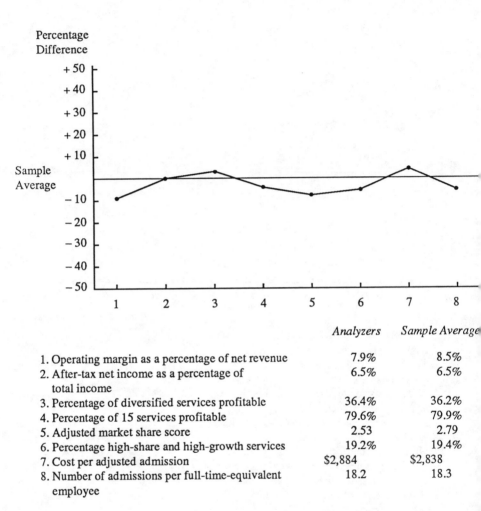

	Analyzers	Sample Average
1. Operating margin as a percentage of net revenue	7.9%	8.5%
2. After-tax net income as a percentage of total income	6.5%	6.5%
3. Percentage of diversified services profitable	36.4%	36.2%
4. Percentage of 15 services profitable	79.6%	79.9%
5. Adjusted market share score	2.53	2.79
6. Percentage high-share and high-growth services	19.2%	19.4%
7. Cost per adjusted admission	$2,884	$2,838
8. Number of admissions per full-time-equivalent employee	18.2	18.3

tiate services, and to create local market synergies. The major difference between the prospector and the analyzer is that the analyzers were seldom first to introduce a new service to the market. On the defender's side, the need to manage costs, to engage in selective differentiation and diversification, and to have some degree of centralized strategic direction and control all

Figure 8.3. Analyzer's Perceived Quality
of Strategic Planning and Control.

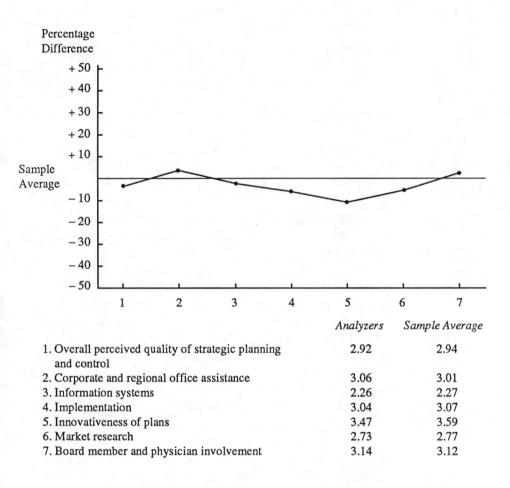

	Analyzers	Sample Average
1. Overall perceived quality of strategic planning and control	2.92	2.94
2. Corporate and regional office assistance	3.06	3.01
3. Information systems	2.26	2.27
4. Implementation	3.04	3.07
5. Innovativeness of plans	3.47	3.59
6. Market research	2.73	2.77
7. Board member and physician involvement	3.14	3.12

apply. As with both prospectors and defenders, analyzers needed to appropriately involve physicians in strategy making. Similarly, the presence of slack resources was an important facilitator, particularly for the prospector component of the analyzer strategy.

But aside from these commonalities, analyzers face some additional requirements:

1. The need to address the complexity inherent in managing two major strategies simultaneously.
2. The need to create synergy between the prospector domain and the defender domain.
3. The need to maximize learning to decide whether and when to enter new markets or develop new services.
4. The need to emphasize new skills and new mind sets for executives and board members.
5. The need to involve physicians in a way that minimizes mixed messages.

Managing Complexity. For many hospitals the analyzer strategy provided the most flexibility in a dynamic, rapidly changing environment. But there were both passive analyzers and active analyzers. The passive analyzers saw their approach as a middle of the road strategy that gave them an opportunity to see, in the words of one informant, "how the dust will settle." They were essentially straddling the fence, looking for cues in deciding what direction to move. Representative statements:

"The old joke around here is that if studying and analyzing the insurance business takes forever but prevents us from losing a lot of money, then we have the authority to study it forever" (vice-president for planning).

"We're big enough to be able to adopt a wait-and-see attitude" (system board member).

"We don't jump in unless we can succeed" (hospital CEO).

The active analyzers appeared more decisive; they knew they wanted to pursue some new markets and services actively (their prospector orientation) while refining and becoming more efficient in providing existing services (their defender orientation). While the passive analyzers more or less backed into their decisions, the active analyzers believed they needed both prospector and defender components to succeed. In the words of one executive, "While we don't necessarily have to be first, we want to position ourselves to take advantage of a number of different types of things."

Although there is some overlap in the operational requirements for both prospectors and defenders, they are sufficiently different to create considerable tension for the analyzer attempting to manage both domains simultaneously. Comments from several informants reflected this tension:

"What we have going is a creative tension within the organization between the commitment to quality, the commitment to the city, and the commitment to sound business practice" (CEO) (Guncheon, 1984, p. M84).

"Approval and review mechanisms can slow down decision making. At times we're very schizoid around here" (hospital planner).

The tensions created by this balancing act were often intensified for religiously affiliated hospitals, who also had to balance mission requirements such as service to the poor with economic realities. As one CEO of a system dominated by analyzer hospitals said, "There is a corridor of reasonableness that we have to operate in. We have to find out how to get these corridors of reasonableness for service and for business to overlap as much as we can. The organization is not committed to providing the largest financial return as possible, and at the same time it's not blindly committed to servicing the poor without a sense of reality" (Guncheon, 1984, p. M84). Thus, for religiously affiliated hospitals the analyzer strategy had to be both market driven and mission oriented.

The components of the analyzer strategy are best summarized in the need to be cost effective. Analyzers had to control their costs, particularly for their more stable basic inpatient services, without compromising quality, while at the same time developing new services based in part on quality differentiation. Unlike defenders, analyzers were more active in their cost-containment efforts. They were much more likely to reduce staff, to consolidate programs and services, to divest services that were not performing well, to initiate productivity and efficiency improvements, and to be more aggressive in reducing patients' length of stay. Their approach to cost containment also appeared to be more long-run–oriented and more strategically directed than either defenders or reactors. In the words of one manager, "Productivity is more than just an approach to management engineering in day-to-day operations. It starts with an organization's ability to chart a direction that will help it maintain a productive future."

Analyzers differed from prospectors in that they were somewhat less diversified and more focused. Their diversification tended to be more related to the core inpatient services, with an emphasis on ambulatory surgery centers, outpatient diagnostic centers, skilled nursing facilities, and alternative delivery and financing arrangements designed to channel patients into the hospital. As expected, analyzers were also somewhat slower than prospectors to respond to market opportunities. One manager's comment, typical of others: "We tend to beat things to death. We analyze and analyze. Others do it quicker."

Being an analyzer also placed significant stress on the relationship between individual hospitals and the corporate office. The stress took two forms, one reflected in what was perceived to be inconsistent messages, and the other in confusion over how much latitude the individual hospitals had. The first stemmed from corporate offices' difficulty in communicating a strategy with two components. On the one hand, hospitals were being told to be creative, to innovate, and to take risks. On the other hand, they were told to focus on basics, cut costs, and, above all, keep the peace with physicians. The problem was compounded by the system's failure to recognize that some hospitals needed to give greater emphasis to the prospector dimension of its strategy while others needed to give greater emphasis to the defender component. There was a tendency to apply the analyzer strategy across the board, aiming for the "golden mean" while missing both of the ends. Insufficient attention was given to local market characteristics and the strengths and weaknesses of each hospital relative to its competition. This caused a number of mostly analyzer hospitals in one system to become disenchanted with the corporate office, leading to some corporate reorganization and reorientation.

The issue of latitude or autonomy arose from the need for disciplined cost control on the one hand but the freedom to innovate and develop new services on the other. As one executive noted, "We have problems balancing central direction and local autonomy." Some degree of centralized direction and discipline was needed to manage the costs, but at the same time local hospital executives, having the most detailed knowledge of their own markets, needed autonomy to develop services for local demand. In the words of one, "We aren't strategic enough. Corporate office is still too inpatient focused." One system CEO expressed the dilemma this way: "These hospitals aren't autonomous, but we try to foster a strong sense of decision making and performance because that's where our productivity comes from. Local hospital management teams must be challenged to respond and achieve results."

Successful analyzers were able to come to grips with this dilemma. They did so by providing overall guidelines and centralized cost monitoring but leaving it to individual hospitals to decide the specific mix of services for their communities. Hospital CEOs were also given the freedom to change strategies in midyear if they consulted with regional or corporate staff. Successful analyzers also recognized that newly diversified services such as ambulatory care and outpatient diagnostic centers often had different operating and managerial requirements from acute inpatient services. These were given the freedom to develop their own personnel policies, patient care practices, and information systems. Finally, the complexity of executing the analyzer strategy was reduced when the corporate guidelines highlighted the need for synergy between the prospector and defender domains.

Creating Synergy. For analyzer hospitals, most of their prospector activities involved creating out-of-hospital services, while most of their defender activities involved maintaining inpatient services. Thus, the trick for analyzers was to develop new services that complemented their inpatient services and to use money that could be gained from efficiency in the delivery of inpatient care to promote new services. This search for synergies was greatly facilitated for systems whose hospitals were geographically concentrated in selected markets. For example, among three systems with a high percentage of analyzers, the two with geographically concentrated hospitals did significantly better financially than the third, whose hospitals were dispersed across several states. This third system faced particular challenges in making improvements in inpatient operating areas in order to fund diversification activities.

Two factors stood out in facilitating prospector-defender synergy. The first was "two-for-one" solutions — a new program or service was not only an additional source of revenue but also helped promote cost containment. The second was the development of carefully targeted market niches where selected services could be bundled together for further development.

Forrest Falls Hospital served as an example of the "two-for-one" approach. Over a period of five years, the hospital developed several ambulatory care centers with relatively sophisticated diagnostic capability. More patients had their prehospital admissions done on an outpatient basis, thus saving the hospital money under the DRG limits while at the same time contributing to greater outpatient revenues. The hospital also developed an extensive outpatient cardiac rehabilitation program as a complement to its inpatient cardiac care programs. The hospital was able to discharge its cardiology patients sooner, again saving money under the DRG payment lids while capturing revenue on the outpatient side.

River Glen developed a similar approach serving a growing elderly population. The hospital was able to get approximately twenty beds designated as "swing beds" to care for patients who required less intensive care than the hospital's acute care but also required some degree of nursing care and medical supervision. The hospital then developed a continuum of "after-care" services, including adult day health care and home care, which facilitated earlier hospital discharge, thereby controlling costs. While the adult day care and home care programs were not net income producers at the time, they did help keep patients within the hospital's network. Some of the patients required subsequent hospitalization, which generated additional revenues.

The passive analyzers and the active analyzers had different approaches to market niches. The passive analyzers were often forced into a market niche strategy by the more aggressive prospectors in their market. The passive analyzers' strategic plans were present oriented, and they were beaten to the market on several occasions. This forced them to consider subsegments of the market. Glen Oaks Hospital, for example, was the third to offer an HMO in a competitive market. In order to survive it targeted the HMO to small employers who self-insured, and it emphasized the "personal caring" features of its physicians. Silverado Memorial was a late entrant into the ambulatory surgery business. But it managed to carve out a successful subsegment of the market by focusing primarily on cosmetic surgery to an upscale clientele.

The more active analyzers placed greater reliance on market research capability to identify *in advance* market segments where they thought they matched up well against their competitors. Moston General, for example, developed several women's health programs aimed at generally younger women. Its service portfolio included health promotion and stress management, weight management , and prenatal delivery and postnatal care involving a variety of alternative birthing options. Decker Hills Hospital identified behavioral medicine as a major market niche. It offered programs for alcohol and substance abuse along with positive self-image seminars, and developed a subniche targeted to adolescents. By creating these types of market niches, active analyzers were often able to preempt competitors that had frequently been first in entering related markets.

Whether active or passive, analyzers took three general approaches to niches: based on market segment, based on program or service, based on geography. The market segment approach centered on defined population groups such as women, children, and the elderly and attempted to package a bundle of services to meet their needs. The primary managerial requirement was for integration and coordination across the service package.

The program or service specialization approach usually began with a defined expertise in a certain area, such as cardiology or rehabilitation medicine, and then a search for markets that needed the service. The primary managerial requirement was to adapt the service to the market.

Less prevalent was the attempt of some hospitals to use their geographic location as a way of carving out a broader niche involving several programs, services, and market segments. In most cases, these hospitals felt that they had strong ethnic or religious ties to the immediate area. They typically had strong cultures emphasizing community involvement and physicians who for the most part lived in the local community and identified strongly with the hospital. These hospitals actively promoted their community identification as a source of differentiation from competitors. This was reflected in the slogan of one hospital: "We have been with you for 100 years. We are with you now. We will be with your grandchildren 100 years from now. Continuity counts. We understand your needs."

Maximizing Learning. While learning is important for any organization, regardless of its strategic orientation, it is particularly important for analyzers trying to decide whether to enter new markets and when. Analyzer hospitals were generally the second or third to enter the market, typically keying off the experience of prospectors as well as some analyzers' own "trial balloon" initiatives. Learning was important for analyzers not only for developing new services and new markets but also for knowing when and how to eliminate services.

We found it important to distinguish between single-loop learning and double-loop learning (Argyris and Schön, 1978), or what others have called first-order learning and second-order learning (Fiol and Lyles, 1985). Single-loop learning involves knowing about the cause and effect relationships associated with a particular decision or event. Double-loop learning involves a fundamental questioning of the underlying assumptions on which the decision or events are based. The decision to develop an ambulatory surgery program based on market size, demographics, financial projections, competitor strengths and weaknesses, and the organizational and operational requirements for running such a program is an example of single-loop learning. These decision parameters need to be studied and "known about" before proceeding. Double-loop learning, however, would question the underlying assumptions on which those parameters are based. For example, the assumptions underlying the determination of market size might include estimates of new technological breakthroughs, physician preferences for doing surgery on an inpatient or outpatient basis, consumer preferences for more convenient accessible care, the likelihood of third-party reimbursement for the service, and so on. All these underlying assumptions determine one's views of market size.

Analyzers needed to use both forms of learning, but those who engaged in the double-loop learning appeared to achieve greater success. Single-loop learning primarily occurred through environmental surveillance activities, observing others, and through attempting to streamline internal decision making to facilitate quicker entry. As one vice-president for planning expressed it, "We need to identify the key functions more quickly. We're too slow. We need to execute more quickly." Environmental surveillance activities centered primarily on secondary industry resources, news clippings, and analysis of secondary data on competitors. This system watched a major competitor system develop a PPO network with multiple clinics — a major threat. To counter this, the system quickly developed its own PPO network incorporating both its own hospitals and others in the area. As one system executive described it, "We did it rather hurriedly with the hopes of tying them [the competitor system] up for a while. We were trying to make it more difficult for them, distract them a bit." This response was based on some immediate perceived cause-effect relationships about PPO competition with relatively little questioning of the underlying assumptions involved.

Double-loop learning primarily involved three dimensions: implementation, market research, and board, management, and physician involvement processes. Analyzers scored significantly higher on these dimensions than defenders although generally not as high as prospectors.

Bevan Hospital used the implementation process to question its assumptions about developing a residential care center for the elderly. While initial data indicated significant projected growth in the elderly market, further analysis revealed that the assumption that they would prefer living in a residential center was problematic. Focus group interviews revealed that many owned their homes and preferred living in them while others had strong ties to local church groups that were beginning to develop their own senior citizen living and support networks. This reexamination led to a markedly reduced senior citizen housing program.

Involving board members and key physicians early in the strategic planning process also helped to surface underlying and often unconscious assumptions. For example, Austerly Memorial Hospital believed that a substantial market existed for an occupational medicine program. Several physicians, however, questioned the need for such a program because of the kinds of problems they saw in their offices. This was information that the hospital had been unable to collect in its initial analysis. The hospital was able to persuade the corporate office to conduct some "trial balloon" learning in outside areas. A more carefully focused program was then developed, one that met a market niche and that was supported by the local physicians. As one physician said, "It helps to make your mistakes in someone else's back yard." Another noted that the experience was also useful "in experimenting with pricing strategies" and learning "what we should emphasize in the way of specific program features." The analyzer, like the prospector, needs to switch back and forth between cost leadership and differentiation strategies, so it can determine how best to be the second or third entrant and how long its initial strategy should be maintained.

In addition to the specifics of single- and double-loop learning, successful analyzers appeared to emphasize a culture of learning, usually through role modeling by the CEO and top management team. They engaged in a wider search for solutions to problems, held more retreats with management, medical staff, and board, made greater use of external consultants, and generally had a tougher questioning attitude toward new ideas and proposals without discouraging their development. As one CEO expressed it, "We're always learning. That's what we're about. We don't have much margin for error so we have to learn as fast as we can."

Developing New Skills and Mind Sets. "Without question our number one problem is within our own minds. We need different ways of thinking about our world, and some of our people just aren't there." These comments of one system CEO captured the common need for many hospital executives and board members to change their mental maps from a pre-1983 internally oriented caretaking attitude, to the more externally oriented risk-taking mentality required by the post prospective payment environment. While this need was perceived by all archetypes, it posed special challenges for analyzer hospitals who needed to protect stable inpatient service domains while becoming more aggressive in their outpatient domains.

Board members and executives making the transition faced several barriers: (1) risk taking had not been needed or rewarded in the past, (2) a premium had been placed on avoiding conflict with physicians, and (3) the inherently conservative clinical mentality — not making a mistake and therefore erring on the side of diagnosing someone as ill rather than missing a diagnosis, resulting in a possibly negative outcome — also carried over into managerial decision making. Comments such as "our board moves too slowly," "we don't know how to deal with risk," and "we're still operating in the 1960s" were heard from a number of respondents.

For the investor-owned and, to a lesser extent, the secular not-for-profit systems, risk taking and entrepreneurship were comparable activities; this was not true for the religiously affiliated hospitals. For many of them, risk taking also involved providing more programs and services to the poor with no economic return, which put a heavier burden on other activities intended to subsidize the commitment to the poor.

To promote a more entrepreneurial, risk-taking management mind set, analyzers tried several approaches: management development programs, better linkage of financial planning and strategic planning, better linkage of human resource planning and strategic planning, adoption of incentive compensation practices, development of a marketing orientation, board reorganization and board development, and selective use of outside consultants.

"Our managers are a little slow. We need better managers. We need to be more creative and visionary." Several analyzer hospitals, reflecting these comments, initiated management development programs designed to foster a broadened sense of vision and encourage creativity. Corporate offices delegated more responsibility to individual hospital executives and their staffs. One system CEO said of his subsidiary corporation executives, "These people are presidents, and I want them in every sense of the word to be developing and managing their corporations. I'm very willing and interested in sharing the operational responsibilities with the subsidiary presidents. Part of the future success of this organization will depend much more on what these people do than on what I do" (Guncheon, 1984, p. M84). In this system, the corporate strategic planning staff was intentionally kept small, and deliberate efforts were made to push strategic thinking down to the individual hospital CEOs and their staffs.

A number of analyzer hospitals were handicapped in their implementation efforts by the lack of integration between financial plans and strategic plans. Often strategic and program plans would be developed in relative isolation from the financial planning until the final stages of the process. More than a few analyzer hospitals found themselves at that point with a list of high-priority programs and services and desired new technologies that could not be funded by the available capital. As a result, changes were made in the planning process to link financial and program planning from the beginning, providing a framework for developing priorities and addressing problematic tradeoffs throughout the process.

While all orientations require a close linkage between human resource planning and strategic planning, analyzers found such linkages particularly challenging. Many of their human resource plans, ranging from wage and salary administration to performance appraisal, were not strategically driven. This was particularly true with the lack of management succession planning at almost all levels of the organization. Most analyzers recognized the importance of this linkage and took steps to bring it about. This included the redesign of performance appraisal systems to reflect the hospital's strategic priorities and the development of "skill banks" by position level needed to support the strategic priorities.

In the process of linking their human resource plans to their strategic plans, many analyzers also initiated incentive compensation arrangements to reward risk-taking behavior. At Altamore Hospital, for example, 40 percent of individuals' pay was based on the achievement of group goals, 30 percent on the achievement of system goals, and 30 percent on the achievement of individual goals. At Bonner Hospital, executives received 10 percent of the profits of new ventures. At many of the investor-owned hospitals, rewards included stock ownership to help ensure the long-run growth of the firm.

"Some of our CEOs are marketing virgins." These words of one system staff member aptly described the need for greater marketing sophistication on the part of many analyzer hospital CEOs. Marketing skills and tools were less important than inculcating a market mentality throughout the organization. Some hospitals put their executives through marketing training programs, including visits to such market-oriented organizations as Procter & Gamble.

Most important was getting across the need to recognize multiple customers, to define market segments, to study how these segments perceived their needs (as opposed to what the hospital thought their needs were), and then to design program packages that best met these needs. Corporate offices and individual hospitals engaged in a great deal of experimentation on how best to structure the marketing function. This ranged from centralizing most marketing activities at corporate office to decentralizing most functions at the individual hospital level. As of 1988, most analyzer hospitals had arrived at intermediate relationships, whereby advertising and marketing research support was provided by corporate or regional office while local hospitals were assigned primary responsibility for identifying their own market opportunities and deciding how best to address them.

To make decisions more quickly, analyzers saw the need to streamline their corporate and hospital boards as well as to establish subsidiary boards to launch new ventures. In the process, some made hospital boards advisory only rather than policymaking. Almost all invested heavily in board development.

Many corporate and even individual hospital boards had grown to between twenty-five and fifty members in the early 1980s, resulting in unwieldy and cumbersome decision making. Many analyzers reacted by trimming their boards to ten

to fifteen members. Small subsidiary boards of five to seven people (including several managers) were established to help support some of the new entrepreneurial activities. In all cases,
members were chosen carefully to fit the strategic needs of each
subsidiary. The more visionary and broad-gauged thinkers were
placed on the corporate board. The more entrepreneurial minded
were placed on some of the new-venture subsidiary boards. At
the same time, some of the not-for-profit systems made the
difficult transition to "downgrading" their individual hospital
boards from policymaking status to advisory only, a policy that
has existed for years among the investor-owned hospitals. This
gave the corporate office greater control over the overall strategic direction of the system and helped to facilitate the development of strategic roles for each hospital within the system.

In regard to board development, one system started a
trustee development fund, giving each trustee $1,000 for con-
ferences and books. Most formed board orientation programs
and had requirements for continuing education. Some developed
mentoring programs, where an experienced board member
served as an adviser to a new member. Most also developed
formal criteria for evaluating individual performance as well as
overall board performance. All these initiatives emphasized the
hospital's ability to compete successfully, and the board's role
in helping the hospital achieve sustainable competitive advantages on both cost and quality criteria.

Finally, many analyzer hospitals made effective use of outside consultants to facilitate a more aggressive, risk-taking mentality. These ranged from facilitating board, management, and
medical staff retreats, to developing strategic plans, to orches-
trating major multiyear programs involving fundamental cultural change.

Analyzer hospitals were beginning to realize the fruits of
these efforts. For example, one system was able to close down
a money-losing hospital it had been carrying for years and
reallocate the resources to other areas of strategic importance.
A religiously affiliated system recognized the need to seriously
consider divesting a hospital in a community that it had served
for more than fifty years. A third system recognized the need

to continuously examine new opportunities not only by watching others but by initiating some pilot programs of its own. And perhaps most important, a growing number of analyzer executives came to the realization that, in the words of one, "strategic doing is more important than strategic planning." Nonetheless, analyzers, like everyone else, were still left facing the physician factor.

The Physician Factor. "On the one hand, the hospital is telling us that we need to cut back on costs, and on the other hand, we see them developing all these new programs." A major problem faced by analyzers was sending such mixed messages to their physicians, reflecting the analyzer's dual orientation. In some cases, hospital efforts were stymied because of physician opposition to such diversification opportunities as the development of urgent care centers, outpatient diagnostic centers, and primary care group practices. In other cases, local hospital efforts to initiate activities with their physicians were complicated by corporate office objectives that ran counter to local interests. For example, one hospital's successful hospital-sponsored HMO was "taken over" by the corporate system with the intent of diffusing the model to other hospitals in the system. Local hospital executives and physicians, however, saw it as disruptive; the decision placed considerable strain on what had been a strong, trusting relationship between the hospital and its physicians. In other cases, some physicians felt the hospital moved too slowly in implementing new programs and services. A perceived lack of followthrough threatened management's credibility with medical staff members. All these situations reflect the complexity inherent in the analyzer strategy.

By far the most successful tactic used to deal with these challenges was involving physicians early on in the decision-making process, particularly in strategic planning. Many physician complaints were not with the outcome of the decision per se but with what they considered inadequate input. To remedy this situation, one East Coast hospital began formulating its diversification strategy by surveying medical staff members about the hospital strengths and weaknesses, the need for new programs, and the physicians' own practice plans. From this survey, the hospital identified three areas for possible new-program development: an outpatient magnetic resonance imaging center, an outpatient cardiac rehab program, and a home health care agency. Since each program also had its detractors, a joint hospital-physician committee was appointed to explore the pros and cons of each activity. After much study and discussion, system leaders decided to pursue the magnetic resonance imaging scanner as a fifty-fifty economic joint venture between the hospital and physicians. They allowed all active staff members to invest in the venture rather than limiting it to those who would directly benefit. Cardiac rehab plans were temporarily shelved pending recruitment of an additional cardiologist. An agreement for joint ownership of a home health care agency with a neighboring hospital was approved by physicians with the understanding that they were not required to refer patients to the agency. Referrals would depend on the quality of services provided by the agency. The hospital appointed two physicians to the home health care agency board.

In a second situation, a West Coast hospital and its physicians decided to form a joint venture corporation *before* considering any specific diversification opportunities. Both parties were at economic risk and had equal involvement in governance and management (five hospital staff and five physicians served on the board, with a physician executive selected to manage the corporation). Criteria were developed for evaluating specific proposals consistent with the new corporation's mission. Among these criteria were the extent to which specialists would benefit through increased referrals from programs designed to increase primary care physicians' practice and the extent to which primary care physicians would benefit through increased institutional prestige from programs designed to enhance specialists' capabilities. After four years the corporation has developed a successful preferred provider organization with several outpatient diagnostic centers, one ambulatory surgery center, and a successful practice management program.

While these represent success stories, greater involvement of physicians in the strategic planning process was not without risk. Many physicians were ill equipped to participate, because their focus reflected narrow clinical interests rather than a broad view of the multiple forces affecting the institution. Others found it difficult to rise above their own personal interests in searching for the common good. In a few cases, executives felt constrained in sharing information with the strategic planning committee for fear that the physicians on the committee might leak it to neighboring competitor hospitals where they also practiced. In at least one case, the administration feared that the physician himself would steal the idea and develop the service in his multispecialty clinic. In most cases, however, these kinds of problems were overcome by judicious selection of physicians who had a primary loyalty to the hospital, were known for their broader view of health care issues, and also enjoyed the respect and credibility of their peers. In a number of larger hospitals, these relationships were also facilitated by paid medical directors or executive vice-presidents for medical affairs.

While corporate offices sometimes complicated individual hospital relationships with their medical staffs, in many cases they played a positive role by raising the visibility of the issues throughout the system. For example, three systems with a high percentage of analyzer hospitals established corporatewide medical affairs offices or divisions headed by physician executives. These offices generally had four major purposes: (1) to develop programs to better link physicians to their individual hospitals and to the system overall; (2) to develop, coordinate, and oversee opportunities for hospital-physician joint ventures and related alternative delivery system initiatives; (3) to develop and oversee systemwide quality assurance efforts; and (4) to ensure an increased physician role in management and governance throughout the system. The overall thrust was best captured in the words of one physician executive: "Our philosophy is to involve the doctors and let them come up with some of the ideas for systemwide application."

Guidelines for Managing the Analyzer

Based on these insights and lessons, we suggest the following guidelines for successfully managing an analyzer.

- Analyzers must be expert at managing complexity. If they are not, a more consistent prospector or defender strategy may be appropriate.
- To manage complexity, flexibility must be designed into the strategic planning and management control process. Disciplined systems are needed to control costs, and some degree of autonomy is required to stimulate creativity and innovation.
- Emphasis must be given to the cost effectiveness of programs, balancing cost containment on the one hand with effectiveness on the other hand.
- Particular emphasis should be given to creating synergies between the prospector and defender domains. This can be accomplished by emphasizing "two-for-one" solutions and developing market niches.
- The analyzer strategy places a premium on organizational learning, particularly learning that derives from questioning underlying assumptions. It is important to learn to divest as well as to create.
- Promoting a marketing mentality, developing marketing skills, and strengthening information systems are needed to promote organizational learning.
- Continuing investments in board and management development programs are needed to develop the mind sets and skills required to execute an analyzer strategy.
- Close linkages between financial planning and strategic planning, human resources planning and strategic planning, and incentive compensation and strategic plans are required to help execute an analyzer strategy.
- Consideration may need to be given to board and organizational restructuring at both system and individual hospital levels, to facilitate synergies between the prospector and defender domains of the analyzer strategy.
- The danger of sending mixed messages to clinical professionals must be mitigated by involving them in strategic planning early on.
- Consideration should be given to organizational designs that facilitate professionals' involvement throughout the corporation. A complex strategic orientation requires more complex organizational arrangements.

9

Managing the
Reactor Orientation

"We can't continue trying to be all things to all people."

The Reactor: Two Mini-Cases

Walden Memorial was the jewel in the crown of its hospital system. Financially successful for many years, the hospital had a high-quality medical staff and was generally regarded as one of the leading hospitals in its largely suburban metropolitan area. It was, however, the highest-cost hospital in its market. The hospital recognized the need to develop a stronger financial management focus and a stronger management information system. It also had some difficulty differentiating itself as the leader in technical quality of care because of the presence of a nearby university teaching hospital and other high technology–oriented competitors. In sum, it lacked a clear strategic orientation to the market.

The hospital responded to the cost-containment pressures represented by prospective payment by initiating a flurry of new programs, from ambulatory surgery to satellite clinics to home health care to health promotion. Individually each of the programs was reasonably well planned, but little attention was given to their relationship to one another or to inpatient services. As a result, the ambulatory surgery center caused conflict among the surgical staff over which clinical procedures should be performed there rather than in the hospital and who should be permitted to operate at both sites. This conflict, in turn, spilled over into other areas, causing wider physician concerns about the hospital's intentions.

While these efforts were being launched, the hospital also attempted to control its costs by consolidating selected inpatient services and making staff reductions. This was viewed by many as a deemphasis on inpatient care, which historically had been the hospital's strength. Many saw the hospital's strategy as one of diverting resources from inpatient care to a highly uncertain and unproved array of outpatient services. One observer described the hospital's reaction to the new environment as like "an outbreak of measles." In an attempt to gain greater control over its future, the hospital was mending fences with key physician leaders by developing mutual decision-making forums.

Baker General offers a second example of indecisiveness that affected its relationship with physicians. A member of an investor-owned system, Baker was caught by the short-run emphasis on profits, to the relative neglect of longer-run considerations. As a result, it often prematurely dropped programs and services that did not immediately generate profits.

Baker was fortunate in being located in a growing market, which enabled it to develop a number of new programs and services. But, like Walden's, these efforts were, in the words of Baker's CEO, "far-flung and not well related to each other." He felt that this was as much a reason for "pulling the plug" on these services as their lack of short-run profitability.

Baker's lack of clear strategic focus was also influenced by the system's strategic planning process. Within the system, there was very little linkage between individual hospital plans and corporate office plans. Furthermore, programmatic or service-based planning was done by a different group, not those involved in market planning. The net result was that Baker received little guidance or direction from corporate office, and the advice that was sent was often contradictory.

Baker's problem was compounded by the fact that it was one of several system hospitals in a rather large geographic market. Baker would sometimes wait before initiating a new service, based on the rationale that the service probably would be better offered by one of the other system hospitals in the area. When this did not occur, Baker's entry into the market was often too late. In the words of one system assistant planner, "We don't tend to look at things as a whole. We do a lot of brainstorming but there isn't much monitoring of the plans." The situation reached its most critical point where the system started a number of ambulatory surgery centers that competed with ambulatory surgery centers developed by its own hospitals.

The system recognized the problems it was creating for Baker and its other hospitals, and moved to develop a more integrated strategic planning process built around hospitals in selected markets of importance. It divested its ambulatory surgery centers and several other related businesses to focus again on acute care hospitals, hoping in the process to help provide them with a clearer strategic focus.

The Reactor's Performance

Of all the archetypes, we know the least about reactors. They are commonly treated as a residual category lacking a consistent strategic orientation, and are generally thought to be less successful.

As Figures 9.1 and 9.2 show, however, reactor hospitals in the present study perform reasonably well, clearly better than defenders. Figure 9.1 suggests they are somewhat less likely to provide uncompensated care and charity care but do spend more on quality assurance activities than the sample average. This is consistent with Chapter Five's finding that reactors give high emphasis to trying to differentiate their services based on technical quality of care. This is, in part, reflected by the fact that they have slightly fewer Joint Commission contingencies than the sample average.

Figure 9.2 indicates that they perform above the sample average on most measures of financial performance, particularly in operating margin as a percentage of net revenue. These find-

Figure 9.1. Reactor's Performance Profile — "Doing Good."

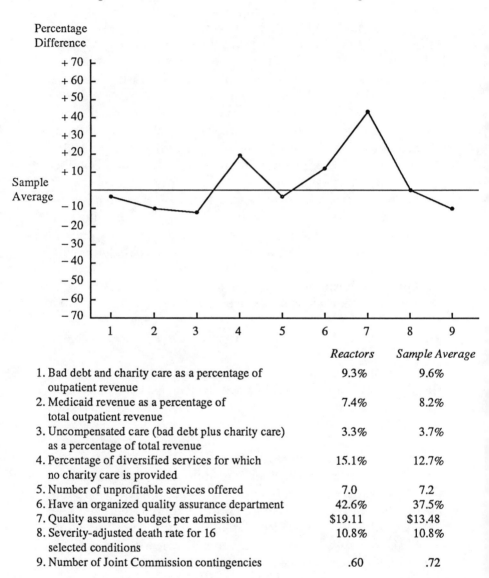

	Reactors	Sample Average
1. Bad debt and charity care as a percentage of outpatient revenue	9.3%	9.6%
2. Medicaid revenue as a percentage of total outpatient revenue	7.4%	8.2%
3. Uncompensated care (bad debt plus charity care) as a percentage of total revenue	3.3%	3.7%
4. Percentage of diversified services for which no charity care is provided	15.1%	12.7%
5. Number of unprofitable services offered	7.0	7.2
6. Have an organized quality assurance department	42.6%	37.5%
7. Quality assurance budget per admission	$19.11	$13.48
8. Severity-adjusted death rate for 16 selected conditions	10.8%	10.8%
9. Number of Joint Commission contingencies	.60	.72

Figure 9.2. Reactor's Performance Profile — "Doing Well."

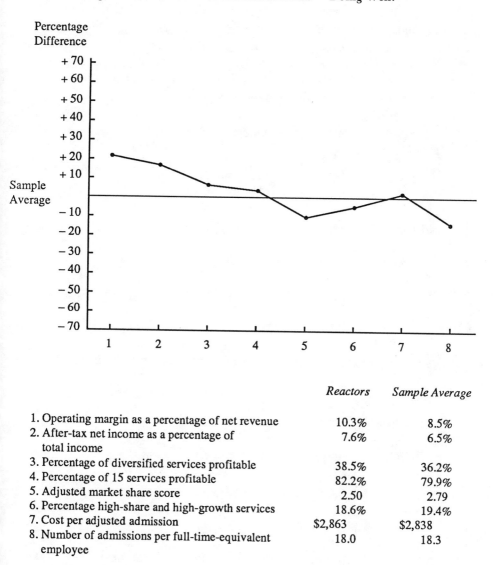

	Reactors	Sample Average
1. Operating margin as a percentage of net revenue	10.3%	8.5%
2. After-tax net income as a percentage of total income	7.6%	6.5%
3. Percentage of diversified services profitable	38.5%	36.2%
4. Percentage of 15 services profitable	82.2%	79.9%
5. Adjusted market share score	2.50	2.79
6. Percentage high-share and high-growth services	18.6%	19.4%
7. Cost per adjusted admission	$2,863	$2,838
8. Number of admissions per full-time-equivalent employee	18.0	18.3

ings are consistent with those of Snow and Hrebiniak (1980), who found that reactors in the air transportation industry outperformed prospectors and defenders. That industry, like health care, is undergoing rapid and radical change. It may be that in such industries, a reactor strategy is not dysfunctional, at least not initially. A reactor strategy may result in better outcomes than a poorly executed defender strategy.

Figure 9.3 indicates that, for the most part, reactors' strategic planning and control systems are perceived to be of similar

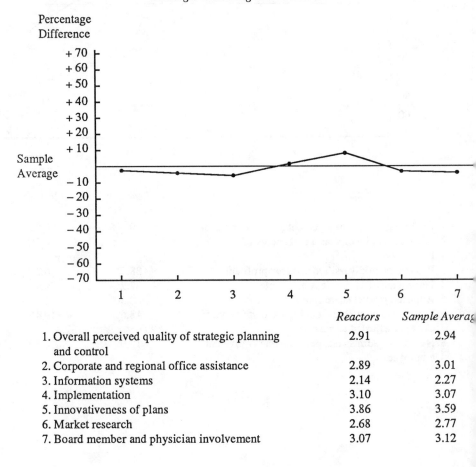

Figure 9.3. Reactor's Perceived Quality of
Strategic Planning and Control.

	Reactors	Sample Averag
1. Overall perceived quality of strategic planning and control	2.91	2.94
2. Corporate and regional office assistance	2.89	3.01
3. Information systems	2.14	2.27
4. Implementation	3.10	3.07
5. Innovativeness of plans	3.86	3.59
6. Market research	2.68	2.77
7. Board member and physician involvement	3.07	3.12

quality as the overall sample average. The major exception is that the reactors' plans, like the prospectors', are perceived to be more innovative than those of analyzers or defenders. However, reactors had a less disciplined strategic planning and control process. Their need for greater discipline and the underlying leadership implied are two of the principal issues in this chapter.

The Reactor's Challenge

On the surface the major problem facing the reactor is the need for stability. The reactor needs to stick with a set of plans long enough to accumulate experience, to see what works.

The major underlying source of instability is the lack of consistent leadership. Keep in mind, however, that while stability and consistent leadership represent major challenges facing the reactors, overall they did very well on most performance indicators and particularly well on selected financial viability measures. A major issue, however, is the extent to which reactors can sustain such performance over the long run. Reactors also shared some of the managerial requirements of the other three archetypes. Like prospectors, reactors needed to understand the difference between related, unrelated, and partially related diversification. Many reactors' diversification strategies were unfocused. Also like prospectors, reactors needed to understand the need for constant differentiation of services. But unlike most prospectors, most reactors did not stick with a given service long enough to enable a differentiation strategy to succeed.

Like defenders, reactors needed to manage their costs carefully. But their cost-containment strategies were generally ad hoc and piecemeal and were not strategically driven. Also like defenders, reactors required more centralized and disciplined strategic planning and control.

Like analyzers, reactors needed to emphasize learning from their mistakes and were particularly handicapped in this regard by relatively poor management information systems. As a result, many reactors behaved like "unstable analyzers." Finally, like all the others, reactors needed to develop effective working relationships with their physicians. Reactors, more than the other three groups, had the most strained physician relationships.

In sum, while not unique, the primary managerial requirements of the reactors' strategy were:

1. To develop consistent leadership.
2. To develop more focused diversification strategies that recognized the various forms of relatedness.
3. To stick with a service long enough to reap the benefits of differentiation.
4. To develop strategically driven cost-containment strategies.
5. To develop more centralized and disciplined strategic planning and control processes.
6. To improve the process of learning from their mistakes.
7. To develop more positive and productive physician relationships.

Consistent Leadership. The reactors' lack of consistent leadership was not primarily the result of executive turnover. Reactor hospital CEOs had been in their positions as long as analyzer CEOs and longer than defender CEOs, although not quite as long as prospector CEOs. Reactor CEOs had also been with their systems approximately as long as prospector and analyzer CEOs and longer than defender CEOs. Rather, the leadership problems centered around the inability to articulate a consistent vision or mission for the institution, without which it was difficult to develop a coherent strategy.

Reactor hospitals often found themselves faced with too many choices. Some large reactor hospitals with slack resources aspired to becoming tertiary care medical centers. Others wished to remain more community focused, but at the same time were faced with regulatory and cost-containment pressures that forced them to consider service alternatives that they knew little about. Many faced what one reactor CEO termed "an institutional identity crisis."

Eastwood Hospital represented one example of a reactor hospital trying to develop a more consistent strategy. In the words of one management team member, "Our management in the past was too reactive." The hospital hired an outside consultant to help develop a strategic planning process. The process began with a retreat for board, management, and medical staff designed to identify the core values of the organization and translate them into a mission statement. They perceived the need to thoroughly analyze their competitors and identify some centers of excellence for themselves.

Westview Memorial Hospital found itself struggling to develop a more proactive diversification strategy. In the words of its chief planner, "Our strategic directions are too present oriented. They aren't particularly creative." With outside assistance, the hospital engaged in several brainstorming sessions among its top management team and began to build scenarios of alternative futures. The CEO also recognized the need for stronger middle managers and a new incentive program to encourage innovation.

Gateway Hospital was the classic reactor, having shifted in and out of several services over the years. "Something's always happening, which in a way is good. But we're not sure what it's adding up to," commented one manager. One example of the hospital's indecisiveness and frustration was captured in the words of another staff member: "Do we want to be in the psychiatric business or don't we? Do we want to get ——— or do we want to be respected in the morning?" Gateway had not yet developed a clear conception of itself, its strengths and weaknesses, its competitors, or the marketplace.

Hortonville Memorial thought that part of its problem was lack of direction from the system corporate office. It felt the system did not know which way it wanted to go. Hortonville did not understand its strategic role in the system's overall plan. In the words of one CEO, "We can't move as fast as we should. We're not on top of the health care environment as much as other systems. One of our biggest problems is the deadwood in corporate office."

Given the dramatic changes occurring in the health care environment, the need for clear, consistent leadership was particularly pronounced. Many reactor hospitals had been reasonably successful in the past and did relatively well in the mid-

1980s. But more than the other archetypes, they appeared to be suffering from indecisiveness and lack of overall direction. This was also reflected in their new-service development and cost-containment approaches.

Unfocused Diversification. "We can't continue trying to be all things to all people." This comment of one hospital planner aptly expresses the problem that many reactors had with their diversification strategies. For many, the attempts to diversify were not part of a *conscious* strategy but merely random attempts to increase revenues. Sometimes reactor hospitals were the first to initiate a particular service, and sometimes they represented a response to what others had done. When they were first, they were seldom able to take advantage of being "first mover" (unlike many prospectors) because they did not fully understand the market or the need to follow up the initial advantage with ongoing support and service differentiation. When they were the second or third entrant, their response was typically "knee jerk" rather than a considered, deliberate approach more characteristic of the analyzer.

Some of the problems reactors faced with their diversification efforts grew out of attempts to develop joint ventures with their physicians. Reactors saw such joint ventures as opportunities to increase their revenue base and to decrease their reliance on acute inpatient care, which was being increasingly squeezed by the prospective payment system and other third-party payors. The major problem was that many reactors developed physician joint ventures on a one-by-one "first-come, first-served" basis. There was little or no attempt to fit them into an overall strategic plan or even to create linkages among the joint ventures themselves.

This approach is illustrated by Carswell Medical Center. Operating in a heavily populated state, Carswell saw the need to get as many services as possible on an outpatient basis and was open to discussing possibilities with selected physicians. It was first approached by a group of surgeons interested in obtaining capital for an ambulatory surgery center, then, several months later, by two internists interested in opening a high-tech outpatient diagnostic center. Shortly thereafter, the hospital was approached by its lab director about developing a free-standing outpatient laboratory. Decisions were made to go ahead with the first two projects but not the third. Different criteria were used in each case, and the hospital was viewed by most medical staff members as simply being "opportunistic." The lab director, in particular, was upset by the negative response to his proposal, accusing the hospital of double dealing with the outpatient diagnostic center physicians, who subsequently established fairly extensive laboratory services in their center. After two years, the joint ventures were below their financial projections and had contributed to considerable conflict with the hospital's medical staff. As one administrative staff member commented, "We were simply reacting to isolated physician requests. We did everything totally wrong."

Contrasting examples were provided by some prospector hospitals that first established the role that joint ventures would play in the overall strategic plan. As discussed in Chapter Six, this involved an assessment of how much diversification was to be pursued, the extent to which the new efforts would be related to the organization's current experience and expertise, and examination of the best ways to approach the new service or new market development, including whether a joint venture strategy was the best way to go. If joint ventures were seen as compatible with the hospital's strategic objectives, a group of hospital and physician representatives established criteria for reviewing each proposal. As in the case of the West Coast analyzer hospital described in Chapter Eight, this sometimes involved establishing a hospital-physician joint venture corporation with equal representation of the hospital and physicians. The criteria that one such hospital developed included the following:

1. Analysis of the amount of capital required, recognizing that many joint ventures are seriously undercapitalized.
2. Specific criteria for return on investment.
3. Specification of the risk-reward relationship on the part of both physicians and the hospital.
4. Detailed examination of short-run and long-run reimbursement considerations.

5. Overall analysis of the ability to sustain the service in the long run.
6. A realistic assessment of management capability and time required by the new service, including assignment of managers who understand physicians and physician practice, development of a strong management information system capability, and development of market research and promotion capability.
7. Specification of clear roles and expectations regarding reporting and accountability.
8. Resolution of the exclusivity issue: what physicians can invest in the venture even if they are not directly a part of the venture itself.
9. Accurate assessment of the regulatory environment and how it might affect the new venture.
10. Organizational structure for the joint venture.
11. Specification of the quality assurance system and the perception of quality in the mind of key stakeholders.

As we will discuss later, the unfocused and disjointed nature of physician joint-venture strategies also became a major source of hospital–medical staff conflict for reactors.

Sticking with a Service. Some reactors deleted a new service shortly after it was started. One hospital started a home health agency only to withdraw from it eight months after starting operations; a second hospital got out of the urgent care center business a year and a half after startup; and a third hospital dropped out of joint venture sponsorship of an HMO after one year. In some cases, these were attempts to cut losses early because the initiatives had been poorly planned, reflecting the reactors' tendency to jump on the bandwagon. In other cases, however, the decision appeared to represent poor judgment, pulling the plug too soon on new ventures that were promising but required more time to demonstrate their profitability or positive synergy with other services. Losing ventures can often be identified within two years, but it may take five years or more to determine the winners. Reactors had problems living with the uncertainty and ambiguity associated with the intervening years.

As a result, some reactor hospitals never had an opportunity to continue to differentiate their services (unlike their prospector counterparts) to capture greater market share. In some cases they also failed to capture learning-curve advantages, largely because the new services were not part of a coherent overall strategic plan. Top management had few checkpoints against which to measure progress or to determine the services' contribution to overall hospital goals and objectives.

To those inside the organization, the apparent inability to stick with a service resulted in a "two steps forward, one step back" management approach, with all its associated frustrations. To the external world and particularly to competitors, it reflected a degree of unpredictability, which ironically gave some reactors a short-run advantage. As the CEO of a competing hospital noted, "You never know what they [the reactor hospital] are going to do, which is upsetting but, on the other hand, they never seem to stick with anything long enough to make a go of it."

Haphazard Cost Containment. Many reactor hospitals' attempts to cut costs were poorly planned and, once again, were not generally part of a coherent strategy. For example, Nartan Memorial Hospital made 20 percent across-the-board cuts in personnel (including nursing), paying little attention to which services were more or less profitable and more or less needed by the community. Administration incurred the wrath of both the medical and nursing staffs, and some of the cuts were eventually restored.

In the case of Pangor Hospital Corporation, management decided to downsize its marketing and planning staff on the assumption that these cuts would be less noticed by physicians and nurses or viewed as symbolic. But, at the same time, the hospital was trying to diversify into a number of new outpatient programs that were greatly dependent on planning and marketing staff skills. The cuts seriously undermined these efforts. The administrative "fat" was not in the planning and marketing areas but in the management of inpatient services, where opportunities existed to consolidate programs and reduce administrative staff without making reductions in direct patient care personnel.

In a third case, Rinaldo Medical Center waited far too long before making any staff reductions. Rinaldo operated in a highly regulated state and a fairly competitive market, so incentives to manage costs existed even before the prospective payment program was introduced. Most hospitals in the area had undertaken severe cost-cutting initiatives, ranging from program consolidation to staff deletions. Rinaldo, however, had done well financially over the years and had accumulated a surplus of funds, and so did not immediately feel the pressures. At the same time, new management had introduced a consensus-style decision-making process greatly favored by physicians. As competitive pressures grew, however, and in particular the hospital's percentage of Medicare and Medicaid patients increased, Rinaldo found itself with its first operating loss in history. Only then, nearly two years after competing hospitals, did Rinaldo initiate cost-cutting programs.

Need for Disciplined Planning and Control. Like the defender, many reactors lacked a disciplined, systematic strategic planning and control process. One system that included a moderate number of reactor hospitals had a planning system that had been in a state of flux for several years. One year, the planning process would be highly decentralized; the following year, it would be centralized. Reporting formats and data requests varied from year to year. One corporate planning staff summarized, "We are moving too fast. Too much, too fast. We are spread too thin. Our roles and responsibilities aren't clear." The system was not without overall direction, as the system CEO was described as a person with "tremendous vision." But the vision could not be translated down to the hospital level because of the inconsistent strategic planning process.

In many cases, reactor strategies seemed to emerge as a reaction to the market rather than as a planned effort to influence the market. As one executive noted, "There isn't much staff analysis of strategies." While emerging strategies (see Mintzberg, 1978) are not inherently dysfunctional, they are less likely to be successful if the organization does not have an overall game plan or context in which to recognize their potential.

Reactors were particularly handicapped by the lack of integration between their programmatic plans and their financial plans. Programs would be developed that included their own financial projections and requirements but did not consider the financial requirements and projections of some other programs. In the case of Kemper Union Hospital, a number of new programs requiring considerable capital were developed before it was recognized that the hospital lacked the capital to fund them. After-the-fact attempts to prioritize created dissension and conflict between management and medical staff, resulting in lost time responding to market opportunities.

Most reactors came to the realization that if they wanted to remain competitive they needed to upgrade their strategic planning process. For one system, this meant providing better overall strategic direction and guidelines within which individual hospitals were charged with developing their own plan in consultation with corporate staff. They also developed more standardized reporting formats while at the same time involving individual hospital CEOs in corporate planning discussions.

Learning from Mistakes. Lacking a disciplined strategic planning process, and unable to stick with services long enough, reactors had particular problems capturing the learning available from their mistakes. This was a key difference between reactors and prospectors and analyzers. Having initiated many programs without sufficient analysis meant that there was no framework or data base within which to interpret results. Deleting services too quickly meant the learning experience was truncated. In addition, many reactors failed to engage in much analysis of why programs did not appear to work. They no sooner dropped one initiative than they started another. In brief, they were indeed moving too fast.

An underlying reason for the reactors' inability to learn from their mistakes was the poor quality of their clinical and management information systems. While nearly all hospitals faced the challenge of upgrading these systems, the problem was particularly acute for reactors, and they seemed to be less far along in the process. As a result, they often did not know how well or how poorly a program was doing, which explains why the plug was pulled on some programs that were in reality doing relatively well. The lack of a good information base also hindered planning activities in developing new programs. At Kemper Union Hospital, the home health care program was started without sufficient information on the demographics and family support systems available in the area. Demand failed to meet expectations. The hospital was fortunate in being able to merge the program with a larger, areawide agency providing services to the elderly.

From a system perspective, the lack of good information systems made it more difficult to transfer learning from one hospital to another. This resulted in missed opportunities and a loss of one of the principal advantages of hospital systems: the ability to capture the benefits of experimentation and diffuse successful programs to other sites.

The Physician Factor. More than any other strategic archetype, reactor hospitals had difficulties working with their physicians. There were three main reasons for this: (1) the heavily regulated external environment placed additional strains on the hospital-physician relationships; (2) the unpredictable and rash strategic moves made by reactors; and (3) insufficient physician involvement in management of the institution.

In addition to the prospective payment pressures, many reactor hospitals existed in states with stringent rate-review requirements and certificate-of-need laws. These programs often put the hospitals in the middle, playing the "bad guy" in implementing the regulations. This usually meant having to cajole, persuade, and otherwise influence medical staff members to discharge patients sooner and to use fewer and less costly tests, exams, and other treatment inputs.

In areas where HMO competition was also dominant, physicians themselves were beginning to feel the economic crunch. A natural outlet for their frustration was blaming the hospital. At the same time, hospitals often added fuel to the fire by opening up ambulatory surgery centers and ambulatory care centers, which some physicians saw as openly competing with their practices.

Reactors often added to these problems by what one physician described as "rash moves"—developing programs and services and then dropping them for no reason that medical staff members could see. The inability to send a clear signal eroded physicians' trust in the institution and its management. Physicians saw the hospital as "opportunistic," "drifting," and "incompetent." Some physicians actively worked to sabotage hospital initiatives. In one hospital's new HMO, physicians changed their referral patterns so that those physicians that signed up with the HMO received no patients.

Further contributing to the reactors' problems was the relative lack of appropriate involvement of physicians in the management and governance of the institution. While reactor CEOs were no more or less likely to report appropriate involvement of physicians than prospectors or analyzers, interview data suggested that physicians themselves were less satisfied with their involvement, particularly in the important decisions facing the institution.

Halston Community Hospital illustrates the problem. Halston operates in a state with a stringent process of rate review and certificate of need. As a result, the hospital has been quite forceful in implementing a strong utilization review program. The hospital had also angered its physicians by starting two ambulatory care centers, which were perceived as a threat by some primary care physicians. The hospital claimed it had made "first offers" to staff physicians but had been turned down. Only then did the hospital help recruit other physicians. The physicians, however, felt that the offers were made only to "a select few."

The hospital believed it was making progress in promoting greater involvement in decision making. For example, two physicians were voting board members (out of fifteen) in addition to the president and vice-president of the medical staff, who served as nonvoting members. Three physicians were members of the hospital's newly formed strategic planning committee. The hospital had also lengthened the terms of office for the president of the staff to two years to provide greater continuity. From the physicians' perspective, however, these changes were primarily cosmetic. They felt hospital board meetings were still dominated by administration. Ideas for new programs and strategic directions appeared to be well developed before they even reached the strategic planning committee. In brief, medical staff members did not feel that they were involved early enough in planning and decision making or that their views were really heard. A "we versus they" culture continued to persist.

The ongoing conflict was coming to a head over the hospital's interest in hiring a full-time medical director who would serve as liaison between administration and medical staff. The staff actively resisted the idea on the grounds that the medical director would be "captured" by administration and would not properly reflect medical staff interests. Nonetheless, the staff recognized that its own leadership structure was insufficient to deal with the new challenges. The hospital continued to be mired in indecisiveness.

A contrasting example was presented by Morietto Hospital, which faced many of the same issues as Halston — a regulated state with previous hospital-physician competition over services, lack of clear strategic focus, and a perceived lack of relevant physician involvement. Morietto responded to the challenges by establishing a separate ten-member steering committee made up of five physicians, three hospital executives, and two board members. The goal of the committee was to identify areas of overlap in which both hospital and physician interests could be represented. At the time the study was completed, Morietto was moving closer to an analyzer orientation, developing a few focused outpatient programs that most physicians could support while continuing to maintain a strong inpatient identity.

Guidelines for Managing the Reactor

Because reactors are viewed as not having a coherent strategy, it may seem incongruous to suggest guidelines for managing the reactor. However, as the present data and other findings show (for example, Snow and Hrebiniak, 1980), being a reactor is not automatically associated with poor performance, particularly in volatile environments. Also, a reactor orientation may be a transitory strategic state for some organizations in their search for a more consistent, coherent strategy. Defenders in their attempt to become analyzers or prospectors may first behave more like reactors. Suggestions for managing the reactor, either for short-run success in a turbulent environment or to facilitate transition to a more coherent strategic orientation, seem relevant. Based on the present experience we offer the following suggestions.

- Successful reactors require some degree of slack resources and a forgiving market.
- Leadership must articulate a clear strategic vision that provides direction for specific service developments and must be willing to stick with new services beyond their initial stage of implementation.
- Greater efforts must be made to integrate new services with each other, whether they are developed independently or through joint ventures.
- Cost-containment efforts must not be ad hoc or piecemeal but must be part of a concerned effort that supports the strategic direction.
- In multidivisional organizations, reactors need a more disciplined strategic planning and control process to provide guidance and direction to individual divisions. Division plans need to be integrated with corporate plans, and financial plans need to be integrated with programmatic plans.
- Stronger management information systems must be developed to facilitate learning from false starts and to help transfer learning from one division to another.
- Partnerships with professionals must be developed to overcome "we versus they" relationships. To do this, it is necessary to involve professionals thoroughly in the planning and decision-making process. Professionals must have a substantively important role and their legitimate interests and aspirations must be recognized.
- To develop stronger partnerships with professionals, new structures may be needed (task forces, parallel organizations, and so forth). Current structures and decision-making bodies may be inefficient or may carry too much negative "excess baggage" to be useful.
- A reactor may be a useful, short-run strategic orientation but is unlikely to help the organization achieve a long-run sustainable competitive advantage or identity.

These guidelines can be used to help guide the reactor to a more coherent strategic orientation over time.

Part Three

Ensuring Hospital Success: Lessons and Future Directions

10

Sustaining
a Competitive Advantage

The previous four chapters provided a behind-the-scenes look at what it means to manage a prospector, analyzer, defender, and reactor in a rapidly changing industry. In this and the next chapter, we take a few steps back to consider some of the more generic lessons learned and their implications for the future.

We believe the key to success lies in sustaining a competitive advantage over time. This is as true for health care organizations as it is for firms in other industries. There are many different approaches for attempting to sustain a competitive advantage, but the common denominator is the ability to add greater value for the customer than competitors. Chapters Ten and Eleven are essentially concerned with how to add value through managing strategic choices.

Lessons for All Strategies

As we examined the experiences of the four strategic archetypes, it became apparent that some of the lessons learned were applicable for all four. The most important were the need for some degree of carefully managed diversification, the importance of slack resources, the need for market research to facilitate learning, the need for a flexible strategic planning and control system with simultaneous properties of centralization and decentralization, the importance of working effectively with physicians, and the general need to stay within the organization's strategic comfort zone. The exact form of these factors varied, but they were common to all.

Diversification. Contrary to conventional wisdom, all strategic archetypes, even defenders, require some degree of diversification, at least in rapidly changing industries characterized by turbulent environments. The logic for diversification is most easily understood for prospectors who, by definition, are continuously involved in developing new services in new markets. Their major challenge lies in understanding the requirements of each diversification effort, particularly in market and technological relatedness. Entry strategies must match the diversification requirements. For hospitals, the greater the extent to which the new venture is related to inpatient care, the greater the advantage of providing it oneself. The further removed the activity is from inpatient care, the greater the advantage of working out joint ventures or related interorganizational networking strategies. Increasingly, the partners in these approaches are physicians on the hospitals' medical staffs (Shortell, Morrison, and Hughes, 1989).

Prospectors also need to develop an appreciation for *timing* in first-mover strategies. The ability to know whether you should be the first to offer a new program or service depends on both market research and a highly developed sense of intuition. Key ingredients are the ability to estimate or guesstimate market size and the ability to package program features that will make it difficult for competitors to enter. At the same time, the organization needs to think ahead to what it will do if competitors do enter. This involves developing an ability to switch strategies, such as from a quality differentiation focus to a cost leadership emphasis.

Unlike prospectors, the defenders' need to diversify represents a supplemental strategy designed to facilitate their primary focus on protecting current domains. To protect current domains, it is necessary to develop a few new programs and services that are highly related to and synergistic with the current domain. For some defender hospitals this included aftercare services (for example, home health) that helped the core inpatient business achieve greater efficiencies by discharging patients sooner. Small-scale diversification efforts also help defenders use personnel resources more efficiently. For example, development of an outpatient physical therapy department enabled one defender hospital to increase patient volume and referrals without adding additional staff. The key to the defenders' diversification strategy is that it must be a component of an overall thrust to become more technically efficient and to protect current domains. Diversification becomes a protective ring for core services. This is particularly important for defenders operating in highly competitive markets.

For analyzers, selective diversification is a way of linking the prospector and defender domains. The key lies in establishing market niches with careful analysis of competitor strengths and weaknesses. While for prospectors the diversification strategy is often based on first-mover assumptions, for analyzers it is more frequently based on looking for and exploiting the weaknesses of the first mover. This might involve targeting a different market segment (for example, the young-old rather than the old-old) or adding a different service feature, such as followup prenatal care to a package of maternity benefits. Analyzers particularly benefit from diversification efforts that will help to contain costs (their defender domain) while at the same time generating new revenues (their prospector domain). Outpatient rehabilitation programs served as a "two-for-one" solution for several analyzer hospitals.

Reactors are inevitably involved in diversification activities, but they tend to be scattered across many different markets and areas. Reactors need to refocus these efforts by emphasizing services that bear greater relationship to each other. For example, rather than attempting to appeal to both the young and elderly markets, reactors would benefit from a focus on one or the other. Rather than trying to develop "centers of excellence" across the board, reactors would be better off targeting one or two areas of potential competitive advantage. Such targeting is a critical component of the reactor's search for a more coherent strategic vision and more consistent strategic orientation.

The industry has learned that diversification must be a part of each hospital's strategy regardless of its specific strategic orientation. That means that hospitals in the 1990s must be more than just acute inpatient care institutions. They must evolve into *relatively* diversified health care organizations responsive to the demands of the new environment.

Slack Resources. Hospitals require different types and amounts of slack resources depending on their strategic orientations. Slack resources are particularly important for prospectors, to promote innovation and risk taking. Not all new ventures succeed, and capital funds must be available to support the losing efforts on the way to discovering the winners. Slack is also needed to help the prospectors switch back and forth from differentiation to cost-containment strategies over the product/service life cycle.

Defenders require a more modest amount of slack resources to mount their smaller-scale diversification efforts. Lacking experience, defenders may need to spend some resources on outside consultants. Analyzers require slack to create synergy between the prospector and defender domains. In particular, this requires investment in market research and management information systems. Finally, reactors require slack so they can afford the mistakes of their false starts. Slack resources help reactors buy time to discover who they are and who they want to become. Without it, some may not survive.

Nearly all archetypes made one common mistake (although prospectors less so): underestimating the capital requirements of their diversification activities. Another mistake made by some involved the failure to integrate financial and strategic planning functions, resulting in a lack of resources to execute strategic plans.

Another challenge that nearly all hospitals faced was understanding and being willing to commit to their strategic role within the system's overall strategic plan. For example, some hospitals needed to accept the fact that some of the slack resources generated would be used to subsidize other hospitals in the system. This was generally facilitated when the corporate office understood the concept of a strategic portfolio of hospitals involving a mix of prospector, defender, analyzer, and, perhaps, reactor hospitals and was able to communicate to each hospital its role and the associated overall rewards. But, as we have seen, this sometimes proved to be problematic.

Market Research and Learning. Significant environmental change means that current sources of information are usually outdated and the current means for acquiring information perhaps outmoded. This is a particular problem for hospitals, which spend only about 2 to 3 percent of their budget on management information systems as compared with 7 percent in other industries (Reep, 1988). Not only does this make it more difficult to learn about the new change, but it also creates problems in interpreting the significance of the change. Particularly important is learning what the change means for customers (including physicians) and markets, underscoring the importance of market research.

Prospectors have perhaps the greatest need for a strong market research capability because of their emphasis on developing new products and new markets. Assessing potential first-mover advantages and following up with various differentiation strategies are critically dependent on good market information. Market data were also needed to help distinguish among services that were more consumer driven, such as health promotion, sports medicine, and occupational health, versus those that were more professionally driven, such as cardiology, oncology, and renal dialysis, versus those with fairly equal components of both, such as obstetrics.

Defenders also have a high need for good market research capability to effectively differentiate their core business — for hospitals, acute inpatient care services. Differentiation is needed to both protect and enhance market share for these services. Because defenders cannot generally compete on technical quality alone, they need market research on other characteristics important to consumers, such as service, convenience, access, comfort, and involvement. Good market research also helped defenders in their selective diversification efforts.

Learning through market research is particularly important in helping the analyzer manage the complexity of its dual strategy. Since analyzers are seldom first movers, they require good data collection and analysis capabilities to discern what remaining markets to enter or whether market share can be taken away from an early entrant. This frequently requires double-loop (Argyris and Schön, 1978) or second-order learning (Fiol and Lyles, 1985) in which underlying assumptions are challenged and often reframed. For the analyzers, this approach is as important for protecting their inpatient services (the defender domain) as it is for launching their new initiatives (the prospector component). It also helps them remain sufficiently "comfortable" and capable of managing the complexity inherent in the analyzer strategy.

Reactors require market research as an important means of acquiring more systematic knowledge about their customer base. Reactors need to do a better job of learning from their mistakes. Market research data assist in this process and help reactors avoid jumping on the bandwagon of every new program that comes along. Developing an effective market research capability is an important part of the reactor's search for a more coherent and consistent strategic approach to its marketplace.

The health care environment of the 1990s will be unforgiving for those who do not know their customers, their customers' characteristics, and how best to reach each segment. Those who learn quickly will have an initial competitive edge. Those who keep on learning may achieve a sustainable competitive advantage.

Flexible Strategic Planning and Control. Among the more complex and subtle findings of the study was the need for flexibility in strategic planning and control systems, particularly in regard to centralization of specific strategic planning functions. A culture that supports flexibility, experimentation, and change is also required.

The need to strike a balance between centralization and decentralization was particularly important for prospectors, who faced the challenge of trying to integrate local market planning with corporatewide strategic planning. Granting too much autonomy or too little autonomy proved dysfunctional. In the long run, a middle ground approach appeared to work best: local units were given primary responsibility for identifying markets and working jointly with physicians to serve these markets within overall corporate guidelines. At the same time, financial control and ultimate accountability resided with the corporate office. The net result was a "guided autonomy" approach.

For defenders, the balance needed to be struck more toward the centralization end of the continuum. In a less turbulent environment, a decentralized strategy may be effective. But in a turbulent environment such as that experienced by the hospitals studied, defenders were slow to react to the changes and, lacking strong centralized strategic planning and control, many floundered. Such direction, however, is not inconsistent with delegating *implementation* responsibilities to the individual unit; the corporate office stops short of actually running the day-to-day operations.

The analyzer, having both a prospector and defender component, requires both some degree of centralized direction as well as a good deal of autonomy. The principle of guided autonomy applies, but with perhaps a somewhat greater emphasis on the "guided" dimension. The complexity involved in an analyzer strategy requires a strong linkage between financial planning and strategic planning activities, human resource planning and strategic planning, and incentive compensation systems and strategic priorities. Where these linkages exist at the corporate level, greater autonomy can be delegated to individual units.

Reactors have a particular need for a more disciplined strategic planning and control system, perhaps even more so than defenders. However, reactors are more handicapped because they lack a coherent strategic vision on which a planning and control system can be based. Thus, until leadership can articulate such a vision, developing a more disciplined strategic planning and control system becomes largely an academic exercise. Once such a vision is developed and committed to by relevant parties, it is critical that a system be established to translate the vision into operational reality. Then a disciplined process that integrates individual unit plans with the corporate vision and links programmatic plans with financial realities begins to pay off. Once the vision is articulated, reactors are able to learn more quickly from their mistakes and make the transition to a more clearly defined strategic state.

The level of experimentation among the systems in structuring planning and control relationships was striking. For the most part, the prospectors and analyzers recognized the need for a balance between centralization and decentralization, control and autonomy, and the need to remain fluid in the process. Defenders and reactors had greater needs for a disciplined process, which often required greater centralization but not without the cost of losing local autonomy. The problem was further complicated by the differences in the strategic orientations of individual hospitals themselves. Each system was a mix of prospector, defender, analyzer, and reactor hospitals, each with its own requirements of the corporate office (Govindarajan, 1988). Thus, a guided autonomy strategy might work very well for a system's prospectors and analyzers but less well for its defenders and reactors. Conversely, a more centralized disciplined process might be appropriate for the defenders and reactors but dysfunctional for the system's prospectors and analyzers. Knowing how and where to strike the balance proved to be a major challenge. The need to be ambidextrous and experimental in approach appears to be an important ingredient for succeeding in the health care environment of the 1990s.

Working Effectively with Physicians. Perhaps the most prevalent issue facing all strategic archetypes was working effectively with physicians to meet the challenges posed by PPS and the related changes in the health care environment. Strategy implementation depended importantly on the cooperation and in many cases active involvement of physicians. (Although the primary emphasis was on physicians, a similar argument can be made for nurses and other health professionals as well.)

For prospectors the major challenge lay in the need to involve physicians in meaningful ways in the hospital's diversification plans. Physicians were often suspicious, sometimes seeing these plans as direct competition with their own interests. The most successful efforts sought the common ground that married hospital and physician interests. This required involving selected physicians early on in the planning process; identifying physician practice needs and interests; and working daily to create an overall climate of trust, openness, honesty, and consistent communication. Successful joint venture activities were characterized by consistency with the hospital's mission, joint financial risk by both hospital and physicians, joint governance, clear specification of roles and responsibilities, detailed business plans, and preestablished mechanisms and forums for managing conflict.

For defenders the major challenge was involving physicians in cost-containment activities and smaller-scale diversification efforts. Physicians feared that hospitals' efforts to contain costs might alter their practice style and invade their clinical autonomy, possibly resulting in a lower quality of care. Hospitals that successfully dealt with these issues worked on many fronts at once. They involved physicians in task forces that identified cost-cutting opportunities that did not compromise quality. They provided incentives by which some of the savings accrued by staying under the DRG limits could be used for medical education, research, and upgrading of technology. They were careful to initiate budget cuts in areas other than patient care. They also cultivated key physician leaders who positively influenced their colleagues to assist the hospital in its cost-containment efforts.

Effective communication with physicians was particularly important for analyzers operating in both prospector and defender domains. Keys to success were early involvement of physicians and involvement at multiple levels: the board, strategic planning committees and task forces, and technology and equipment purchasing committees. In many cases, a full-time or part-time medical director or vice-president for medical affairs played a key role in moving projects along. Sometimes, assistance would also be provided by corporate office staff through a systemwide office for medical affairs.

The challenge of effectively involving physicians was perhaps greatest for reactors. The lack of a consistent strategic vision often resulted in unpredictable behavior that was upsetting to the medical staff. The hospital-physician relationship was often further strained by a more stringent regulatory environment that frequently placed hospitals and physicians in conflict with each other. A "we versus they" mentality developed. Most reactor hospitals found the current medical staff structure unable to deal with the issues, and several developed alternative structures ranging from steering committees, to professional practice associations, to joint physician/hospital organizations designed to facilitate closer linkages around common economic issues. In more than one case, the strategic direction for the institution came out of the deliberations of these alternative groups, representing a classic illustration of emergent strategy making (see Mintzberg, 1978).

The need to develop effective partnerships with their physicians was a dominant theme for all eight systems and their member hospitals as they prepared for the 1990s. The challenge is in creating a mutual understanding of the economic interplay of the two groups. When both perceive their economic and professional futures as closely intertwined, a climate exists where structures, processes, and incentives can be designed to promote effective collaboration.

Knowing Your Comfort Zone. A basic thesis of the model of strategic adaptation outlined in Figure 2.1 was that organizations operating outside their strategic comfort zone would perform more poorly than those operating within. As it turned out, there is little evidence to support this thesis. We believe that this is at least partly due to the short time frame of the study.

The insights, however, derived from the qualitative analysis presented in Chapters Six through Nine provide general support for the validity and utility of the strategic comfort zone concept. Reexamination of the numerous comments made by system executives, planners, hospital CEOs, and management staff members indicated their levels of comfort and discomfort with the various strategic orientations adopted by their organizations. Some felt their organizations were moving too fast, others saw them as moving too slowly. Some felt they had bit off too much and were spread too thin, others thought they had not bit off enough. Some thought they were moving in the right direction, others questioned the wisdom of recent choices. The comments reflect the organizations' struggle not only against inertial forces but also with the process of determining the "correct" strategic response.

Summary. As a group, the common lessons reflect the three themes set forth in Chapter One about the paradigmatic shifts occurring within the industry: (1) the shift from a product orientation to a market orientation; (2) the shift from a caretaking mentality to a risk-taking mentality; and (3) the shift from a focus on operational management to an emphasis on strategic management. Learning how to diversify, how to use slack resources, the need to emphasize market research, the need to balance autonomy and control, working effectively with physicians, and understanding the nature of a strategic comfort zone are what these three shifts are all about.

Lessons Specific to Each Strategy

In addition to the common or core lessons, each strategic archetype also had its own set of specific lessons.

Prospectors. Prospectors needed to consistently differentiate their services, carefully assess first-mover advantages, and create local market synergies. Since examples of each are provided in Chapter Six, only a few additional comments are made here.

To be successful, prospectors must recognize the need to constantly differentiate services *early* in the planning process. One hospital thought it helped to think in terms of three two-year phases for its urgent care centers. The first phase emphasized rapid startup with three centers in well-located areas. Attention was paid to initial marketing and operating efficiencies. The second phase attempted to anticipate competitors by extending service hours and emphasizing the centers' linkages to the high-quality sponsoring hospital. The third phase envisioned additional services surrounding the urgent care centers, including an ambulatory surgery center, a home health care agency, and a sports medicine complex. The key was in recognizing that there would be competitive responses and that the hospital needed to stay one step ahead of the competition.

Whether first-mover advantages existed often could be determined by a careful analysis of the questions posed in Chapter Six. Some successful prospectors, however, also recognized that they might be able to create some first-mover advantages where none existed by having a greater capacity to differentiate the service once in the market. In one case two competing hospital-sponsored HMOs entered the market at the same time, but one was able to gain a greater number of enrollees by offering a more comprehensive maternity benefit and by being known as the hospital with the strongest family practice and "community caring" image. The lesson is that first-mover advantages must always be coupled with the ability to sustain the advantage through constant differentiation.

Successful prospectors also looked for opportunities for synergies among their new offerings. This was particularly important in competitive markets where employers and employees were looking for "one-stop" care and continuity across treatment settings. This placed a premium on developing successful, vertically integrated services, both pre- and posthospitalization, in geographically concentrated areas. Several prospector-oriented hospitals, for example, developed integrated medical campuses composed of multispecialty clinics, ambulatory surgery centers, diagnostic imaging centers, sports medicine, home health care agencies, and related services. These successful prospectors recognized the need to give attention to continued differentiation, to link first-mover advantages to continued differentiation, and to link new programs and services to each other on a continuum of care that appealed to physicians, their patients, and to the employers paying the premiums.

Defenders. More than other archetypes, defenders needed to actively manage their costs, pay greater attention to the overall portfolio of services, and, in particular, require a more disciplined strategic planning and control process.

Active cost management must begin with an overall analysis of the hospital's strategic plan and is therefore tied to paying attention to the overall portfolio of services. What services are being targeted for expansion, modification, or deletion? What services depend on each other? What is the cost structure of each service? Such an analysis reveals areas where cost cuts can be most effective. Across-the-board cuts are seldom effective, even when limited to management areas. Cost cutting must be strategically driven, with a view to the longer-run ability to be competitive in addition to achieving short-run objectives.

In reviewing the service portfolio, defenders must pay particular attention to opportunities for divesting or consolidating services. Sometimes this involves slaying sacred cows, but this is the price of survival in a turbulent environment.

Analyzers. Because of the challenges involved in bridging two domains (prospector and defender), analyzers must place considerable emphasis on being cost effective. This requires synergy between the two domains, learning mechanisms that question underlying assumptions, and close linkages among planning system components, including financial planning, human resource planning, and incentive compensation systems.

In each of these three areas there tended to be a difference between the active and the passive analyzers. The more active analyzers tended to develop new ventures with the goal of making them profitable in their own right. Passive analyzers saw new ventures as a way of protecting the current inpatient domain and channeling referrals to the acute care hospital. In either case, however, there was a need to establish a relationship between the two sets of activities. This was particularly true where resources were constrained and diversification opportunities had to be carefully selected.

The learning by the active analyzers primarily involved a variety of "what-if" scenarios related to new services and programs. Active analyzers also invested in rigorous competitor analysis. Passive analyzers gave greater emphasis to divesting services and rearranging resources so that new diversification could be pursued. They were also more passive in analyzing the competition and emphasized learning *after* others had made mistakes.

For the active analyzers, there was a particular need to link financial planning and strategic planning early in the process and to develop incentive compensation arrangements to encourage innovation. Passive analyzers tended to give greater attention to human resource development issues associated with the rearrangement of service priorities. Overall, however, both types of analyzers saw the need for closer integration of their strategic planning systems with their financial and human resource planning systems and their compensation arrangements. This was particularly true for physician involvement in major capital and technology purchases and for developing staffing requirements for centers of excellence in areas such as cardiology and oncology. Perhaps above all, analyzers required strong information systems.

Reactors. Although we question whether a reactor strategy can be successful in the long run, there are several things reactors can do on the way to developing a more coherent strategic identity. Beyond the obvious need for strategic leadership and vision, these include a willingness to stick with services beyond initial implementation, consistent cost-containment efforts linked to a strategic plan, and stronger management information systems to facilitate learning.

The ability to stay with a new service is greatly facilitated by a strategic vision for the organization as reflected in its strategic plan. Such a plan provides a road map for each service and its place in the overall strategy. Realistic detailed business plans can then be developed for each service. With such an approach, one is less likely to abandon an HMO losing money when the main intent of the strategy is to preempt competitors and give the hospital a toehold in an expanding market.

As with the defender, the reactor's cost-containment efforts must be linked to a strategic plan and vision to avoid haphazard cost cutting. This process is assisted not only by a strategic plan but by a strong management information system that identifies the costs and revenues of major service centers. These systems help reactors develop the greater discipline required of a more coherent strategic vision. Reactors who recognize the ability to stay with selected new services and to diversify while strategically cutting costs are well on their way to becoming analyzers. Those in more competitive markets and with greater slack may lean toward becoming prospectors. Those in less competitive markets and perhaps with fewer resources may opt for becoming defenders. In any case, given a turbulent environment, reactors need to steer a straighter course.

Lessons About Switching Strategies

A major issue facing hospital executives was whether, when, and how to initiate strategic change. Exactly half of the hospitals we studied switched their basic orientations during the study period. Sixty-two percent of analyzers and 40 percent of prospectors did not switch. They felt their current strategies positioned them well for the changing environment. Eighty-one percent of reactors and 75 percent of defenders did change, and for the most part they changed to a more proactive orientation, becoming either a prospector or an analyzer. Some, particularly defenders, believed they had made the switch too late or at least too slowly; others believed they had made it too quickly. Almost all indicated the changes brought major challenges, particularly those who switched outside their strategic comfort zones. One California observer felt the process bore many similarities to surfing. Strategies are like waves. The trick to being an effective surfer (strategist) is in catching and riding the right wave. You need to know when to stay with a given wave and when to abandon it. You can crash if you abandon a wave too soon as well as too late. You need to know when a particular wave is about to play itself out. A smart surfer knows when to abandon a wave even though it may still be possible to get some mileage from it. Surfers (strategists) need to scan the horizon for the developing new wave (strategy) and get some early experience with it to become consistently effective.

Whether and When to Switch

Timing a shift in basic strategic orientation is a tricky business. As suggested by the model of strategic adaptation out-

lined in Chapter Two, there are three dimensions to the issue:
(1) the need to shift, (2) the desire to shift, and (3) the ability
to shift. The need to shift is primarily a function of the organization's perceptions of the changing environment in relation to
current performance, strategies, and capabilities. A common
explanation for structural inertia is that organizations have been
rewarded for behavior associated with successful performance
in the past. This leads to a tendency to continue the behavior
in the future, even in the face of a rapidly shifting environment.
The result may be a decline in performance.

Whether or not there is a need to shift also depends on
the organization's environmental assessment capabilities and
management's astuteness in interpreting the *meaning* of the environment. It did not take much to recognize that PPS and its
associated effects represented a major environmental change in
the hospital industry. But interpreting the significance of the
change was not necessarily simple. Some executives, for example, felt PPS would have relatively little effect on their organizations because they saw a relatively low percentage of Medicare
patients. In contrast, others were greatly concerned, not necessarily because of the percentage of Medicare patients but because
they felt the payment changes would have widespread implications for hospital reimbursement. Perceptions also varied as a
function of how well the hospital was doing financially and the
intensity of competition in the local market. Generally, prospectors and analyzers who did not switch had anticipated the
likelihood of a changing payment environment and had begun
using slack resources to develop diversified programs and services for several years before 1983. These hospitals felt that their
strategic orientations would continue to bear fruit in the new
environment. In contrast, many defenders either failed to recognize the inappropriateness of an exclusively defender strategy
in a rapidly changing environment or were unable to execute
their strategy successfully. Thus, poor past performance, which
often acts as a trigger for change, was actually associated with
strategic inertia for many defenders.

The desire to change also played a role. Rather than structural inertia, in some cases there was a process of "individual

inertia." Some top executives, particularly among defenders, simply did not wish to expend the energy required to change their organization's strategic focus. They hoped that PPS, like the industry's wage and price controls in the 1970s, might be transitory and that other factors (for example, political opposition) might act to mitigate its effects. Some of these executives had been with their institutions for fifteen to twenty-five years and were looking forward to retirement. While they intellectually recognized the need for change, they were psychologically ill equipped to deal with it. Hospital board members were often negligent in failing to recognize the signs and symptoms. Many of these boards were largely controlled by the hospital CEO, who selectively communicated information to them. As a result, some boards did not even recognize the need for change and were not in a position to deal with a reluctant CEO. In other cases, board members were relatively well informed but, having known the essentially caretaking environment of the 1960s and 1970s, were unable to make the transition to the risk-taking environment of the 1980s, particularly without CEO leadership. This was often true for the hospitals that had been doing well for many years.

A third important factor is the organization's ability to change, which is a function of both money and mind set. In addition to the necessary slack resources, all the involved groups — the board, the top management team and staff, middle management, and physicians — have to be personally able to change.

Some executives' desire to change was hampered by a relatively uneducated, passive board of directors. For example, the CEO of Passmore Hospital spent over a year of intensive work trying to sell the board on a more aggressive market stance. In other cases, boards had to be reconfigured and restructured by adding members with greater expertise before headway could be made on new strategic directions.

Executives also had to assess their own and their staff's abilities to manage the change process. In many cases, the top management team lacked the necessary skills in marketing, joint venture development, and strategic planning to make a successful transition to a proactive strategy. The ability of the corporate office to provide such assistance varied. Some hospitals' efforts to change were delayed until the right kind of management team was put in place. In other cases, plans proceeded in "fits and starts" as new initiatives were stalled for lack of appropriate staff support. In a couple of organizations, a single talented individual was spread too thin, trying to manage too many activities at once.

Even when top management staff were available, middle management often represented a significant roadblock to implementing new strategy. Most middle managers of nursing, pharmacy, laboratory, and radiology services, for example, had been rewarded throughout their careers for running departments that kept physicians and patients happy. The transition to more aggressive, entrepreneurial strategies emphasizing innovation represented a major cultural shift. This transition was particularly difficult when the organizations' incentive and reward systems were not changed to match the new emphasis on innovation and risk taking. As one hospital laboratory manager said, "They want us to develop new programs and services and take risks, but they pay us using the same old criteria they've always used." Many hospitals were caught playing "catch up" in upgrading their management development programs and incentive systems for middle managers and key employees.

As we have emphasized throughout, physicians also played a key role in the ability of hospitals to respond strategically to the changing environmental forces. Many hospitals were hampered by their physicians. In some cases, physicians simply did not see the need for change. In other cases, certain powerful physicians saw the new strategic initiatives as directly competitive with their own interests. In most cases, physicians felt estranged from the entire process from which the new strategic directions emerged.

Some hospitals delayed their efforts until a sufficient core group of physicians could be brought aboard. In the process they admitted that "we lost out on a few opportunities, but we decided it was more important to make sure and have physician support." Others plunged ahead, only to find their efforts undercut by physician forces. In still other cases, executives felt they had done a good job involving, educating, and gaining the support of physician leadership only to find the physician leaders were not able to deliver on their commitment because of an inability to attract a sufficient number of followers.

Ironically, in some cases physicians were the catalyst for strategic change, pushing on a somewhat reluctant managerial team. This tended to occur in highly competitive markets where physicians had organized themselves into an independent practice association (or similar arrangement) to permit entering into economic arrangements with managed care plans and undertaking joint ventures with the hospital. They sometimes approached administration with opportunities before administration was willing or able to move. In these cases the timing of strategic change was slowed by management inertia rather than physician resistance.

The Switching Process

From a process perspective, the more successful switchers were those that understood the significance of the environmental change for their own organization, had a personal desire to change, were able to correctly diagnose their organization's capability to initiate the desired change, and could recruit or develop internally the additional abilities required.

It is possible to organize the process elements around four steps: (1) recognizing the need for change, (2) developing a vision of the new desired state, (3) taking the practical first steps to get from the present to the desired future state, and (4) providing continuing support and followup.

Step 1. Creating the Need for Change. People, groups and organizations will generally not change unless they are sufficiently uncomfortable with their current state, or unless the rewards to be gained by the change are very great, tangible, and clearly attainable. Successful executives take advantage of, even create, situations of discomfort to trigger change. In the present study, the change to PPS and the increased competitive forces were often not sufficient by themselves for some hospitals to see the need for change. The fact that many hospitals were *more* profitable after the first year of PPS added to the difficulty. Board members had to be educated on the future implications of the change. Some executives drew on examples from hospitals in highly regulated states (for example, New York, New Jersey, and Massachusetts) to drive home their point. Many sent key board members, physician leaders, and top management staff to conferences and seminars that focused on the implications of the change. Others brought in outside consultants for assistance.

Getting physicians to see the need for change was particularly difficult because the new incentives did not *directly* affect them. The trick was to demonstrate to physicians the negative indirect effect: if the hospital did not do well in the new economic environment physicians would have fewer resources with which to practice medicine and in the worst scenario might not have a hospital available at all. This argument was, of course, weakened in a multihospital community where physicians could play one hospital against another. More successful executives, however, targeted their campaigns on physicians who were high hospital admitters and "loyalists," communicating the basic economic and professional interplay.

In recent years, as the relative increase in physician incomes has declined and managed care plans compete for each physician's patients, physicians' level of discomfort has grown. As a result, they have become more receptive to strategic initiatives to control costs, develop new services, and experiment with new organizational forms. In many cases, however, the pace of change was slower than management desired because they had to wait for physicians to be "hurting enough" to try new approaches. Some were better than others at creating this state, and some were better than others in timing key initiatives such as waiting for the "right" physician to become chief of staff. Others were savvy in encouraging competing physician groups that would bring short-run unrest to the medical staff but in the process would provide a conflict forum around which attention could be focused on the need for change.

Step 2. Creating the New Vision. Once a sufficient number of people in the organization are dissatisfied with the current strategic state, the new vision must be created. In reality, these tend to be simultaneous and parallel processes. Some people do not fully appreciate the dissatisfaction with current strategies until they see the possibilities of a fresh new approach.

Creating a vision is particularly important for reactors. In many cases new leadership is required. Such was the case for McKinley Memorial Hospital, a classic reactor in the late 1970s. Operating in a highly competitive environment, McKinley had always enjoyed an outstanding reputation for the quality of its medical staff and for its clinical programs and services. It had suffered, however, from weak management and lack of board leadership, and had been drifting for several years. A scandal involving a member of the medical staff finally precipitated the resignation of the CEO and several board members. A new CEO and several board members were brought in to articulate a new direction. The new CEO, a firm believer in strategic planning, quickly mobilized a nucleus of ten to fifteen key physicians with whom he charted the strategic direction for the institution. After assessing available resources and strengths and weaknesses, they set a clear prospector strategy with an aggressive approach to the marketplace. New initiatives were undertaken, involving urgent care centers, ambulatory surgery centers, outpatient diagnostic imaging, and decentralized integrated medical campuses featuring a wide array of outpatient treatment centers and physician offices in a single setting. Strong medical staff, management, and board leadership resulted in a clear understanding of the need for the direction and thus widespread support. Key individuals throughout the organization came to understand what the vision meant for them in their daily work, rather than in the abstract.

Step 3. Taking the First Steps. Some executives are very good at moving from mountaintop to mountaintop in articulating the goals and dreams of their organization. They are less good, however, at filling in the valleys, the hard work associated with taking the practical first steps toward implementation (Peters and Tseng, 1983). Successful strategic change requires a lot of "valley fillers."

The need for practical first steps is well illustrated by Prosser Medical Center. Like McKinley, Prosser had been a drifting reactor for several years. A slow decline in market share, a presence of a new competitor, and the retirement of the incumbent CEO were the precursors to recruitment of a new business-oriented CEO. Like McKinley, Prosser was also blessed with an outstanding medical staff, and the CEO created a new vision and a strategic direction based on this strength. The organization chose an essentially analyzer strategy of solidifying its acute inpatient business by developing centers of excellence while selectively diversifying into outpatient areas to better position itself for cost-containment forces and managed care programs. The new direction was supported by detailed implementation plans, ranging from recruiting different types of new board members who would support the new thrust, to appointing several multidisciplinary task forces of physicians, board members, and managers to work out the details.

Taking the practical first steps lets everyone in the organization know that the new direction is for real. Taking the practical first steps energizes people. Taking the practical first steps increases people's confidence in the attainability of the new strategic direction.

Step 4. Providing Ongoing Support. Successful strategic switching requires persistence. Once the new direction is started and the plans develop, ongoing support is required. Things never stay the same and the best-laid plans often go astray. Management must be willing and able to step in with additional resources as needed, providing ongoing encouragement and support, and be flexible in entertaining alternative or modified pathways to the goal. The failure to provide ongoing support was many hospitals' downfall in their attempts to diversify. The need for additional resources was not contemplated, and several of the early projects were understaffed.

Ongoing support is particularly important in developing joint programs with physicians. Physicians usually operate on shorter time frames than managers. Physicians are less comfortable with "soft" data and information. Most have little experience in group dynamics and group decision making. In many cases, their objective for a particular program may be much narrower. These differences mean that management must be ready to educate and inform continually, to model desired behavior, to be creative in developing fresh approaches to problems, and to be sensitive to physician needs and interests while at the same time communicating the hospital's goals and objectives.

The need for ongoing support of strategic change is well illustrated by Angston Hospital. Angston was a defender hospital in the process of becoming an analyzer. It was attempting to develop selective centers of excellence that would anticipate the future of medical practice in its community. But, rather than leave the implementation details to chance, Angston developed a multiyear special project of ongoing support jointly funded by the hospital, its medical staff, and an independent physicians' practice association representing the hospital's major admitters. The project represented a bold "two-for-one" decision that would provide ongoing support for change and help refine the organization's future vision of itself and its environment.

Executing the four steps of change is likely to be easier for those who stay within their strategic comfort zone. Those attempting to change outside their comfort zone must recognize the need for a multiyear planned change involving alterations in their basic culture (Bice, 1984). Those who made changes outside their comfort zone had particular problems with steps 3 and 4, and so at times appeared to behave more like reactors. Being a reactor may be a transitory state for some organizations on their way to becoming a prospector, analyzer, or defender.

Lessons for Strategy Switchers

From the analysis described here, we can summarize ten lessons on switching strategy.

1. Past success may predict future success even in a rapidly
    changing environment *provided* an organization's basic stra-
    tegic orientation is able to accommodate the requirements
    of the new environment.
2. Past poor performance should *always* result in consider-
    ing the need for fundamental strategic change, particularly
    in a rapidly changing environment. A redoubling of cur-
    rent effort is not likely to be sufficient.
3. Assessing the need for strategic change and the direction
    of change requires *interpreting the meaning* that the new en-
    vironment holds for the organization. This interpretative
    process is facilitated by strong environmental assessment,
    market research, board and top management staff capabil-
    ities, and enlightened physician leadership.
4. The board and top management staff must be as psycho-
    logically open to the possibility of fundamental strategic
    change as they are intellectually aware of the need for such
    change. If they are not, they should be replaced.
5. The timing, degree, and direction of strategic change must
    take into account the nature of the organization's culture
    and capabilities in relation to the environmental demands.
    The strengths and weaknesses of the board, top manage-
    ment team, middle management team, and physician
    leadership must be assessed and worked on continuously.
6. Before you can consider undertaking significant strategic
    change, you must create an environment of discomfort or
    dissatisfaction with the current strategy among key orga-
    nizational members.
7. The desirability of the new strategic state must be com-
    municated to key organizational members in a way that
    has significant meaning for their professional careers and
    involvement in the organization. To be successful, this
    communication must have both a cognitive and emotional
    component. To sustain change, you must capture both
    people's minds and people's hearts.
8. It is not enough to create a new strategic vision. Practical
    first steps must be taken to lend a sense of realism, mo-

tivation, and confidence that the new direction can be achieved.

9. Continuous ongoing support of many forms must be provided to assure a successful transition. The race does not necessarily go to the swift but to those who persist and endure.

10. It is easier to change strategies if the organization stays within its strategic comfort zone. At the same time, in a turbulent environment, it is the leader's job to continually work on expanding the organization's capabilities so it can move beyond its current comfort zone if necessary.

11

Key Requirements for Success in a Changing Health Care Environment

Chapter Ten summarized the lessons from the study findings. In this chapter we explore the implications of these lessons for meeting future demands. We make six assumptions about the future of the U.S. health care system and, given these assumptions, develop four major requirements for future success. The assumptions and success requirements go beyond the present study to explore issues facing all health care organizations.

Environmental Assumptions

Most of the forces influencing the delivery of health care services in the 1990s are already in place. The six assumptions are:

1. Cost-containment pressures, reflected in both payment rates and managed care programs, will continue to be the dominant factor influencing the delivery of health services.
2. There will be continued concern with what the nation is getting for its health care expenditures, and increased attention will be given to measuring and assuring the quality

of services delivered; hospital payment will be tied to outcome measures.

3. There will be continued growth in new technology but with much greater emphasis given to cost-saving technology that will make it possible to provide more care in out-of-hospital settings such as physician offices and patients' homes.
4. Governmental and private programs will be developed to provide some degree of increased financial support to provide health care services to the elderly, the poor, and the uninsured.
5. There will be increased social morbidity (substance abuse, homicides, accidents) associated with the continued stresses of modern society.
6. There will be increased economic and professional conflict among health professionals (physicians, nurses, and other health professionals) as each struggles for its place in a rapidly changing delivery system.

Cost Containment. The easiest assumption to accept about the future is the continued emphasis on containing costs. All payors — federal and state government, insurance companies, and the employers who pay the premiums — have a strong interest in seeing costs controlled. The federal budget deficit and larger political economic forces underscore this concern. In the 1990s, these forces will extend beyond the acute hospital setting to embrace the entire continuum of health care services, from hospital care to physician care to home health care. The current congressional initiative to use resource-based relative value scales to redistribute fee levels away from higher-paid surgical procedures to lower-paid cognitive procedures (for example, establishing a diagnosis) is likely to be a transitory step on the way to establishing a global cap for physician services (Physician Payment Review Commission, 1989). Managed care plans emphasizing physicians who practice cost-effective medicine will continue to grow across the country, approximating the 70 percent levels that have already been reached in California. In brief, the flexibility within the system to shift costs from one part of the system to another — from hospital care to ambulatory care; from one provider to another, such as from primary care physicians to specialists; from one payor to another, such as from Medicare providers to private insurers — will be greatly reduced if not eliminated altogether. Successful corporations positioning themselves to operate in such an environment are *now* putting together cost-effective continuums of care.

Quality of Care. As the health care system is increasingly squeezed financially, greater attention will be paid to the quality of services delivered. An obvious reason is to assure that the emphasis on cost containment is not at the expense of patient welfare. But another important reason is that health care corporations and their member hospitals will learn that there are limits to the ability to compete on costs alone, and they will see the need to differentiate themselves on quality criteria as well. Clinical and health services research devoted to measuring patient care outcomes and adjusting for differences in patient severity of illness will have made significant advances in the 1990s, permitting the payment of providers based on patient outcomes. The more cost-effective providers (better outcomes for a given cost or lower cost for a given outcome) will be financially rewarded, and those with poorer outcomes will be financially punished.

The successful health care corporations of the 1990s are now developing clinical and management information systems to provide the data needed to adopt appropriate cost to quality strategies and to provide evidence of value added to payors. Corporations that today adopt a mind set of continuous improvement in the quality of care, supported by appropriate organizational and clinical investments in research and development, will be the success stories of the future.

Cost-Effective Technological Growth. Many of the new technologies, ranging from lasers to monoclonal antibodies, will permit extensive growth in out-of-hospital care. It is likely that two-thirds to three-quarters of the surgical operations performed in hospitals today will be done on an outpatient basis within the next decade. What is now tertiary care will become relatively routine secondary care, and what is now secondary care done in the hospital will become primary care done in the physician's office or patient's home. A recent study of hospital systems' use of technology indicated that 97 percent would make use of monoclonal antibodies, 95 percent in-home diagnostic testing, 89 percent laser technology, 84 percent magnetic resonance imaging, 57 percent lithotripsy, 58 percent Cine-CT, and 19 percent powered limb prostheses within the next few years (Arthur Andersen & Co. and the American Hospital Association, 1987).

Underlying these technologies will be the development of sophisticated computerized medical-decision support systems, ranging from computerized drug-dosage dispensers to computer-assisted diagnostic data bases to the computerized medical record. Between 30 and 81 percent of a national sample of hospital systems planned to have these information technologies in place by the early 1990s (Arthur Andersen & Co. and the American Hospital Association, 1987). The successful health care corporations of the future are already experimenting with these new technologies and will look for opportunities for continued experimentation and investment.

Financial Coverage for the Elderly, the Uninsured, and the Poor. The American public is expressing increased dissatisfaction with its health care system. A recent poll showed that 89 percent of Americans believe the system needs fundamental change, far greater than the British and Canadians' dissatisfaction with their system (Blendon, 1989a). The concern primarily focused on inadequate financial coverage for services.

A growing number of elderly Americans, particularly the old-old group eighty-five and over, will place an increasing strain on the health care system and the American economy at large. Government and private-sector programs to insure against catastrophic illness (for example, the Catastrophic Health Care Act of 1988) will grow, providing resources for care of these individuals. Elderly people who can afford to pay some of their care will be required to do so; others will receive increasing amounts of subsidization.

Increased coverage for at least some subsegments of the currently 37 million uninsured Americans will also grow. The group of greatest concern is the approximately one-third of the uninsured who do not have the financial means to purchase insurance on their own or are unable to pay for their medical care. There will be increased coverage for the poor and unemployed, and increasingly they will receive services through managed care plans. For the immediate future, the approaches for raising and distributing the monies are likely to remain pluralistic, involving a combination of increases in general taxes, the use of special "health" taxes (for example, alcohol and cigarettes), mandated employee health insurance, and related federal, state, and local initiatives. To maintain their social and political legitimacy, successful health care corporations will be active participants in these debates and will work with others to fill in gaps. They cannot, however, be expected to do it alone.

Increased Social Morbidity. AIDS is now the fifth leading cause of death among young Americans. Alcoholism and drug addiction continue to be major social problems. Automobile and motorcycle accidents and homicides continue to wreck havoc on individuals, families, and communities. Rightly or wrongly, much of the responsibility for the aftermath of these tragedies will be placed on the health care system. If these issues remain highly visible on the national political agenda (the war on drugs, the National AIDS Commission, and so on), resources will be available to health care corporations to meet these growing needs. Depending on their local environment, the successful health care corporations of the 1990s will position themselves to provide these services as part of their overall market strategy, while at the same time attempting to anticipate newly developing social pathologies.

Conflict Among Health Professionals: Managing Tribal Warfare. Professional groups are always in the process of redefining themselves to extend their domain, with the associated economic and institutional implications. The major sources of redefinition in the 1990s will be new technology, an increasing supply of some professionals, tightened reimbursement, increasingly sicker patients, a chronic shortage of nurses, and changes in the role of women in society. New technology causes conflict over who is most qualified to use it. Battles between anesthesiologists and radiologists, neurologists and radiologists, cardiovascular surgeons and cardiologists, obstetricians and family practitioners, general internists and family practitioners, to name a few, will continue to grow. The growing role of the primary care physician within managed care systems in channeling patients to specialists will add a further tension to the relationships. The technological battles will be fought not only within medical specialties but between medicine and other groups such as nursing, podiatry, and optometry as well.

The increasing number of physicians in certain specialties such as surgery will be a second source of strain. In some parts of the country, many surgeons are already redefining themselves as primary care physicians to attract patients, causing great concern among internists and family practitioners.

Physicians are also beginning to feel the bite of managed care programs and tighter reimbursement. The growth in physician income has slowed and new physicians find it increasingly difficult to build a practice.

The trend toward treating people outside hospitals has meant that patients in hospitals are much sicker than before. At the same time many of the nation's hospitals are ill equipped to cope with the problem because of an acute shortage of qualified nurses. Some units have been closed and patients transferred elsewhere. The situation has resulted in increased tension among physicians and nurses as they attempt to cope with the added responsibilities.

Significantly, unlike earlier nurse shortages, which were mitigated when the economy was depressed and nurses returned to the labor force, the current shortage has deeper structural roots. For example, 80 percent of the nurse labor pool are *already* practicing. The issue is not to attract trained nurses back into the labor force but rather to deal with more fundamental issues, including the changing roles of women in American society.

Increasingly, women are pursuing careers in business, law, engineering, and medicine — all seen as more attractive than nursing. Nursing school enrollments have declined. Nursing leaders are attempting to make the profession more attractive, but they are unlikely to succeed without significant salary increases throughout the career ladder and fundamental change in the working conditions and managerial practices. In many respects, what it means to be a hospital and to provide hospital care needs to be rethought and redesigned (Coile, 1988). These changes will threaten many physicians, hospital executives, and for that matter nurses themselves. The net result is another factor that will increase tribal warfare among health professionals.

The successful health corporations of the 1990s will need to face up to the challenges of managing the tribal warfare. The winners will be willing to try innovative and creative approaches for surfacing and managing the real conflict, for developing overarching goals that different groups can support in their own ways, and for developing partnerships and linkages that have economic and professional advantages for the parties involved (Neuhauser, 1988).

The Four Keys

The six environmental assumptions are interrelated in subtle and complex ways. Health care corporations will need to recognize the interplay between these factors and in the process learn how to put programs together and take programs apart much like tying and untying knots. To accomplish this health care corporations must do four things: (1) develop cost-effective integrated continuums of care, (2) behave like true multidivisional systems or corporations, (3) develop successful hospital-physician partnerships, and (4) engage in programs of strategic leadership development for board members, executives, and physician and nurse leaders. Each is an important dimension of managing strategic adaptation.

Integrated Continuums of Care

Much has already been said about the importance of developing integrated continuums of care. These largely local delivery systems, involving prehospital primary care, hospital care, and posthospital care, are needed to keep patient flow and dollars within the health care corporation's umbrella. The name of the game is regenerating patients. Employers and other third-party payors will also be looking to sign contracts with reasonably comprehensive delivery systems to avoid the coordination and monitoring costs of dealing with multiple provider systems. The advantages for patients are obvious.

Developing cost-effective integrated continuums of service will depend on the corporation's ability to follow the selective diversification and vertical integration lessons discussed in Chapters Six through Nine and summarized in Chapter Ten. As Chandler notes in his study of other industries, "The firms that first grew large by taking the merger route remained profitable only if after consolidating they then adopted a strategy of vertical integration" (Chandler, 1977, p. 315). The same applies to the health care industry in the 1990s.

The selective diversification and vertical integration strategies will work only if they add value in local communities and make sense to the physicians and other health professionals involved in them. Making appropriate use of the new technologies that facilitate out-of-hospital care and the new information systems will help build the required linkages across different levels and components of the system. Also needed are new organizational and managerial practices that focus on managing both *interorganizational* relationships and *transaction costs* within and across organizations. As Mick and Conrad note, "transfer prices must be effectively managed or the advantages of a vertically integrated system will be lost either through inefficient exchanges in comparison to market exchanges or through costly political arrangements created to maintain a workable relationship among all units" (Mick and Conrad, 1988, p. 356). They also note the transaction costs that can occur inside organizations from goal displacement and goal conflict among units; poor communication and distortion of information; weak, inappropriate, or incomplete control systems; inappropriate design structures; managerial incompetence; and ineffective conflict resolution mechanisms.

As discussed throughout the book, most of the health care corporations studied are well on their way to developing integrated systems of care in targeted markets. To derive a sus-

tainable competitive advantage, they must continuously differentiate a network of services relative to competitors. This will, in
turn, depend on the other three keys to success.

Behaving Like a System

To be effective in the 1990s systems will need to behave like
true systems rather than like loose collections of hospitals organized under a corporate umbrella. This challenge is particularly
acute for the newer not-for-profit health care corporations typically
made up of hospitals with a strong tradition of local autonomy
and governance. The corporate office, working with its local hospitals, must determine the best strategic role for each hospital
in the system and the best interface between the hospital and the
system. For example, to build a cost-effective network of services
in certain markets, some hospitals might be asked to give up certain services because they are better provided by another hospital within the system. Other hospitals may be encouraged to
develop new services they had not considered.

Table 11.1 outlines six criteria for assessing the degree
of "systemness" of a healthcare corporation (Shortell, 1988):

1. A common culture shared by all members of the system.
2. Systemwide financial planning and control mechanisms.
3. A formal systemwide strategic planning process.
4. Systemwide human resource planning.
5. Systemwide decision-making and information support
   systems.
6. A systemwide quality assurance program.

In general, health care corporations that have a high degree of
each will be better positioned to meet their own objectives,
to add value, and to sustain competitive advantage. For systems
with hospitals in geographically concentrated areas, these criteria will help facilitate integration of services needed to develop cost-effective continuums of care. In the final analysis,
the ability to develop clinically and managerially integrated services in targeted markets will most influence system success.

Table 11.1. A Typology of Hospital Systemness Based on Relational Attributes and Behavioral Processes.

Criteria	Degree of Systemness		
	Low	*Intermediate*	*High*
Common Culture	Individual hospitals maintain their own cultures, which have little in common with each other or with the system as a whole. Individual hospitals refer to the corporate office as "they."	There is a well-articulated systemwide mission statement, but this mission is not yet fully reflected in behavioral norms shared by each hospital in the system. Participants identify more strongly with the individual hospital than with the system. "What are they doing for us?"	There exists a highly articulated mission statement and set of behavioral norms shared by each hospital within the system. Participants identify at least as much if not more with the system than with the individual hospital. "What are we doing to help the system succeed?"
Financial Planning/ Control	Each hospital retains its own profit (loss), handles its own cash management, and develops its own financial controls. Budgets are approved locally.	Profit (loss) is shared between the hospital and the system; individual hospitals are granted some latitude in cash management and development of their own financial controls. Corporate office provides budgetary guidelines, but budgets are largely approved locally.	Profits (losses) are shared systemwide. There is systemwide cash management, and systemwide financial control policies and incentives. All capital acquisition is done systemwide. Corporate office approves all budgets.
Strategic Planning	Each hospital develops and implements its own strategic plan with little or no input from regional or corporate offices. Local hospital board maintains strong policy-making authority.	Corporate office sets guidelines, but each individual hospital continues to develop its own plans and is free to depart from corporate guidelines. There is relatively little interaction between and among hospitals, regions, and corporate office. Local hospital board retains most of the authority.	A formal, systemwide strategic plan is conducted with input from all hospitals and a high degree of interaction between and among hospitals, regions, and corporate office. The local hospital board, while active in the process, is advisory only.

Table 11.1. A Typology of Hospital Systemness Based on Relational Attributes and Behavioral Processes, Cont'd.

Criteria	Degree of Systemness		
	Low	*Intermediate*	*High*
Human Resource Planning	Each hospital determines its own staffing needs, recruitment policies, performance appraisal systems, and reward systems.	Corporate office sets system guidelines, but individual hospitals largely develop their own human resource plans with relatively little interaction between and among hospitals, regions, and corporate office. Some coordination exists in recruitment and labor representation but no common salary or fringe benefit policies have been developed.	There is a systemwide plan for the identification of staffing needs, clinical and management development of personnel, recruitment policies, performance appraisal, and rewards. Uniform salary and fringe benefit policies exist, with deviations permitted only to the extent that local market conditions dictate.
Decision and Input Support Systems	Each hospital has its own management information system, local resources for market research, freedom to purchase from local suppliers, etc.	System guidelines and consultation are provided, but individual hospitals largely develop their own management information support systems, marketing research capabilities, etc.	A systemwide management information system is used by all hospitals, systemwide market research and analysis capability exists, systemwide guidelines exist for new product and new service development, and systemwide bulk purchasing arrangements are used by each hospital.
Quality Assurance	Each hospital has its own quality assurance plan and physician credentialing.	The system sets quality assurance and physician credentialing guidelines and offers assistance, but each hospital largely develops its own quality assurance and physician credentialing plans. There is relatively little interaction between and among hospitals, regions, and corporate office.	A systemwide quality assurance plan is used by all hospitals. Efforts are made for systemwide credentialing of medical staff and health personnel, review of privileges and reappointment, and disciplining of staff members. Explicit quality assurance improvement targets and objectives are established for all hospitals within the system.

Source: Shortell, 1988. Reprinted by permission of Health Administration Press.

Exhibit 11.1. "Systemness" Rating Scale.

In regard to each of the following characteristics, where do you place your organization on the scale?

1. The extent to which your organization's hospitals and other health care organizations share a common culture.

   1   2   3   4   5   6   7
   Low   Medium   High

2. The extent to which there is systemwide financial planning and control

   1   2   3   4   5   6   7
   Low   Medium   High

3. The extent to which there is integrated, systemwide strategic planning.

   1   2   3   4   5   6   7
   Low   Medium   High

4. The extent to which there is integrated systemwide human resource planning.

   1   2   3   4   5   6   7
   Low   Medium   High

5. The extent to which there are integrated systemwide decision and input support systems (market research, management information systems, etc.).

   1   2   3   4   5   6   7
   Low   Medium   High

6. The extent to which there is an integrated systemwide quality assurance program.

   1   2   3   4   5   6   7
   Low   Medium   High

7. The extent to which clinical services between and among facilities are coordinated and integrated with each other.

   1   2   3   4   5   6   7
   Low   Medium   High

8. Overall, the extent to which your organization behaves as an integrated system.

   1   2   3   4   5   6   7
   Low   Medium   High

Exhibit 11.1 provides a simple rating scale that systems can use to assess where they stand on these criteria.

In pursuing systemness, health care corporations will continue to face the issue of simultaneous centralization and decentralization. A recent study of home office functions in forty-five leading British companies helps to sharpen the relevant questions that American health care corporations should be asking (Cresap, 1988). What core tasks can be performed only by the corporate office and cannot, therefore, be delegated? What functions and services might be best provided by the corporate office based on cost-effectiveness criteria? What functions and services might best be provided by the corporate office because they add greater overall value than if they were provided by subsidiary units?

To answer the first question, nondiscretionary tasks would include defining the overall corporate mission, philosophy, and global objectives, selecting and monitoring overall financial targets and setting investment policy, conducting external relationships and managing key external stakeholders, including those involved with capital markets and the larger political economy surrounding the industry, meeting legal statutory requirements, and managing senior executive resources, including succession planning.

The second set of tasks to be determined on cost-effectiveness grounds might include such activities as centralized purchasing, insurance and risk management, marketing research support staff, and a labor relations office. These activities could be done by individual units but would be more costly than if provided centrally. Also, central provision might create greater expertise and faster learning.

The third set of value-added tasks might include establishing a systemwide office of medical affairs, quality assurance, technology transfer, research and development, an office of prepaid plans, or an office of HMO and PPO contract negotiations. These activities enable the corporate office to provide a wider range of short-run and long-run potential benefits to the entire system on issues that cut across individual units.

The British study also identified four styles of corporate office–individual unit interface: hands off, guiding, directing, and running (see Figure 11.1). In the hands-off model, corporate staff act only as functional experts and consultants to division and unit managers; individual divisions have maximum autonomy. In the guiding model, activities that add value to the operating units are emphasized. The corporate staff primarily serve as coordinators and help to establish interdivisional and interunit linkages. In the directing model, corporate staff are more directly involved in operating and decision-making responsibilities, particularly through cost-effective central services such as purchasing, marketing, and related support systems. Corporations using this model often recruit corporate staff from

Figure 11.1. Activity Allocations Between the
Corporate Office and Hospitals for Various Models.

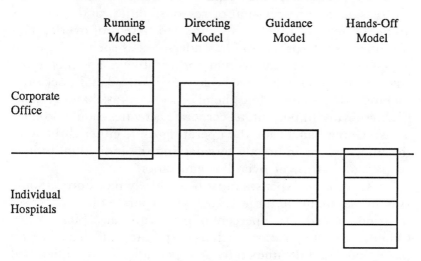

Source: adapted from Wrigley, 1970.

among managerial ranks, and there is a good deal of exchange
between the operating units and the corporate offices. In the
running model, the corporate office becomes directly involved
in the day-to-day management of the operating units.

Most of the health care corporations studied were in a
guiding stage, with some moving toward a more active directing stage. This is supported by other recent national data in-
dicating that by 1995 over 90 percent of the corporate
headquarters of hospital systems will provide "guidance" activities
in the areas of information systems and in-house management
training, while over 50 percent will provide clinical consultation. In addition, over 90 percent will provide "directing" activities such as purchasing and procurement, insurance and risk
management, personnel and human resources support, marketing and advertising support, labor relations, HMO and PPO
contract negotiations, and prepaid health plan development (Arthur Andersen & Co. and the American Hospital Association,
1987). This is in addition to the nondiscretionary core tasks
reserved for corporate management.

Regardless of the approach taken, it is important that all involved, particularly the hospital operating units, understand the reasons for the division of responsibilities, and that roles and expectations are clearly delineated. Areas of overlap and "fuzziness" or "gaps" should be understood as such and viewed as opportunities for innovation and creativity. For this to occur, the operating units must be actively involved in the decision-making process, including the allocation of tasks and responsibilities. Most important, all corporate activities should produce a discernible benefit for the operating unit, either directly to the unit itself or indirectly by enabling the individual unit to be part of a stronger overall organization.

Corporate expenses must be carefully monitored. Some systems set financial targets, such as corporate office expenses must not exceed 3 to 5 percent of gross revenues (Bice, 1989). Others set staffing ratios, such as corporate staff should be no more than .02 full-time-equivalent per adjusted occupied bed or twenty corporate staff for a 1,000-bed system (Green, 1989). Finally, it is important to remember that each corporate office model requires a somewhat different set of staff skills. For example, a directing model requires greater operational skills and experience than a guidance mode, which relies more on support skills. In either case, the skill mix must be matched to the model selected (of course, the selected model may be determined somewhat by the availability of existing skills). The winning health care corporations of the 1990s will work on achieving these matches as a necessary requirement for behaving like a true corporate system.

Hospital-Physician Partnerships

The previous chapters have highlighted the importance of developing effective hospital-physician partnerships across all strategic orientations. These relationships are currently in a state of flux. Some hospitals are modifying their current medical staff organization structures by extending the terms of office for the president and president-elect to assure greater continuity of leadership; by adding additional members to the medical executive committee to provide broader input; by allowing younger physicians to participate as nonvoting members, to cultivate future staff leadership; by adding additional physicians as voting members of the board of trustees; by increasing physician input into strategic planning; by adding full-time or part-time medical directors or executive vice-presidents for medical affairs to play key communication and liaison roles between board, medical staff, and management; and by adding full-time and part-time paid section chiefs to provide better oversight of quality assurance activities.

Others have moved beyond these changes to develop parallel organizations of physicians to deal with the economic issues facing both hospitals and physicians (Shortell, 1985). These organizations take many forms: independent practice associations (IPAs), professional practice associations (PPAs), common provider entities (CPEs), and more recently joint physician-hospital organizations (PHOs). They are typically a subsegment of a hospital's medical staff, representing the more loyal, higher admitting physicians. Their purpose is to negotiate managed care contracts with purchasers, to protect both physician and hospital economic interests. Sometimes they also develop and oversee specific joint ventures between the hospital and selected physicians. The more effective ones typically involve selecting the most cost-effective physicians on the staff, strictly monitoring physician use of resources, and reviewing compliance with quality assurance indicators. In some cases, an independent group of physicians provides services to the hospital.

Most of these relationships have resulted in a relatively neat separation of roles and responsibilities between the hospital medical staff and the parallel organization. The medical staff concentrates on hospital issues related to credentialing, termination of privileges, continuing education, and quality assurance. The economic transactions and relationships are the responsibility of the parallel organization. However, as the parallel organizations continue to grow and take on added responsibilities for supervising their members, including many of the quality assurance and utilization functions currently performed by the medical staff, the neat demarcation between the two could blur.

Currently the responsibilities for quality assurance are separated on the basis of inpatient care (medical staff's responsibility) versus ambulatory care (parallel organization's responsibility). However, it is likely that the more integrated delivery systems of the 1990s will require corresponding integrated quality assurance and credentialing systems.

The net result is that the balance of power and influence may shift to the physicians associated with the parallel organization. If they are also the hospital's medical staff leadership, few problems may exist. But if they diverge, executives will have an additional conflict situation to deal with. What do you do, for example, when the current chief of your medical staff not only does not belong to the alternative parallel physician/hospital organization but was actually turned down by it? This is not merely a hypothetical question. It is the situation currently facing one executive. And it will occur more frequently throughout the 1990s as strategic power relationships are realigned (Carper and Litschert, 1983).

One thing appears clear: both hospitals and physicians will be choosing their "first team." While many physicians, particularly specialists, will continue to hold appointments at two or three hospitals in an area, economic pressures will force them to develop a primary identification with one. Similarly, hospitals with a medical staff of 400 to 600 will be forced to select a smaller group of 150 to 200 or so loyal physicians with whom they will actively work as partners for mutual economic and professional survival. For both sides, there will be winners and losers, good choices and poor choices. And the consequences of having made the wrong choice will be increasingly high.

To help ensure that the "right" decisions are made, the winning hospitals and the physicians associated with them are likely to adhere to the following guidelines.

For Hospitals

- Select and develop physicians whose practice habits and career goals are consistent with the hospital's strategic orientation. Prospectors must place greater emphasis on entrepreneurial-oriented physicians willing to innovate and to take on some degree of risk. Defenders must make sure that they have a nucleus of cost-conscious physicians committed to helping the hospital maintain its market share. Analyzers require some of both, and reactors require physicians who can tolerate a great deal of ambiguity and what appears to be random experimentation.

- Develop a short-run and long-run human resources plan for medical staff recruitment and physician practice development linked to the institution's strategic orientation. Determine the number and mix of physicians by specialty needed to accomplish the institution's goals in the short run and in the long run. Also, determine the number and mix needed to gain a sustainable competitive advantage.

- In considering physicians for the "first team," look beyond the high admitters. Make sure to target physicians who may not be the highest admitters but may bring in high dollar volume, such as cardiologists and cardiovascular surgeons. Make sure to consider physicians who may be low-volume admitters but who are big channelers of referrals to others on the staff. Make sure to consider physicians who may be neither high admitters nor referral sources but who act as important "brokers" between the two by serving as consultants. Make sure to consider politically influential physicians whose support may be particularly helpful in working out economic transactions. Most importantly, make sure to consider selected younger physicians who are likely to emerge as tomorrow's high admitters, high revenue generators, referral sources, brokers, or political influentials.

- Be careful about playing in the medical superstar wars. Stealing a nationally known high revenue-generating physician from a competing hospital poses at least four potential problems. First, make sure you have the support staff, equipment, and related resources to sustain the superstar in the long run. If you are not willing or able to make a long-run commitment beyond the initial recruitment package, think twice. Second, be prepared to deal with the jealousies and hurt feelings among existing staff members who are either passed over or who resent having so much of the hospital's resources spent on one individual. The contribution of the superstar to the well-being of other physician practices and to the overall well-being of the institution must be communicated clearly and demonstrated persuasively. Other physicians must recognize the value-added potential of the superstar. Third, be prepared for the competing institution to make a counterattack on some of your own stars, particularly those who feel they were passed over in the process. Finally, be prepared to counterattack any subsequent offers for your newly acquired star. Having jumped once, he or she may jump again for an even better opportunity. A fair number of academic medical center–affiliated hospitals around the country can attest to this experience.

However, if you have an opportunity to significantly improve your competitive position by acquiring a superstar, do it. But do it with your eyes open and with full recognition of the costs involved as well as the rewards. Most importantly, be sure that it is consistent with the hospital's overall strategic orientation and be prepared to work hard to make sure that the temporary advantage is turned into a long-run sustainable competitive advantage.

• Do not ignore chemistry. Select physicians who work well with each other, who trust each other, who can disagree with each other while maintaining respect, who are willing to do the same with hospital management, who are willing to learn new things, and who are willing to pay at least some of the price for succeeding in the new environment. At the margin, be willing to trade off a high-volume, troublesome physician for a lower-volume physician who is a team player. In many sports, the winners are often those with the best team, not necessarily the best raw talent.

For Physicians

• First, figure out what you want from your professional career, both in the short and in the long run. How do you want to practice medicine in the 1990s? Do you want to be practicing medicine in the year 2000?

- Once you have figured out what you want from your career, choose a hospital whose short-run and long-run strategic interests are largely compatible with your own. In particular, look at who your medical colleagues will be, by number and specialty, and evaluate how much they will help you practice high-quality medical care.
- Commit to a hospital that is financially strong and that is a major player in its market, including involvement in managed care plans. This will help to assure that it will be able to keep up to date technologically and will be able to recruit the best available nurses and ancillary professional staff.
- Commit to a hospital that has strong strategic board and executive leadership. In many respects this is the most important criteria, because if this exists, all the above will follow — financial strength, strong market presence, technological sophistication, and high-quality support services. Look for a board and executive team that understand modern medicine, appreciate the challenges facing physicians, and want to work with you in offering better health care to the community within the context of realistic economic objectives.
- Commit to a hospital that will give you a voice in its management and governance and provide you with reasonable control over your destiny. Select a hospital where physicians are actively involved at the governing board level and in the strategic planning and implementation processes of the institution, and where physician input is sought early in the decision-making process.
- Select a hospital with a reputation for strong medical staff leadership in its executive committee, a strong commitment to continuously improving the quality of medical care, and strong clinical and management information systems in support of cost-effective care.

Above all, the first team physicians and the first team hospitals will recognize that they are in a relationship for the long run. Like a good marriage, there will be setbacks and squabbles, but they will also discover the tools needed to deal with them effectively. Over time, the relationship will become more attractive than available alternatives. They will learn to keep moving on together.

Strategic Leadership Development

Today's hospital industry must learn to think and behave strategically. Underlying all the lessons and suggestions for sustaining a competitive advantage in a new environment is the need for strategic leadership by hospital board members, top executives, and physician and nurse leaders. By *strategic leadership,* we mean the ability of these groups to work together to develop the skills needed to make a multidivisional health care corporation really work. A recent survey of multihospital system CEOs indicated that the most important skills were in leadership, strategic planning, financial planning, board relationships, and interpersonal skills (Arthur Andersen & Co. and the American Hospital Association, 1987). Based on the current study and taking a somewhat different cut, we spotlight the skills involved in managing change, negotiating, managing networks of organizations, managing markets, and managing quality.

Managing Change. Board, management, medical staff, and nursing staff must master the four steps of creating effective change discussed in Chapter Ten: create discomfort, articulate a new desired vision, take practical first steps, and provide ongoing support. Learning these skills requires training. In particular, the four groups must develop a sensitivity to the *pace* of change, learning when to speed it up and when to slow it down. Some of the steps may need to be revisited throughout the change process. At various points, key people may need to be reminded of the discomfort and disadvantage of retreating to the prior state. The advantages of attaining the new desired vision may have to be repeated many times along the way. Small, tangible successes should be celebrated and reinforced. In brief, leadership skills among health care corporations in the 1990s must be centered around the ability to manage change.

Negotiating. In the era of multidivisional organizations, alliances and consortia, alternative delivery systems, parallel organizations, joint ventures, and managed care contracting, a premium will be placed on the ability to negotiate. At least three-fourths of the health care executive's job will involve negotiation. Negotiation will come to be viewed as the art and science of bringing together financial, marketing, and strategic planning skills to obtain what is needed from the organization's stakeholders in order for the organization to meet its objectives. All the marketing, strategic planning, and financial expertise in the world will go for naught if individuals do not put it together to achieve the organization's goals. Negotiation becomes an important lens through which to view the health care dynamics of the 1990s.

Managing Networks. The challenge of the 1990s lies not so much in managing individual organizations as in managing networks of organizations. Leaders need a willingness to give up some autonomy to achieve larger advantages; a willingness to consider alliances with organizations different from one's own; an ability to establish planning, marketing, financing, and information systems that cut across organizations; and a thorough understanding of external and internal transaction costs. Health care corporation board members must see the broad picture, not just the individual parts. They must understand the needs and demands of a vertically integrated health care system, not merely the operational needs of individual units. Individual hospital executives must consider their organization's welfare within the larger context of the corporation's overall welfare. CEOs may need to subjugate what would be best for the individual hospital to what would be best for the vertically integrated system in a particular market area or region. The challenges of managing networks will place a premium on communication and negotiation skills and on people's creativity in developing alternative organization designs.

Managing Markets. Even if the trends and assumptions outlined earlier in this chapter are only approximately correct, the health care corporation will find itself primarily managing markets—not individual patients, products, or services. Managing markets means dealing with the entire continuum of services, ranging from health promotion to posthospital rehabilitation and followup home care. The markets will be determined not only by consumer and physician preferences and by location but also by major employers, who will channel patients to more cost-effective providers through various alternative delivery and managed care arrangements.

The potential interrelatedness of different segments such as the elderly and youth must be understood and managed accordingly. This requires insight and imagination. For example, a hospital not in the current study learned through focus groups that both the young and elderly in its community had a considerable interest in horseback riding, dog racing, and related activities. While it had many programs designed to appeal to the young and old segments individually, the hospital found an additional common interest in these outdoor sporting activities. As a result, the hospital is giving strong consideration to developing a specialty area in veterinary medicine and health care. The initiative is viewed as strange by many both inside and outside the hospital. The hospital's analyses to date, however, indicate that not only will a veterinary health care program pay for itself in the long run, it will also help attract new patients (human patients) both young and old. Most importantly, such a specialty, because of its very strangeness, is not likely to be imitated by others, so it probably represents a *sustainable* competitive advantage. Being somewhat strange in the 1990s will be a good thing to be.

The ability of new technology to disrupt existing markets and to create new markets must also be understood and, where possible, anticipated. Managing such markets requires skills on both sides of the patient care transaction: knowledge of the product or service characteristics needed to meet consumer needs and preferences and knowledge of where the market forces are driving consumer needs and preferences, in order to anticipate future shifts. A "managing markets" perspective also enables one to see possibilities of combining services in novel ways and, thus, to gain further advantages.

Managing Quality. Quality management goes beyond the technical proficiencies of physicians, nurses, and other health professionals directly involved in providing patient care. It extends to all aspects of the organization. As one CEO said, "We are all *directly* involved in providing patient care here, from the housekeeper to the neurosurgeon." The winning health care corporations of the future, regardless of their strategic orientation, will need to differentiate themselves to some extent on quality features — either technical, or those more closely related to patient access, comfort, convenience, and service. Evidence from other industries indicates a generally positive relationship among high quality, market share, and profitability (Buzzell and Gale, 1987), and there is preliminary evidence suggesting the same for health care (Binns, 1989).

A true commitment to quality, of course, must begin at the top — the board, top executive team, and physician leadership. It must permeate the strategic vision. It must be reflected in the standards the leaders set for the organization and for themselves. It must be reflected in the criteria for recruiting and orienting physicians, nurses, and all those associated with the institution. It must be reflected in the organization's human resource policies, performance appraisal mechanisms, and reward systems. It must be modeled on a daily basis. It must be reflected in the pressure professionals exert on each other to be better. It must not be compromised. It must be behavior and not just intention, reality and not just talk, fact and not fiction.

In the 1990s health care organizations increasingly will be rewarded based on the quality of their patient outcomes. Those achieving better outcomes will be rewarded with greater payment and additional patients. Those with poorer outcomes will suffer lower payments and fewer patients. Further, as health care organizations put together integrated systems of care in local and regional markets, they will increasingly be held accountable for the *health status* of the population in their areas (Seay and Sigmond, 1989). While the 1990s will see the evolution of organizational outcome indicators (for example, condition-specific severity-adjusted mortality), the first decade of the twenty-first century will see the development of organizational accountability based on population-based indicators (for example, the functional health status of community residents). The winning health care corporations are already preparing for such an event.

Taking Care of Immediate Needs: Developing the Board

The need for bold, enlightened hospital executive leadership that forges new effective partnerships with physicians is exceeded only by the need to strengthen the governing boards of America's health care corporations and hospitals (Delbecq and Gill, 1988; Kovner, 1985; Griffith, 1987; Shortell, 1989). In the current study, we could count on one hand the number of times hospital governing boards played a key leadership role in initiating strategic change or even in reassessing the hospital's strategic direction. In most cases, the impetus came from the corporate office or individual hospital executive leadership. In more than a few cases, these efforts were actually thwarted by a weak governing board. In a few cases, the initiative came from physician leaders who had to overcome the inertia of both the board and hospital executives.

Too many hospital boards remain too large, too representation oriented, lacking in relevant expertise, too process- and consensus-oriented, too conservative, too operationally oriented, and, in a few cases, too lazy. They must become smaller, expertise-focused rather than worried about representation, decision-oriented and results-focused and less process-oriented, quicker acting, more strategic, more visionary, more risk taking, and, simply put, more energetic. In the process, more CEOs will become board chairs (similar to other industries), more board members will be paid, and accreditation standards will require more rigorous board self-evaluation. Some boards have already made these changes, and many are in the process of doing so (Alexander, Morlock, and Gifford, 1988). But a fair number still have a long way to go. Sadly, in at least a few cases, by the time they get there they will no longer have an institution to govern.

Particularly important to the success of health care corporations in the 1990s will be the working relationship established between the corporate and individual unit boards. The simultaneous need for centralization and decentralization will serve as a useful guideline. To develop integrated systems of care and respond quickly to national changes in the environment, corporate boards will need to have considerable authority in developing and overseeing corporate policy and holding individual units and divisions accountable. Corporate board members must have great abilities to generate alternatives and to understand the implications of national health policy for their own region of the country. They must understand health care as broadly defined and recognize the interdependency of its various components.

Increasingly, individual hospital boards will become advisory rather than policymaking in nature. Their primary goal will be to help assure quality of care in the local area, to assess local market needs, to provide strategic guidance and direction to local hospital and physician leaders, and, in the process, to help assure that the local hospital is playing its strategic role effectively for attaining corporate objectives.

In all board development efforts, the need for clinical input will increase and so, therefore, will the need for greater involvement of physicians and nurses. In all board development efforts, linkages with the boards of the newly merging parallel or alternative physician-hospital organizations will need to be made. Above all, they will need flexibility. In this sense, flexibility is like a rope, made up of interwoven strands of board, management, and medical staff and nursing staff leadership. Of course, you can also hang yourself with a rope. But the four groups will need to take the risk.

Summary

Health care corporations and their member hospitals will continue to be tested in the 1990s in both performance and values. The most important and informative lens for viewing the action will be the institution's strategy-making process. The key to success will be the ability to first identify and then sustain competitive advantages. Organizations that can develop an appropriate set of diversified yet integrated services in defined markets; can behave like a true system (that is, like a true corporation); can forge effective working partnerships with physicians; and can engage in strategic leadership development have the best shot at success. Perhaps the most fundamental lesson to carry into the 1990s is that the ability to sustain a competitive advantage involves a process of continual renewal.

12

The Model Revisited: Directions for Further Research

The model presented in Chapter Two was intended to provide a reasonably compact and yet realistically comprehensive framework for the analysis of strategic adaptation. Although the model is based in the current literature, large parts of it were derived from the experience of the present study, which contributed four primary insights: (1) a deeper understanding of why some organizations faced with a significant environmental jolt change their strategies and why some do not; (2) evidence suggesting that not all strategies are necessarily equally viable in a given environmental state; (3) a greater elaboration of the administrative domain of what it means to manage a prospector, defender, analyzer, and reactor; and (4) the development of certain "switching lessons" to guide organizations changing from one strategic orientation to another. The study also provides some understanding of the role that ownership (for-profit versus not-for-profit) plays in the strategic adaptation process. Each of these is highlighted below, followed by suggestions for further research involving (1) the relationship among strategic fit, organizational life cycles and environmental shifts; (2) the relationship between strategic fit and sustaining competitive advantages; (3) the relationship between strategic adaptation and the top management team; (4) the issue of strategic adaptation in multidivisional organizations; and (5) the relationship between strategic adaptation and interorganizational networks.

To Change or Not to Change?

"Should we change too?" That is the question facing the top management team when presented with a significant change in the organization's environment. We found that the answer depended on management's assessment of whether the *current* strategy could deal with the environmental shift and whether the organization was *able* to implement strategic change if change seemed desirable. Overall, approximately half of the hospitals studied changed their strategies, and half did not.

We found that analyzer hospitals and prospector hospitals were least likely to change their strategies in response to the introduction of PPS in 1983, and defenders were most likely to change. Because the nature of the environmental shift was to encourage lower-cost, out-of-hospital treatments, greater competition, and alternative revenue sources while controlling in-patient costs, most analyzer CEOs felt that remaining an analyzer (with both a prospector domain, emphasizing some diversification, and a defender domain, emphasizing cost containment and operational efficiency) best positioned them to meet the environmental demands. Nearly one-third of the prospectors felt that sticking with their strategy made the most sense. Interestingly, of those prospectors that did change, 77 percent became analyzers; none became defenders. In contrast, most executives of defender hospitals felt that the defender strategy was inappropriate in the new environment. Of the 83 percent that switched, 75 percent became analyzers.

In addition to assessing the correctness or appropriateness of a given strategy, executives had to assess the *feasibility* of implementing a change. We found that this involved considerations of the organization's strategic comfort zone—the demands that the new strategy would place on current skills, knowledge, experience, resources, and ways of doing things. Not only might these considerations prevent desired changes from being made, but more importantly, they might channel the nature of any change undertaken. For the most part, we found that the desirability of making certain strategic changes was stronger than considerations of implementation problems.

Nonetheless, the concept of a strategic comfort zone largely governed the direction in which the strategic changes were made. Overwhelmingly, the majority (65 percent) of the changes took place within the organization's comfort zone. Going outside the comfort zone requires deeper changes in basic culture, not merely changes in peripheral properties. Thus, it appears that executives who initiate strategic changes in the face of significant environmental disruption do so within a zone of relative compatibility with existing organizational resources, knowledge, and skill base. While there were relatively few performance differences between those who stayed within their comfort zone and those who did not, the few differences that existed generally favored those who stayed within their comfort zone. One issue requiring further research is the extent to which such differences might become more pronounced over time.

Are Some Strategies Better Than Others?

Based on present findings, it does not appear that all strategies lead to the same desired performance outcomes. Contrary to suggestions in the current literature (Miles and Snow, 1978; Hambrick, 1981), not all strategies are equally viable. It appears that in rapidly changing industries such as health care, proactive strategies such as the prospector and analyzer, which emphasize experimentation, innovation, risk taking, diversification, and continual differentiation of new products and services, are likely to be more effective. The present evidence indicated that prospectors and analyzers consistently outperformed defenders on most key performance dimensions. Defenders appeared to recognize the inappropriateness of their strategy: the majority shifted to another strategic state, most becoming analyzers. It is possible to argue that a well-executed defender strategy with a disciplined strategic planning and control process and strong cost-containment practices can succeed even in a turbulent

environment. In fact, defenders who had more disciplined planning and control and who enforced strict cost-containment practices did appear to do better, but were still not as generally successful as the prospectors and analyzers. Also we found that the
more successful defenders had begun to develop some diversification initiatives and so resembled analyzers, if not prospectors.

The finding that a more prospector-oriented strategy appears to be more successful in rapidly changing environments
opens anew the investigation of the environment-strategic fit relationship (Venkatraman, 1986). It may be that prospector
strategies are favored only when the environmental change supports (or demands) innovation, diversification, and risk taking,
as, for example, in deregulated industries. For instance, studying the airline industry Cheng and Kesner (1988) found that
prospectors responded more forcefully to deregulation than other
strategic archetypes (although performance was not examined).
Studying small manufacturing firms in turbulent environments,
Covin and Slevin (1989) found a positive relationship between
a prospector-oriented strategy and performance. In contrast,
when the environmental change involves reregulation or stricter
regulation, a defender-oriented strategy, emphasizing operating
efficiencies and cost containment, may be more effective. Where
the pace of environmental change is slowly evolving, an analyzer
strategy, which straddles the fence and covers one's bets may
be preferred. The current findings, suggesting that certain environmental states may indeed favor specific strategic orientations, could be extended with additional research that linked
specific environmental characteristics such as the rate, uncertainty, and complexity of change to the performance of specific
strategic orientations.

Elaborating the Administrative Domain

There has been little research on what it means to manage
a prospector, defender, analyzer, or reactor. Miles and Snow
(1978) identify some general characteristics likely to be associated
with the different strategic archetypes — for instance, prospectors should engage in broad rather than intensive planning and

defenders should engage in intensive planning with centralized control—but these have gone largely unexamined.

We found that for prospectors the major administrative challenge was to coordinate their diversification activities in a way that created market synergies. Usually this was accomplished through a "guided autonomy" approach in which local units identified market opportunities and assumed operational responsibility for meeting market needs but did so within a framework of overall corporate guidelines, mission, and philosophy. There was simultaneous centralization and decentralization of strategic planning functions and decision processes. Using this approach, prospectors had greater overall perceived quality of strategic planning, market research, and implementation capability and also scored highest on plan innovativeness.

For defenders, the major administrative challenge was to develop sufficient discipline to pursue cost-containment initiatives, including consolidating or divesting selected services. This appeared to require a greater degree of centralization of strategic planning processes than existed. But contrary to conventional wisdom, defenders also had some need for selective diversification and differentiation for which a strong market research capability was important.

The major administrative problem facing analyzers was the need to coordinate their prospector and defender domains. This may require some administrative restructuring. But, most importantly, analyzers have great need for second-order learning that challenges underlying assumptions. For this to occur, analyzers need considerable investment in their information systems and board and management development programs.

The major administrative problem facing reactors was the need for strong, consistent leadership to articulate a strategic vision that key stakeholders support. This must be accompanied by a disciplined strategic planning and control process that gives some emphasis to both cost containment and new services and new markets.

In addition to these somewhat strategy-specific requirements, we also uncovered a number of administrative requirements that cut across all strategies. All archetypes need to (1) be able to manage some degree of diversification; (2) have slack resources available to pursue new initiatives and to implement current strategies; (3) emphasize market research as an important means of organizational learning; (4) make use of both centralized and decentralized planning and decision-making processes ranging along a continuum involving various degrees of guided autonomy; (5) develop mechanisms for effective involvement of key professionals; and (6) assess and generally work within the organization's strategic comfort zone. These findings suggest some characteristics of administrative domains that may be common to all strategic archetypes in addition to the unique requirements currently highlighted in the literature (Miles and Snow, 1978).

Switching Lessons

Unlike Smith and Grimm's (1987) findings for the railroad industry, we did not find consistent performance differences between those hospitals that switched strategies and those that did not. Partly this is because a number of hospitals *remained* analyzers and prospectors, strategies fairly well suited to the environmental changes occurring. Thus, the first switching lesson is, refrain from jumping the ship too soon. Carefully assess the requirements of the new environment and the current strategy's ability to meet them. This involves consideration of such inherent features of strategic orientations as diversity, divisibility, reversibility, and complexity — features that must be taken into account in assessing the organization's strategic comfort zone.

But several other lessons also emerged from the qualitative interviews. For example, in a frequently changing industry, poor performance in the immediate past should be a signal that a shift in strategy may be needed. A redoubling of current efforts is not likely to win the day. There is also the need for a strong interpretive process (environmental assessment, competitor analysis, and so on) by the top management team; an openness to change; a realistic assessment of the organization's capabilities for change; and a thorough understanding of the change process, from creating discomfort to providing ongoing support.

Finally, from a process perspective it appears to be easier to change strategies if the organization stays within its strategic comfort zone.

The Ownership Issue

We also examined the effect of ownership differences on a wide range of issues, including strategic orientation, the likelihood and direction of strategic change, strategic planning and control practices, and performance. In a service industry undergoing rapid change, such as health care, whether the firm is set up as a for-profit or a not-for-profit organization appears to make little difference on these issues. The major exception is that not-for-profit organizations with a strong philosophical commitment to providing services for which they are not reimbursed (such as hospitals serving the poor and medically indigent) have somewhat less strategic flexibility than competitors without such a commitment. At least two of the not-for-profit systems could not walk away from their commitment to serve the poor without calling into question the very existence of the system. At the same time, however, the longer-run strategic flexibility of the investor-owned hospitals was constrained by the pressure from Wall Street to meet short-run earnings objectives.

There were some ownership differences, however, in selected areas of strategic behavior. Not-for-profit hospitals, for example, were generally more diversified in specific service offerings than their investor-owned for-profit counterparts. Not-for-profit hospitals perceived strategic planning and control as more centralized but expressed greater satisfaction with the strategic planning assistance provided by corporate office than the investor-owned for-profit hospitals, for which strategic planning and control were more decentralized. The investor-owned system hospitals, however, were perceived to do a better job of involving physicians in their strategic planning, management, and governance processes. None of these differences, however, was associated with differences in performance. Investor-owned system hospitals were somewhat more profitable than the not-for-profit system hospitals, but the differences in profit margins were narrowing.

During the study period, many of the not-for-profit hospitals studied, as well as other hospitals in the industry at large, established for-profit subsidiary corporations to better adapt to the new environmental requirements. It may be that in industries experiencing rapid and significant environmental change, ownership forms begin to blur in complex ways. The strategic implications of change in ownership form and ownership "blurring" deserve further attention in the literature.

Areas for Further Research

Strategic Fit, Organizational Life Cycles, and Environmental Shifts. To advance our understanding of strategic change, we must make closer connections among the concepts of strategic fit, organizational life cycle, and environmental change. The idea that organizations must align their strategies with the requirements of the environment has received increased attention in the literature (Ginsberg and Grant, 1985; Gray and Ariss, 1985; and Venkatraman, 1989). The notion of what it means to be "strategically fit," however, has been largely treated in a static cross-sectional fashion, ignoring the dynamic, long-run implications. The recognition that strategic orientations and strategic change may be associated with different stages of the organization's life cycle (Kimberly, Miles, and Associates, 1980) has only recently received attention (Anderson and Zeithaml, 1984; Tushman and Romanelli, 1985; Romanelli, 1988). The influence of rapid environmental shifts or jolts (Meyer, 1982) in relation to the organization's life cycle, strategic orientation, and the concept of strategic fit is largely unexamined outside the environmental selection perspective (Hannan and Freeman, 1977; Aldrich, 1979). In brief, what is needed is a rather ambitious agenda of longitudinal studies involving the examination of firms' strategies over many years, using firms at different stages of their life cycle and operating in a variety of different environments, ranging from stable and predictable to rapidly changing and unpredictable.

Within that agenda, we can ask a number of interesting questions. For example, from a dynamic perspective what does it mean to be "strategically fit"? We might distinguish between short-run and long-run fit. An organization that is fit in the short run may not be fit in the long run; an organization that is fit for today's environment may not be prepared for a radical change in that environment. In other words, in rapidly changing industries the future high performers may be those that are slightly unfit for the current environment because they are anticipating the demands of the future and making appropriate investments.

As shown in Figure 12.1, the organization that is strategically fit today may need to bank on a slowly evolving environment to remain fit over the longer run. The organization that is not fit today needs to bank on the idea that the environment will be radically different tomorrow and in a manner congruent with its orientation and capabilities. This does not rule out the possibility that the organization fit today could adjust to a radically altered environment or that today's unfit organization could not adjust to a more slowly evolving environment (see broken lines in Figure 12.1). But each of these possibilities would mean significant changes in the organization's current strategic orientations.

The above scenarios raise interesting additional questions, such as whether some strategic orientations are better suited to some organizational life cycle stages than others; how organizational life cycles and environmental factors interact to influence strategic orientation; whether organizations moving through their life cycles adopt characteristic strategic profile patterns; whether it is more or less difficult to change from one orientation to another; whether there are differences in the type and amount of learning derived from one strategic orientation versus another; and whether the concept of a strategic comfort zone is equally applicable across all life cycles and environmental situations.

The present research provides some tentative answers to some of these questions. For example, it appears that in rapidly changing environments that require new ideas and new approaches to the market, it is better to be a prospector. A greater richness and variety of learning appears to accrue from adopting prospector and analyzer strategies than defender and reactor strategies. Most changes, even in the face of a significant en-

Figure 12.1. Short-Run Versus Long-Run "Fit."

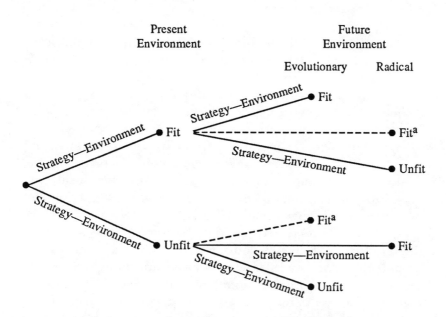

ªRequires significant change in strategic orientation

vironmental jolt, appear to be made within the organization's strategic comfort zone. We assume that in a more slowly evolving environment, changes in strategy would be made less frequently and almost exclusively within one's comfort zone, since there would be less need to consider a more radical jump. These findings, however, are for a very short time period surrounding an environmental jolt, and do not deal with organizational life cycle issues. They only suggest future issues that require exploration.

Of particular interest is the issue of how organizations learn. Burgelman (1987) suggests the need for both induced processes, which come from formal environmental assessment and related strategic planning methods, and autonomous, spontaneously generated internal processes that lead to the development of "emergent" (see Mintzberg, 1978) strategies. The relative degree of emphasis given to induced versus autonomous processes seems to vary with the nature of the environment; it also seems to be facilitated or constrained by strategic orientation. For example, in a dynamically changing environment, autonomous processes would become more important than induced, while in a stable environment the reverse might be true. Similarly, a prospector orientation might facilitate autonomous processes while a defender might facilitate induced processes. In some multidivisional organizations, however, these relationships might be more complex. For example, we found that it was often difficult for some systems to separate strategic decisions from operational decisions because strategies often emerged from the operational decisions made by individual hospitals in local markets. Further examination of how these processes function and how they evolve over time is needed.

A related issue involves the relationship between an individual firm's strategies and the firm's life cycle with that of its industry. For example, what is the relationship between industry life cycles, organizational life cycles, and the firm's strategic orientation? In relatively young industries such as computer technology, for example, are industry leaders primarily prospectors? To successfully enter such an industry, does one need to adopt a distinctly different strategic orientation to find a market niche — for example, to be a passive or active analyzer? In older, more mature industries, such as food products, do analyzers predominate? What would it take to successfully enter such an industry? What happens when an entire industry (as in the case of health care) is affected by an environmental change, compared to situations where only selected firms' local environments change (for example, local demographics, labor supply, or local tax issues)? Do certain strategic orientations predominate by industry? Are industries dominated by reactors an early warning signal of eventual demise? What does it mean to be a strategic leader and a strategic follower in different industries? These questions, of course, can be answered only by cross-industry studies and careful meta-analysis of individual industry studies to infer relevant commonalities and differences.

Strategic Fit and Sustainable Competitive Advantage. In addition to the global issues involving organizational life cycles and macroenvironments, important strategic fit questions can be raised about the firm's local market environment. This is particularly true in industries where what it means to be strategically fit depends primarily on the nature and intensity of local market competition. In these cases, strategic fit is largely determined by the ability to sustain a competitive advantage and vice versa. Given a set of environmental circumstances, the ability to sustain a competitive advantage is at the crux of the debate over strategic choice versus environmental selection. Organizations that will be able to sustain a competitive advantage over the long run will be those that can best meet today's demands and anticipate tomorrow's. The key lies in the ability to anticipate tomorrow's demands and move to meet them more quickly and more competently than competitors. To be strategically fit today says nothing about future ability to sustain competitive advantage and, in fact, may be a constraint on achieving such an advantage if most of the organization's resources are being spent on simply trying to deal with the current environment. In fact, being fit with the current environment may not even be generating any short-run competitive advantages, particularly when competitors are approximately equally fit. The organization may simply be existing in a state of strategic gridlock.

Given the above, an interesting question becomes the extent to which different strategic orientations enable a firm to sustain competitive advantage over time. This ultimately comes down to the organization's ability to provide greater value (cost relative to benefits) to greater numbers of consumers than its competitors. But as Barney (1988) notes, this also depends on the *rarity* and the *imitability* of the strategy. Thus, the key lies in developing strategies that exploit environmental opportunities in ways that have not already been thought of by very many others and that will be very difficult for others to imitate. In brief, the objective is to work toward being uniquely strategically fit.

This suggests that only in very stable industries operating in very stable environments is it possible to sustain a competitive advantage (assuming one has already achieved such a state) by staying with the current strategy. The strategy can be refined, modified, and perfected over time so that the other firms in the industry will always be a little bit behind. In most industries and most environments undergoing a reasonable amount of change, however, sustainable competitive advantage can be gained only by switching strategies. The timing of the switch (early or late), the ability to implement the switch (including the costs involved), and the extent to which the switch creates imitability barriers become the relevant issues.

The present findings shed some light on all three issues but within a very short time frame and within a specific industry setting and environmental jolt circumstances. What are needed are studies of strategic renewal of selected firms within selected industries over several decades. Few firms are known for their ability to manage strategic renewal consistently well (Burgelman, 1987). The key may lie in obtaining a greater understanding of both the induced or formalized planning and learning approaches on the one hand and the autonomous, spontaneous approaches on the other.

How do firms prepare for the future while managing the present? What does one do when it becomes apparent that the future will bear little relationship to the past? How does an organization prepare for discontinuity without self-destructing along the way?

When we consider these questions, the notion of how current strategies facilitate or impede an organization's ability to adapt to the future and the relevance of staying within one's comfort zone emerge as important and potentially helpful guides to further research. Strategies generate a complex web of people, resources, technologies, skills, norms, behaviors, decision-making structure and processes, and rewards. How closely tied to a given strategy is this web? How generalizable is it to new and different strategies? In examining firms in the microcomputer industry, Romanelli (1988) found a high level of persistence in strategies over the course of the life cycle. But when changes did occur, it was always in response to major environmental change. Further work is needed on whether such changes are successful or unsuccessful in both the short and long run and an identification of the key factors that appear to distinguish between the two groups.

Strategic Adaptation and the Top Management Team. There is renewed interest in the role played by the top management team in the strategy-making process (Hambrick, 1981; Hambrick and Finkelstein, 1987; Hambrick, 1988; Daft, Sormunen, and Parks, 1988). While the present study did not specifically address characteristics of the top management team, it was clear that individual hospital CEOs and selected corporate office executives were the primary instigators of most strategic change, as found by others (Peters and Tseng, 1983) — not hospital board members and, with some exceptions, not the hospital's physicians. The CEO and the top management team were also the central figures around which the change process described in Chapter Ten (ranging from creation of discomfort to provision of ongoing support) largely unfolded. It was beyond the realm of the present study, however, to examine the specific role played by managerial characteristics (age, past experience, and functional skill areas), executive turnover, leadership style, or related factors. Of particular interest is the question of whether given strategic orientations (prospector, defender, analyzer, reactor) not only require different top management team background characteristics, as the current literature suggests (Miles and Snow, 1978), but also whether they require different leadership, decision-making, and conflict resolution approaches? Taken at face value, one might assume that prospectors would thrive under a loose, freewheeling, risk-taking leadership style. In contrast, defenders might do better with a more centralized, conservative, and disciplined approach. Can a top management team with a conservative approach change sufficiently to move a defender along the continuum to an analyzer if that is deemed desirable? Can a top management team brought up on running a prospector change sufficiently to move it back down the continuum toward being an analyzer if that is deemed desirable? Can each recognize when the current "strategic wave" has about played itself out and jump off in time? The extent to which these issues may vary as a function of the organization's life cycle, the industry's life cycle, and the envisioned external environment are related issues of importance.

Within the context of rapidly changing global markets, international economies, and continued technological breakthroughs, it appears that organizations' needs for strategic adaptation and ongoing strategic renewal will increase. Increasingly, CEOs and the top management team will focus on initiating and guiding such changes rather than managing steady-state operations. These will involve both planned intervention approaches, such as the comprehensive collaborative approach developed by Greiner and Bhambri (1989), and the approaches that capture the spontaneous learning and opportunities arising out of the autonomous model highlighted by Burgelman (1987). An attractive feature of the comprehensive collaborative approach is its focus on the *dynamics* involved in strategic change; it considers issues ranging from CEO replacement, to the development of strategic consensus, to the implementation of motivational systems to assure consistent work force behavior. The challenge is to move beyond the current largely anatomical description of top management team characteristics to the development of "physiological profiles" emphasizing the behavioral dynamics associated with strategic renewal.

Strategic Adaptation in Multidivisional Organizations. Interest in multidivisional organizations (the M-form) continues to grow. To learn more about them, it is necessary to marry the strategic content literature (Fahey and Christensen, 1986) and strategic process literature (Huff and Reger, 1987) with the industrial organization and organization economics literature (Barney and Ouchi, 1986; Teece, 1987; Williamson, 1979; Williamson and Ouchi, 1981). This is particularly true for issues involving the relationship between the corporate office and individual divisions or units of multidivisional firms (Gupta, 1987; Hill and Hoskisson, 1987; Hoskisson, 1987; Jones and Hill, 1988). Whether a given unit or division should use the market or the hierarchy depends importantly on the nature of the transaction costs and benefits involved in the relationship with the corporate parent.

In considering this relationship, there are two sets of costs and benefits to be examined. The first involves the corporate office's assessment of the costs and benefits involved in conducting market transactions for all its divisions and units versus the internal transaction costs and benefits associated with bringing the function in-house and making it available to all units and divisions. The second set of transaction costs and benefits involve whether the individual unit decides to transact in the external market for itself or bring it inside, taking into account the various costs and benefits associated with each. The extent to which individual units are *free* to engage in the latter is a useful operational measure of the degree of autonomy enjoyed. For example, in the current study, a multiunit hospital system could choose to purchase a quality assurance program from an outside vendor and use it for all its hospitals. Or it could decide to develop its own system in-house and use it for all its hospitals. Or it could decide to let each hospital make its own decision, including whether to purchase from an outside vendor or develop its own system internally.

These decisions are likely to be influenced in an important way by the corporation's overall strategic orientation, the strategic orientations of the individual units, the degree of linkage or relatedness (technological, market, and so on) among the units and between the units and the corporate office (Govindarajan, 1988), the characteristics of the external markets involved, and the nature of the environment in which the firms function. This is a complex set of issues for the multidivisional organization to consider when assessing the need for and capability of strategic change. It requires a thorough understanding of the strategic role to be played by each unit within the corporation and each unit's market and environmental segment. This may mean that different planning and control processes are needed for defender units than for prospector or analyzer units (Simons, 1987). Also, prospectors with an emphasis on aggressive diversification may require greater need for feedforward control systems while defenders may have greater need for feedback features (Schreyogg and Steinmann, 1987). In addition, the pace of change may be different for different units given the different environments faced. This is likely to be particularly true with units that have a greater degree of unrelated diversification. In such situations, a relatively loose linkage to the corporate office may facilitate strategic change by the individual unit. Where the units are characterized by more highly related activities, the corporate office may be in a better position to provide certain services and functions across all units or divisions.

The point to be highlighted here is the need to consider the interplay between strategic orientation, the capability for strategic change, and the nature of multiple sets of transaction possibilities that exist for multidivisional organizations. Not only can internal transaction costs and benefits be reduced (or increased) by organizational and managerial practices within the individual firm (Mick and Conrad, 1988), but they can also be reduced (or increased) by the nature of the relationship between the individual unit and the corporate parent (Golden, 1989). The nature of these relationships, how they operate, and with what effect are all areas for further examination.

Strategic Adaptation and Interorganizational Networks. Increasingly, organizations are looking outside themselves for assistance in coping with environmental turbulence. This is resulting in a variety of interorganizational and strategic networks (see Aldrich and Whetten, 1981; Fombrun and Zajac, 1987; Jarillo, 1988; Nielsen, 1988). The very growth of hospital systems (see Chapter One) is one indicator of this trend. The hospital systems themselves are joining larger alliances and umbrella systems in an attempt to gain still greater economic and political advantages. In addition, most independent hospitals belong to various alliances or consortia to gain specific expertise and economic advantages (Luke, Begun, and Pointer, 1989). Shared service and joint venture relationships are proliferating in the health care industry and in other industries as well.

The growth of these interorganizational networks suggest several promising questions and issues for research: What are the factors behind the growth of such networks? How do such networks form in different industries; for example, what role is played by strategic groups? What are the characteristics of the networks themselves, such as their size, frequency of transactions, major strategic purpose, and so forth? Are there differences in the *organization* of interorganizational networks across different industries? How successful are interorganizational networks in achieving their objectives as a network and in meeting member needs? What are the organizational life cycle dynamics of interorganizational networks themselves, including rates of additions and deletions over time? Can networks replenish themselves? What are the "mega-strategies" of interorganizational networks? Do they have prospector, defender, analyzer, and reactor orientations analogous to those of the individual organizations that make them up? Do prospectors, defenders, analyzers, and reactor organizations have a different propensity to join networks? What specific role does the network play in an individual organization's strategic planning process? Is it possible that an organization that desires to move to a particular strategic orientation but lacking the capacity can gain such capacity through its involvement in a network?

As we can see from these questions, the research agenda includes treating the interorganizational network itself as a unit of analysis, in addition to the individual organization and the dyadic relationship between the individual organization and the network. Advances in our understanding of strategic adaptation will increasingly involve examination of interorganizational networks and even "networks of networks."

Concluding Observations

It is evident that greater attention needs to be given to longitudinal studies, including those of a retrospective, prospective, and processual nature. Time series data and archival data are useful for establishing the timing of significant changes and environmental shifts and for documenting their effect, but are inadequate for understanding the process dynamics involved. For that, primary data collection using questionnaires, interviews, and observation must be used to interpret current and past events and also in prospective studies designed to capture the dynamics of strategic adaptation as it unfolds. Such studies are expensive and time consuming, but are the price that must be paid if our knowledge of strategic change and strategic adaptation is to advance.

Implicit in this recommendation is the need for a triangulated approach to the study of strategic adaptation, involving the use of multiple methods, research designs, and testing of competing theories both within and across studies. Quantitative approaches involving time series analysis, pooling of cross-sectional data, and multivariate modeling of outcomes must be integrated with qualitative approaches emphasizing single case studies and longitudinal comparative case studies to obtain a fuller understanding of the adaptation process and its effects. While quantitative data can tell us something about what happened and with what effect, qualitative data are frequently needed to address issues of how and why things happened as they did. A regression coefficient may tell us that prospectors enjoy greater market share than defenders in a rapidly changing environment but cannot tell us anything about what it means to be a prospector or a defender or how one might move from being a defender to a prospector. For answers to these questions, one must probe through interviews, questionnaires, direct observation, and related methods to look for what is behind the regression coefficient. What does it really mean? The quantitatively oriented variable-based approach inevitably misses this level of complexity and understanding, which can be understood holistically only by looking at complete cases.

Working within the framework of triangulation, Ragin (1987) has recently suggested a novel approach to the analysis of quantitative and qualitative data based on Boolean algebra. His qualitative comparative method is particularly useful for addressing questions about outcomes resulting from multiple and simultaneously occurring causes — precisely the situation in most issues of strategic adaptation. The approach examines cases in terms of *combinations* of variables and compares the cases with different combinations holistically. Cases are in essence assigned to different causal paths. Every logically possible combination of values is examined and then simplified through the use of truth tables to arrive at the necessary and sufficient conditions for explaining a given event or outcome. Although Boolean algebra was not used in the current study, a loose application of the qualitative comparative approach was used. We found, for example, that certain factors appeared to be associated with outcomes across *all* strategic archetypes whereas others were specific only to a particular archetype (see the summary in Chapter Ten). More systematic application of the qualitative comparative method approach holds great promise for advancing the study of strategic adaptation, helping to reconcile the need to examine a relatively large number of cases for purposes of generalizability and statistical robustness with the need for greater understanding and interpretation of the dynamics and complexities of the adaptation process.

A third implication of the research agenda is the need for more sensitive and more diverse measures of strategy outcomes. The *intent* of a given strategic orientation must be understood. Interviews, questionnaires administered before the observation of strategic behavior, direct observation, and content analysis of documents (strategic plans, annual reports, and so forth) are needed to measure intent. Measures can then be developed to examine whether the objectives are achieved. These may or may not involve the typically used measures of profitability, return on equity, and market share — at least not when used exclusively at the firm level. For example, a more appropriate measure of the success of a prospector whose intent is to increase its diversification activities might be to assess the profitability and market share of those *specific activities* and not firmwide measures. Alternatively, one could look at the relative contributions of the new activities to firm-wide performance measures.

Measures also need to distinguish between the short run and the long run and take into account reasonable time periods for implementation before one would expect to observe a performance effect. For example, evaluating the financial effects of a change from a defender orientation to an analyzer orientation might most appropriately be done two to three years after the shift. In the meantime, intermediate process measures might be used, such as an increase in the number of new products, programs, or services offered or an increase in research and development expenses as a percent of revenues. Again, the need to understand the intent of a given strategy can help to distinguish between short-run and long-run indicators. For example, the decision to diversify into a new business line might be based on the intent to create long-run barriers to entry. To measure the success of such a strategy based on short-run financial ratios and profit margins would miss the point. The more appropriate measure would be the number of new competitors entering the business over time and their relative degree of success in taking away market share.

Finally, there is a need to study a wider variety of industries and firms of both a profit-making and voluntary nature. The present findings and the further questions that have been raised need to be examined in other industries. While data availability, the ease of access to field sites, and related considerations understandably govern much of what we do, a systematic approach to the selection of firms, industries, and research sites is needed. The selection should be based on theoretical considerations tied to gaps in the current literature as well as significant managerial and public policy decisions facing society. Organizational life cycles, industrial life cycles, and the rapidity of environmental change should be explicitly considered. In some cases the unit of analysis ought to be interorganizational networks or fields rather than individual organizations alone. Increased attention also needs to be given to the rapidly growing service industries and to the roles of professionals within them. This study represents an example of one effort in that direction, and it is hoped that others will follow.

13

Crafting Health Policy in the 1990s: Strengthening the Ties Between Industry Leaders and Policymakers

"We have taken about eight years off in addressing some important health care policy issues."
—W. J. McNerney

The previous chapters have examined the changing nature of the health care environment, and the ways hospitals have changed their strategy in response, and have highlighted the implications for both hospital management practice and future research. It would be easy to end the book at this point. But we believe that the study findings have important implications for public policy. Some of these deal with how health policy could be improved if there were greater understanding of the strategic composition of the industry and the strategic orientations of the firms within the industry. Others are concerned with suggestions for improving the policymaking process itself by structuring a more effective interface between the industry and governmental policymakers at all levels.

As a broad generalization, most health care policy in the United States has been based on the assumption that government enacts and institutions react. The history of public-sector health planning legislation over the past fifteen years provides ample evidence for this assertion (Foley, 1981; Kirkman-Liff, Lapre, and Kirkman-Liff, 1988). Alternatively, in the absence of government action, organizations pursue their own self-interest. This pursuit may or may not meet society's needs, particularly in areas such as health care where free-market principles operate imperfectly. A major problem, of course, has been that institutions have often acted or reacted in ways that scuttled the original policy intent (for example, cross-subsidization of hospital costs) or otherwise compromised desired outcomes. We believe this comes largely from a lack of understanding of industry and market structure, a lack of understanding of the strategic behavior of health care organizations, and a lack of appreciation for the health care organization's role as an active shaper of its local environment.

In addition, we need a policymaking process that can address the challenges posed by the current reorganization of the health care system, including the horizontal and vertical integration activities of the corporate systems examined in previous chapters. Brown has concluded that "the role that public policy can play in these matters is problematic" (Brown, 1985, p. 38). But we strike a more hopeful note.

Health Policy Themes in the 1990s

In broad terms, over the last quarter century health policy in the United States has moved from the expansionary policies of the 1940s through the early 1970s (growth in hospital facilities, personnel, and increased financial access to care) to the cost-containment and resource-restriction policies of the late 1970s to the present (rate-review programs, certificate-of-need programs, prospective payment, and managed care initiatives). In our recent concern for controlling costs, McNerney (1988) reminds us that we have forgotten or ignored the fact that we never fully delivered on our rhetoric of providing a basic set of health benefits for everyone. In the meantime, we have experienced a rapid increase in the percentage of elderly in addition to such "social surprises" as the AIDS epidemic. Also, the nation faces a federal budget deficit which will have a marked impact on all domestic social programs, and health care in particular.

National polls show that 89 percent of Americans believe the U.S. health care system needs fundamental change, far more than British or Canadian respondents believe about their systems (Blendon, 1989a). Sixty-one percent of Americans favor a system similar to Canada's government-funded insurance program but with free choice of doctors and hospitals. Thus, as we enter the decade of the 1990s there are simultaneous pressures to expand and retract the health care system; to expand services for certain groups such as the elderly, the uninsured, and the poor while keeping costs within general inflationary pressures and, at least, from eating into the country's larger public policy agenda.

The two major health policy themes in the 1990s will be (1) making tough choices based on value added (that is, greater perceived quality and improvement in health status for a given cost or lower cost for a given level of perceived quality and improvement in health status) and (2) holding individuals, organizations, and systems *accountable* for their choices. Given the budget deficit and the growing fiscal uncertainty, resources flowing to the health care sector will be carefully scrutinized. Within these resource constraints, should more money go to provide basic services for the uninsured and poor or to extend coverage for the elderly? Should more revenues go for maternal and infant child care (particularly for minorities in inner-city areas) or to the elderly? On what basis should the latest available technology be allocated to communities? Who should pay for it? How much should we invest in a cure for AIDS versus expanding resources for current treatment? Which hospitals should stay open, and which should be closed? How much are we willing to pay to attract more women and men into the nursing profession? The list of questions is almost endless, and each one raises ethical, economic, and social conundrums. The "answers" to these questions will vary depending on who is asked. But, if public opinion polls are any guide, the public would resist cutting care for the elderly and would not support explicit rationing but rather would limit care to the poor in other ways, freeze hospital charges and physician fees, limit the diffusion of medical technologies, and attempt to reduce inefficiencies (Blendon, 1988). Although no one wants to make these choices, the need for tradeoffs is clear.

Above all else, the 1990s will be the decade of accountability at all levels — federal, state, and local, and in both the public and private sectors. The new accountability player is, of course, private industry. Purchasers have gained greater power relative to providers. While this may be new to the current generation of health care leaders, it is not so different (except in scale) from what existed in the early 1900s when the railroads, mining, and lumber companies contracted with providers for medical services on a retainer or salaried basis (Light, 1987-88). Under such systems, thousands of physicians and other health professionals worked on a salaried basis.

Private payors will join with government payors in holding providers accountable for both the cost and overall quality of care provided. Providers will increasingly be paid on performance criteria, emphasizing value added. The data underpinning such systems will come from an agenda of patient outcome, treatment effectiveness, and quality of care research now being launched in a vigorous fashion (Blumberg, 1986; Wennberg, 1984; Ellwood, 1988; Brook, 1989). Medical practice guidelines and standards will become commonplace. Large employers and coalitions of small employers will have employee-specific as well as aggregate data on diagnostic-specific outcomes and costs. They will use these data in negotiations with providers. Federal and state governments will have similar data on which to base their purchasing decisions. The ability of providers to deliver the goods will become transparent.

How active will the federal and state governments be in dealing with the tough choices, and what role will they play in regard to accountability? Governmental health care policy will continue to be characterized by a combination of regulatory and competitive approaches. Competitive approaches alone, as we have learned over the past five years, will not touch the indigent care and uninsured issues, and regulatory approaches alone will not contain overall system costs. But it is also clear that those involved in marketplace competition will be held to strict standards of performance accountability. While some degree of disequilibrium may be tolerated in certain markets in the short run, it will not be tolerated in the long run. Government's role will be to set broad guidelines and establish financial and performance targets within which systems of providers can respond as they wish in organizational structure, strategy making, networking, and staffing. Providers' failure to produce, however, could bring on more invasive strategic and operational regulation — to avoid such an event, everyone needs to better understand the changing nature of the industry and some of the lessons from the present study.

Understanding the Industry

If the mid-1940s to the mid-1970s were characterized by expansionary health policies and the past decade by policies of constraint, the coming decade will be characterized by policies best described as *refocusing* and *renewal* — refocusing in the sense of establishing a basic set of benefits for all Americans; renewal in terms of recognizing what will be required of provider organizations and health care professionals to make the system work. This refocusing and renewal must begin with an understanding of the changing nature of the industry.

A Macro Framework. Porter (1980) provides a useful and widely recognized framework for analyzing industries (see Figure 13.1). The major dimensions to consider are (1) the bargaining power of buyers; (2) the bargaining power of suppliers; (3) substitutes for one's product or service; (4) the threat of new entrants; and (5) the nature and intensity of competition among firms within the industry. The potential utility of Porter's framework for health care policymaking lies in the attention it gives to considering the interdependencies among these five dimensions. These interdependencies can be examined at both a systemwide level and at the level of a specific policy intervention.

At a system level, the bargaining power of buyers (employers, health care coalitions, state and federal purchasers) in many ways has increased more than providers. One reason for hospitals consolidating into alliances and systems is to offset the

Figure 13.1. Forces Driving Competition.

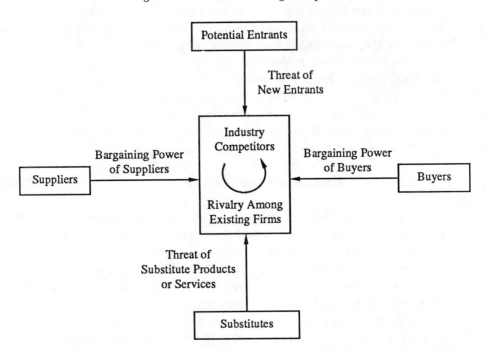

growing power of buyer groups. In fact, the growing influence and pressure of buyer groups may ameliorate somewhat antitrust concerns related to hospital mergers and consolidations. The ability of a more concentrated market to set higher prices will be mitigated by strong buyer demands for cost-effective care.

The bargaining power of suppliers (pharmaceutical, biomedical, and hospital supply companies) is in a state of flux. But, again, hospitals that join alliances and systems may find that they are in a better position to negotiate discounts with suppliers and, in some cases, to have greater access to technology.

There are a growing number of substitutes for acute inpatient hospital care as technological advances, cost-containment pressures, and consumer preferences all push for delivering more care outside the hospital. The ability to continuously differentiate a product or service, which was such an important factor in successful diversification for prospectors and analyzers (and even defenders), is essentially an attempt to stave off substitute products or services. In essence, differentiation is the process by which the organization creates its own substitutable products and services. Hospitals can be expected to continue to diversify and vertically integrate to remain competitive.

Another characteristic to consider is the threat of new entrants into the market. While study hospitals did an increasingly good job of analyzing current competitors, many lacked sufficient realism and imagination about likely future competitors, particularly in ambulatory care services. It is possible that at least half of the competing organizations in health care over the coming decade will be new to the industry. They will be drawn to the industry by relatively low barriers to entry, a growing demand for less expensive and more accessible out-of-hospital services, by a continuing interest in health promotion and overall fitness, and by more favorable payment rates for providing care to the elderly.

Some of these competitors may come from overseas as Japan and western European nations make advances in experimental therapies and related technological breakthroughs. At the same time, changes in European health policies toward experimenting with private market competitive forces, similar to the United States, may open up opportunities for U.S. hospital systems. For example, Britain's plan to provide incentives for general practitioners to choose the most cost-effective consultants and hospitals may result in a significant growth of hospital systems if they are able to achieve greater economies in providing care than freestanding hospitals.

Finally, competition among hospitals and health care organizations within the industry has intensified. Hospitals are selecting subgroups of loyal, cost-effective, high-admitting physicians for joint arrangements. Physicians with multiple appointments are beginning to identify with a single primary hospital. In effect, both hospitals and physicians are selecting their "first team" partnerships.

To illustrate the utility of the framework, let's assume the federal government provides incentives to enroll Medicare subscribers in HMOs for a fixed price, a policy designed to contain costs while providing a reasonable range of needed services. The question is, how will the industry respond to this policy?

First, the policy obviously increases the government's bargaining power, for although local delivery systems can refuse to enroll Medicare beneficiaries in HMOs, they will be hurt financially if they do. It also has a secondary negative effect on suppliers. Because HMOs have incentives to keep costs at a minimum, they will shop for the least expensive supplier who can meet established quality guidelines. Incentives will also be created to offer substitutable lower-cost services to enrollees, and HMOs will have to constantly be on guard against the possibility of substitutes for their services. In some areas, we can also expect a number of new entrants into the market, depending on the size and health status of the Medicare pool of beneficiaries.

Finally, all these considerations will be influenced by the degree of existing competition within the market. Where the competition for Medicare patients is high, we can expect the following conditions: (1) bargaining power of providers will be lower relative to the purchaser; (2) the bargaining power of suppliers will be somewhat higher (that is, the providers can be played off against each other); (3) the incentives to create substitutable products or services will be higher; and (4) the attractiveness of the market to new entrants will be somewhat lower. Where competition is less intense, the opposite conditions are likely to prevail. The important point is that the framework provides a way for policymakers to consider the likely actions and reactions of all the key groups involved—buyers, suppliers, current providers, and the likely future competitors.

Future Significance. Porter's framework takes on added significance when we consider the changing nature of the industry itself. Approximately 45 percent of the nation's hospitals already belong to a formal system, and another 30 percent or so belong to alliances or networks. Over the coming decade, the number of hospitals belonging to systems and the number of systems themselves will grow, particularly hospitals in medium-sized communities seeking greater local market power to deal with employers and managed care arrangements (Shortell, 1988). Subsequently, there will be some degree of system consolidation largely along regional lines. By the turn of the century, the composition of the industry will resemble roughly that shown in Figure 13.2, with about 80 percent of the nation's hospitals being members of a formal system. As a result the industry will be much less fragmented than it is today, but nonetheless stratified. Like good geologists, policymakers will have to understand the characteristics of the different organizational strata. National systems will be most concerned with achieving financial economies across different markets. Regional systems will attempt to link support services across markets within the

Figure 13.2. The Hospital Industry as Organizational Strata.

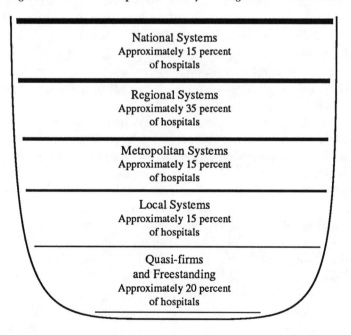

Source: Shortell, 1988. Reprinted by permission of Health Administration Press.

region. Metropolitan and local systems will focus on clinical integration of services in local markets and the erection of barriers to entry. The freestanding and quasi-firms (for example, hospitals belonging to alliances) will attempt to maintain their competitiveness while retaining their autonomy. Because of systems, the policymakers' task is reduced from having to deal with thousands of individual hospitals to several hundred health care systems with identifiable characteristics.

The relative power of buyers and sellers, substitutes for products and services, the threat of new competitors, and the degree of competition among existing firms can be overlaid on the five organizational strata. For example, national systems are likely to have a wider variety of hospitals in terms of bed capacity, service mix, and locations than metropolitan-based systems. Regionally based systems will be much more affected by policies involving the addition of new technology or policies affecting rural residents' access to health care. Metropolitan systems, on the other hand, will be heavily affected by policies involving the reimbursement of teaching costs and policies dealing with care for the uninsured and medically indigent. For each stratum the implications about relative bargaining power, substitutable products, and the threat of new entrants will be somewhat different.

For all strata, public policy implementation will be heavily influenced by the structure and intensity of local market competition. Existing research suggests that the amount of competition — whether a hospital is a sole provider, or one of two or three in a given area, or one of a dozen or more hospitals in an area — affects the number and types of services it offers (Shortell and others, 1986; Starkweather and Carman, 1987); the levels of charity care provided (Shortell and others, 1986); the level of technology used (Luft and others, 1986; Robinson, Garnick, and McPhee, 1987); and staffing ratios (Luft and Robinson, 1988). And while most competition to date has been based primarily on services and amenities rather than price (Robinson and Luft, 1985; Robinson, Luft, McPhee, and Hunt, 1988; Friedman and Shortell, 1988), recent evidence suggests that some price competition may be occurring, as evidenced by lower costs in more competitive markets (Melnick and Zwanziger, 1988). The ability to compete on both price and quality criteria is likely to be most important in the more competitive markets, particularly for metropolitan-based systems, for selected local systems, and for pockets of regional and national system hospitals.

These issues will also be greatly affected by the specific ownership and strategic configuration of hospitals in a given market. A three-hospital market, with one secular not-for-profit hospital, one religiously affiliated not-for-profit hospital, and one investor-owned hospital, is likely to behave differently than a three-hospital market composed of one not-for-profit secular, one investor-owned hospital, and one public hospital. In charity care, for example, we would expect (other things being equal) a more equal distribution among the three hospitals in the first market than in the second. To take another example, a community hospital operating in a market with a nearby teaching hospital will behave differently than a similar community hospital in an area without a major teaching hospital. In this case, other things being equal, we would expect both hospital costs and total costs to be higher in the first market than the second.

To date, most public policy has been based on attributes of the industry related to hospital bed size, ownership, teaching status, geographic region, and location (urban versus rural). We suggest the need to add to this list system size, organizational strata, and the specific characteristics of local markets, including the number and types of other hospitals and health care organizations in the market and the nature of competition among them. In addition, it is important to consider the strategic orientations of the major firms within the industry.

Understanding Strategic Orientations

Strategic orientations — and hence the likely response to changes in public policy — cannot be inferred from structural characteristics alone. What we need are *market biographies,* an accumulation of knowledge over time of the behavior of organizations in local markets.

Developing market biographies involves pooling and organizing different data sets by market area. Most but not all of the needed data already exist. Relevant items include (1) sociodemographic data on the community pertaining to age, sex, education, income, family size, median value of home, employment, mix of employers, and so on; (2) changes (additions and deletions) in the number and types of hospitals, HMOs, group practices, nursing homes, home health agencies, insurers, and related health care organizations; (3) data on hospital admissions, patient visits, and related utilization statistics; (4) the number and type of services offered; (5) personnel ratios; (6) cost, profit margins, return on equity, uncompensated care, debt to equity ratios, bond rating, and related financial indicators; and (7) data on patient outcomes and patient satisfaction. Initially, these data might be collected for a sample of major metropolitan and suburban health care markets throughout the country and selected rural markets, to experiment with different definitions of what constitutes a health care "market" (Garnick, Luft, Robinson, and Tetreault, 1987). Such data could be supplemented from time to time by in-depth selected case studies and occasional larger-scale studies such as reported in this book. Policymakers and others could use the market biography and related information to construct "what if" simulations of the likely consequences of various decisions.

Using these kinds of behavioral indicators makes it possible to develop some understanding of health care organizations' strategic orientations in given markets throughout the country, and thus extend the analysis begun in this book. Based on current findings, it is evident that most hospitals are moving away from a defender orientation to an analyzer or prospector orientation, although a significant minority are reactors. Hospitals are diversifying in a more selective fashion in attempting to continuously differentiate their services in their search to achieve some sustainable competitive advantages. They are choosing their first team of physicians and building business and professional partnerships to deliver services more cost effectively under the incentives created by managed care. For the most part, hospitals appear to be making changes within their strategic comfort zones of knowledge about their own capabilities and capacities for change. What does all this portend for public policy? What is the likely reaction of the different strategic archetypes to proposals to increase coverage for the uninsured and medically indigent? To provide catastrophic coverage for the elderly? To extend DRG-based payment principles to ambulatory care? To merge part A and part B of Medicare into a single payment? To develop a resource-based relative-value physician fee schedule? To develop incentives for enrolling Medicare beneficiaries in HMOs? To develop incentives for converting selected rural hospitals to alternative health care facilities? Answers to these questions require some knowledge and understanding of what it means to be a prospector, defender, analyzer, or reactor, in terms of both the content of such a strategy and what it takes to manage such a strategy.

Knowledge of the strategic orientations of hospitals, of other health care organizations, and of systems in given markets adds a new dimension to Porter's framework by specifying the strategic configurations of competitors within the market. For example, we found prospectors were more prevalent in more competitive markets than in less competitive markets. If a governmental policy is intended to stimulate new ideas for delivering care, markets dominated by prospectors might be targeted; defenders will have particular problems responding to such initiatives. If the goal is to achieve better linkages between inpatient care and outpatient care, markets dominated by analyzers might be targeted; some prospectors may have problems achieving such linkages. On the other hand, prospectors are likely to be most sensitive to technological obsolescence and the threat of substitute products and services. Analyzers are likely to give great attention to potential new competitors in trying to decide whether and when they should make their move into given markets. Defenders may have particular problems in dealing with managed care buyers because defenders do not have the range of services desired by the managed care purchasers. Markets dominated by reactors may be particularly ripe for new entrants and, at the same time, will be problematic for policymakers because reactors do not signal a consistent or clear strategic intent.

We can readily add to this list of possibilities. Porter's framework, combined with knowledge of the strategic orientations examined in this book, can be used to help policymakers ask a wide variety of relevant questions — which is as important as the answers. The likely outcome of this process is the realization that there are no single answers that will meet the needs of health care markets throughout the country. There can only be approximations and modifications. But these approximations are likely to be closer to the target and the modifications better anticipated if the firm's strategic orientation is considered along with market structure characteristics. It is perhaps pertinent here to re-emphasize that hospital strategic orientations contributed more to the explanation of differences in performance than such variables as geographical location or urban versus rural distinctions.

From this discussion we can derive six characteristics of the health care executive's mind set that policymakers must recognize when developing new policies.

1.   For the most part, health care executives take a local market perspective (at times, regional) on health care policies, not national. The concern is with how it will play in Peoria because, for the manager, that's where the action is.
2.   Unlike most policymakers who focus on a single policy of interest at a time, health care executives have to work with the *interdependencies* and *interplay* of *multiple* policies as they affect the organization in the local market. Some policies create incentives that move the organization in the same direction, while others are contradictory and create incentives for inconsistent behavior.
3.   Aside from the interests represented by policymakers, health care executives have multiple and often diverse constituencies to satisfy.
4.   Health care executives must work to implement public policy with a group of professionals (physicians) who are largely beyond the executives' direct control. The situation is further complicated when the public policy is aimed at hospitals but not physicians (or vice versa) or when competing incentives are established between each group.
5.   Unlike policymakers engaged in creating new legislation, health care executives have to *keep things going today* plus deal with the future. There is a business to be run.

6. Health care executives are emotionally as well as intellectually involved in their organization's mission and strategic orientation, and so are reluctant to shift gears to a new
policy without compelling reasons. Policymakers need to
think through the incentives and disincentives of a given
policy for encouraging or discouraging changes in strategic behavior.

From an organizational and strategic perspective, developing policies that promote cost-effective care becomes a question
of how federal, state, and private-sector health policy can best
promote selected diversification and effective hospital-physician
partnerships in bringing about integrated systems of care in local
markets that are accountable to the purchasers and consumers
of those services. The 1990s are likely to be neither the age of
the managerial imperative to contain costs (Brown, 1985) nor
the entrepreneurial imperative to expand services, but, rather,
of the accountability imperative to be *judicious innovators.*
To facilitate a policy of judicious innovation, industry and
government must develop a somewhat different relationship.

Developing a Productive
Government-Industry Interface

The increasing consolidation of hospitals into systems
makes it possible to develop a different kind of government/
industry interface than presently exists. No longer is one constrained to working primarily through the lobbying process with
industry and professional associations such as the American
Hospital Association, American Medical Association, and various state hospital and medical associations. While these groups
will continue to serve important and useful functions, the field
is now broadened to open up new possibilities. Certain industry-
strategic groups exist, represented primarily by the kinds of hospitals and health care systems studied, on which more targeted
and refined public policy can be developed. Various consumer
and employer groups, such as the American Association of
Retired People (AARP) and the business coalitions for health,
should be included. The national trade and professional associa-

tions remain appropriate forums for addressing across-the-board issues such as the need for increased coverage for the uninsured and a basic set of benefits for all Americans. But issues that divide various constituencies, such as urban versus rural payment differentials, physician reimbursement, and health manpower policies, may be better handled through input from local and regional health care systems and alliances and their umbrella organizations, such as the American Health Care Systems and the Voluntary Hospitals of America. In addition, these groups should participate in thinking through the implementation issues associated with proposed legislation involving the across-the-board issues. Understanding the nature of the industry, the structure and dynamics of local markets, and the strategic orientation of the major players in those markets will be of great assistance in improving the quality of public policy dialogue among the groups involved.

We propose that government and the health care industry develop a relationship analogous to the more effective corporate office–hospital unit relationships found in the present study. In brief, like the corporate office, government's role is to establish a *vision* for the American health care system consistent with the country's values, and within that vision to establish *broad policy guidelines*. Federal and state governments should also be important players in the financing of the system and in establishing standards and processes for accountability. But, like individual hospital units in the corporate office–hospital relationship, the actual organization and delivery of services should be left to the industry—the individual hospitals, group practices, nursing homes, other health care organizations and systems working with health care professionals, and consumer-employers in local markets. While the accountability issues that this strategy raises may have been very difficult to deal with ten to fifteen years ago when the industry was largely organized around thousands of individual hospitals and independent practitioners, it becomes much more feasible with the emergence of health care systems, alliances, and physician groups. The systems and alliances can serve as major sources of intermediate accountability and planning and provide public policy input and review. The situation is rather like building a new college campus and waiting to pour the concrete sidewalks until students, staff, and faculty have created their own natural pathways through the lawns. The organizational pathways of the American health care system have now been largely revealed and, to some extent, simplified. They are ready for increased two-way traffic between the public policy community and the practitioner community.

In structuring the interface, guiding criteria should include *maximum flexibility* and *early involvement*. Federal and state policy must recognize the value of local market experimentation. As Kinzer notes, "Participating systems will need to be given maximum flexibility in developing their management and governance structures and in the organization of their clinical services. The great diversity of our country in health status, practice styles, and public expectations make this seem necessary" (Kinzer, 1988, p. 32).

The need to involve systems early on in the public policy process is analogous to this study's finding regarding the importance of involving physicians early on in the hospital's strategic planning process. There needs to be joint planning and development of public policy and not merely after-the-fact lobbying for or against initiatives that have already been largely developed. Again Kinzer notes, "the most effective regulatory strategy is to spend lots of time on consultation with the regulatees before promulgation and, once promulgated, be very deliberate and painstaking with any and all efforts to change the regulation" (p. 23).

A Proposal

To illustrate how the above guidelines might be implemented, we suggest that a government/industry employer steering committee be established to deal with near term (one to three years) policy issues. (Such a relationship is similar to joint committees that exist between the Japanese government and the Japanese business community to promote industrial growth.) In addition to the Health Care Financing Administration (HCFA), the National Center for Health Services Research and Health

Care Technology Assessment (NCSHR/HCTA), the Government Accounting Office (GAO), the Secretary's Office of Health Policy and Planning, legislative staff, and other key governmental representatives, there would be representatives of the major industry trade and professional groups (American Hospital Association, American Medical Association, Health Insurance Association of America, the American College of Health Care Executives, and so on), representatives from the major systems' umbrella organizations, and representatives from several of the major systems and alliances themselves. There would also be representation from labor, business, and major consumer groups. The overall steering committee might well be twenty-five to thirty people. Their main goal would be to structure the debate surrounding the major issues at the time and to establish a work agenda to be carried out by existing governmental and private agencies and by some newly created work or study groups. The study groups would report directly to the steering committee. The National Leadership Commission on Health Care serves as a partial example of this approach.

Some elements of the work agenda, particularly those involving the need for new or additional research and analysis, would become the responsibility of such existing organizations as HCFA, NCHSR/HCTA, GAO, the Office of Health Policy and Planning, the Institute for Nursing Research, selected components of National Institute of Health, the Institute of Medicine, university policy and health services research centers, and various private health policy think tanks. Other elements of the agenda, particularly those involving more immediate issues around which a reasonable body of knowledge already exists, would be assigned to various work groups composed of no more than seven or eight people from relatively diverse perspectives but with knowledge and expertise on the given topic. There would be no more than four or five work groups at one time. Each work group would have a full-time staff professional as a facilitator. The task of the work groups would be to make recommendations to the steering committee on the issue at hand, with emphasis on implementation issues designed to anticipate second-order and unintended consequences of proposed initiatives. After discussion and further refinement by the steering committee, recommendations would be passed on to the appropriate decision-making and policymaking bodies within the public and private sector.

This approach does not deal with a number of specific issues but represents an example of a forum by which a more productive interface between government and the industry could be structured. A particular challenge would be to balance the industry supply-side interests of hospitals and physician groups with the demand-side interests of employers and consumers. It would obviously exist in parallel with many other forums and would probably do little to deter current lobbying initiatives. What it would achieve, however, is an *ongoing forum* by which the relevant groups would meet together and around which a *common information base* and knowledge base would be generated for debating the issues. It would provide a way for governmental policymakers to learn more about the nature of local market structures and local market dynamics and the strategic orientations of firms within those markets. It would provide industry representatives, labor, management, and consumer groups with the opportunity to work with rather than against policymakers in fashioning the legislation or in proposing alternative approaches to meet the intended objectives. It would also provide a forum in which disagreement about goals and objectives (as opposed to the means of achieving them) can be surfaced early in the process. Its ultimate effectiveness would depend on the quality of the ideas put forth and the ability of its members to influence relevant policymaking and decision-making groups inside and outside of government. This committee would report through the Public Health Service to the Secretary of Health in the Department of Health and Human Services. This type of interface takes on added importance if one makes certain assumptions about where policy is headed. One such scenario is suggested below.

A Public Policy Scenario for the Year 2000

There are three main features of the proposed scenario: (1) the establishment of both *fiscal* and *clinical* accountability for care provided to a defined geographically based population; (2)

the overall allocation of resources based on a given population's health needs and the internal allocation of resources within an area based on provider's performance; and (3) explicit up-front bargaining, discussion, and negotiation among all relevant provider, purchaser, and consumer groups about what services will be delivered to what people at what price.

Establishing Fiscal and Clinical Accountability. Given the changes that have been occurring over the past five years, it is not implausible to imagine a system of increasingly centralized control over resources with distribution of those resources based on performance. *The only sure way to control health care expenditures is to cap them.* Thus, one can imagine a scenario in which federal and state governments, private insurers, and employers are involved in establishing a fixed pool of dollars to provide for the health care needs of defined geographical groups. Each area will have a global budget along with established ranges for expected patient outcomes and health status indicators, both objective, physiological indicators and subjective measures of consumer satisfaction.

Under such an arrangement, the federal government (on the basis of recommendations of the joint government-industry-employer-consumer steering comittee previously described) would establish a minimum set of mandated benefits for all Americans. The benefits will be "costed out" according to the demographic, epidemiologic, and health status characteristics of the area. Employers and individuals would be free to go beyond the basic benefit package, but these too would be costed out. Consideration will also be given to the capabilities of providers in the area with an understanding of local market structure and the strategic orientations of the firms within the market. The dollar estimates will be adjusted for area differences in the consumer price index and manufacturing wage index. A separate budget will be established for each area's capital needs.

With the advice of the steering committee, the country would be divided into health promotion and accountability regions (HPARs), which will assume fiscal and clinical performance accountability for the budgeted pool of resources for their regions. A less populated state may have only one HPAR; a more populated may have several. The HPARs will be made up of the major purchasers (federal and state government, private insurers, and employers) plus representatives from labor, community groups, and hospitals, physicians, nurses, a bioethicist, other health care professionals, and health care executives. Purchasers and providers will be required to participate in the HPAR arrangement as a condition for Medicare reimbursement. Each HPAR will have a technical resource staff to analyze and interpret financial, quality, patient outcome, health status, and patient satisfaction data, which will be reported to the public at least once a year. The resource staff will "risk rate" its population according to health needs, as proposed by Enthoven and Kronich (1989), and health plans will be allowed to charge higher prices for the care of people in the higher-cost, higher-need groups. The HPARs will report through the Public Health Service to the assistant secretary of health in the Department of Health and Human Services.

Performance-Based Allocation of Resources. Having established the budgetary limits and expected performance ranges, the purchasers will then grant considerable autonomy to the local delivery systems to organize themselves any way they wish. They may be built around health care systems similar to the health care corporations originally envisioned by the American Hospital Association's Ameriplan proposal (American Hospital Association, 1970) or around Kaiser model HMOs or large multispecialty physician groups. (The Rochester Area Hospitals Corporation (RAHC) represents one example. A group of nine hospitals worked with the local Blue Cross, Medicare, and Medicaid offices to develop an experimental payment project that placed all providers under a communitywide revenue cap; Hartman and Mukamel, 1989.) Competitive forces will be allowed to play themselves out within areawide global budget limits. Systems that can provide greater added value will gain more patients. Systems that cannot will suffer the losses. Some may choose to emphasize staff model HMOs. Others may choose looser network models, and still others may stick with Independent Practice Association models based on fee-for-service arrangements. Under a budget cap, establishing resource-based relative-value physician fee schedules is up to the purchasers and providers in that area. What will be politically acceptable in one area may not be in another. But, ultimately, the area's purchasers and providers will have to work out solutions that are economically viable given the budget cap. *The objectives and incentives are to link clinical responsibility with fiscal accountability for a given package of services for a defined population.*

To give full force to the incentives involved, we propose that each provider/delivery system be allowed to retain approximately 75 percent of any surpluses generated for its own use, with the remaining 25 percent going to the HPAR for continued development of technical support resources and overall area needs. Losses would also be borne primarily by each provider/ delivery system. To assure that no patients go without needed care, each HPAR would have a reinsurance pool to draw from. Such a mechanism is particularly important in the early years until greater experience is gained in risk rating and assessing the population's health needs. The reinsurance pool could also be drawn on in the event of a natural disaster or to take into account greater than expected utilization resulting from an influx of people from another HPAR.

Up-Front Negotiation. The third key feature of the scenario is that all relevant parties are at the table in advance to decide their respective responsibilities to various populations. Some providers, whether by philosophy or geographic location, may choose to specialize in providing care to the poor and medically indigent, since the dollars assigned to provide such care are based on the needs of those groups. Other providers may focus on other population subgroups suited to provider capabilities. Issues involving care for people who move in and out of various insurance plans, employee turnover, and coordination of benefits must be considered in advance. Mechanisms for allowing cross-provider transfer of funds to follow patient preferences and mobility must be worked out. The bottom line is to eliminate after-the-fact cost shifting and abdication of responsibility for providing care to various population segments.

Advantages. There are five key advantages of this arrangement. The first is that it will help payers build stable, predictable, ongoing negotiating structures with providers (Brown, 1985). Public and private purchasers are forced to *work together* in assessing the health needs of a given region and developing a total lump sum budget to meet those needs. Cost shifting between and among purchasers must be explicitly addressed at the outset; so too must the likely flow of consumers who will gain or lose employment and thus become the responsibility of one or the other purchaser. The net result is that needs are related to resources.

The second advantage is that dollars are allocated to provide a continuum of health care services from prehospital primary care to posthospital restorative care. It is a comprehensive *health care* budget, not a budget to pay hospital care, home health care, hospice care, ambulatory surgery care, and physician bills separately.

The third key advantage is that the ultimate level of dollars allocated to the region will depend on that region's *performance.* In turn, each region is free to pay its various delivery systems or health care corporations based on achieving performance targets that will enable the region to meet its overall performance goals. *Accountability is driven by performance at all levels.* Strong incentives exist to provide only the most effective, appropriate care (Brook, 1989). Thus, the need to contain costs and control resources is married to the need to safeguard quality, protect patients, and promote health.

A fourth advantage is that it *combines features* of free enterprise competition with social responsibilities, to provide some level of services to all Americans within an overall fiscal budget tied to defined geographic needs. The proposed scenario promotes clearer accountability while preserving local delivery system options and autonomy. Flexibility is allowed for variable risk rating, based on the needs of different population subgroups. This addresses some observers' concerns that competition between firms for markets will leave some markets (specifically, the less desirable) untouched (Kane, 1989). Further, many of the existing systems are of sufficient geographical scope to serve the geopolitical boundaries on which the HPARs are likely to be based.

The final advantage, of course, is the *discipline* imposed by the budget cap. Everyone's feet are held to the fire and, in this respect, the approach is generally consistent with Enthoven and Kronich's consumer choice plan (1989): a total budget is set in advance; a basic set of benefits is established; and providers are rewarded based on the delivery of cost-effective care.

Disadvantages. It is also important to recognize the potential downside of the proposed scenario. Without question, the process involves several difficulties.

Determining the relevant HPAR geopolitical regions is complicated by the many existing layers of state governmental health planning and welfare agencies. In some states, the areas served by the old health system agencies may be a useful starting point. In other cases, new demarcations may be needed. In addition to political considerations, guiding criteria should take into account the size, needs, and composition of an area's residents relative to the size, characteristics, and capabilities of the area's delivery system and providers. Knowledge of local market structure and the strategic orientations of organizations in the market should be part of this determination.

Choosing the right membership for the HPARs is critical to their success. Like many housing authorities and school district boards, the HPARs could become overly politicized and "underexpertised." The greatest weight should be given to *expertise*. Community advisory groups should be formed to provide additional relevant input.

The ability to assess the population's health status needs and meaningfully to measure severity-adjusted patient outcomes is currently as much an art as a science. Thus, in the early stages variances and errors must be allowed for, and appropriate adjustment made. Even where severity-adjusted patient outcomes can be made in a meaningful fashion, there are problems in attributing substandard performance to the behavior of health care providers and organizations alone. Patients' health status or achieved level of outcome is also dependent on their own behavior, that of their support network, and, in some cases, human service agencies other than those directly involved in providing health care. These considerations need to be taken into account by the HPARs in making payment decisions based on outcomes and in deciding what contracts to renew.

These measurement issues also pose a general problem associated with allocating resources based on performance. Substandard performance could result from underestimating the health care needs of the population served by a given health care corporation, errors in severity adjusting patient outcomes, or ascribing to providers responsibility for behavior not under their direct control. This complicates the process of making retroactive adjustments as well as planning for the subsequent year's budget and performance targets.

Finally, under such a scenario it is likely that at least two levels of care will continue to exist — a basic benefit package that will cover those with fewer resources to purchase health care service and a more comprehensive package for those with greater resources. Nonetheless, providing at least a basic set of benefits reduces the significant variance that currently exists between those with financial access to the system and those without. Developing a basic set of mandated benefits will not be easy, but it is possible to learn from Oregon's experience in developing such benefits for its Medicaid recipients. In addition, developing medical practice guidelines and payment based on outcomes achieved is likely to reduce differences in the *quality* of care provided within a given benefit package. Thus, differences in levels will be related primarily to the *scope* of services or benefits provided, rather than to different degrees of quality per se.

Implications. While recognizing these limitations and imperfections, it is important to note that significant strides have been made in both health status assessment (Lohr and others, 1986) and patient outcome measurement (Blumberg, 1986; Brook and Lohr, 1985). Further, a considerable national investment has been made in an ongoing program of patient outcome and quality assurance research, which is likely to bear important dividends over the coming decade. A major advantage of the proposed HPAR framework is that it provides an ongoing structure and set of systematic incentives for continuous improvement in measurement methodology. Although it is not without problems, we believe the HPAR proposal is a workable and reasonable scenario for the 1990s — one which combines some features of the British and Canadian systems with Americans' desires for local autonomy.

Based on present study findings, the scenario holds several important implications. Most obvious is the importance of systems developing integrated continuums of care (from prehospital to posthospital) in local and regional markets. Only those that have reasonable control over the entire delivery channel will be able to perform well. Or, put differently, those that have such control are likely to have a comparative advantage in negotiating with their HPARs. With appropriate differentiation over time, such systems may be able to sustain the advantage and gain major repeat business year after year. This will require that systems be of sufficient size and have sufficient geographic presence in a given market. This is precisely why many local hospitals are consolidating to form their own systems and why some of them will further consolidate in the years ahead to achieve an even wider market presence.

A second implication is the need for health care corporations to develop integrated financial, managerial, and clinical information systems for reporting performance data. These systems should include data on patient outcomes, patient satisfaction, and costs in such a way that the organization will have an ability to compete on both price and quality. These information systems will need to be more than hospital based. They must also include the primary care and long-term care components of the system. Ultimately these data will become input for population-based health status indicators.

The third implication, underscored throughout this book, is the need for hospitals, physicians, and other health professionals to develop effective economic partnerships for delivering care. The organizational forms for these partnerships can vary, from loosely coupled (for example, separate physician and hospital organizations that contract with each other) to tightly coupled (for example, joint physician-hospital organizations), but they must be able to provide technically competent, accessible care along the continuum of desired services—hence the potential utility of such concepts as the integrated medical campus or the "hospital without walls" (Goldsmith, 1989).

Whether one believes in the scenario in all its details is not important. What is important is that it contains elements of current trends that are likely to continue over the coming decade. The scenario, in other words, is approximately correct. It is in the general direction of the way health policy in the United States is evolving. The incremental steps are being taken. The ability of providers to help shape this future may well depend on developing the kind of government-industry-consumer interface discussed here.

The message is that the buck has to stop somewhere. Financial and quality performance standards will be developed and linked to defined geographical groups to establish clearer channels of accountability. The strategic transformation of the American health care industry into systems and alliances now makes this possible. The ultimate success, however, will be measured in terms of value added, aggregated up from local markets to regions to the country at large. This, in turn, will depend on the freedom health care organizations have to manage strategically within the guidelines established. Based on the findings and lessons of the present study, the winners and losers will become apparent and will be rewarded accordingly.

Resources

Resource A

The Strategic Planning Survey

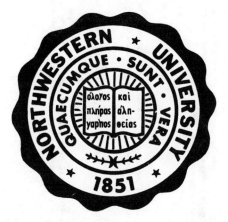

STRATEGIC PLANNING SURVEY 1986

Center for Health Services and Policy Research
Northwestern University

Principal Investigator: Stephen M. Shortell, Ph. D.

Senior Investigators: Bernard S. Friedman, Ph. D.
Edward F.X. Hughes, M.D., M.P.H.
Susan L. Hughes, D.S.W.

Project Director: Ellen M. Morrison, M.A.

Executive Summary

This survey has been designed to measure your perceptions about your hospital and your hospital system. It represents the final request for information from your hospital for this study. The Northwestern University study team is working closely with the corporate office staff of your system to assure the quality, usefulness and confidentiality of the data collected. **Your responses will not be released to anyone, including your own system's corporate headquarters.** Information from this survey will be reported to your system's corporate staff in aggregate form ONLY. Your corporate staff will be able to use this information to measure its management effectiveness and to improve services and support it offers to you as a member hospital. For our purposes, your responses will be integrated with other data already collected, and included in an analysis of organizational strategy, structure and performance.

General Instructions

— Sections I (Market Share), II (Market Growth) and III (Service Profitability) should be completed by the person(s) most knowledgeable in each area. In addition to the CEO, these persons may include your hospital's CFO, Vice President for Planning or Marketing, or Assistant Administrator.

— Sections IV (Service Specific Strategies), V (Decision Making), VI (Hospital's Market Response) and VII (Planning Process) should be completed **ONLY BY THE CEO.**

— Choose the **SINGLE MOST APPROPRIATE RESPONSE** of the alternatives provided. If actual data is not available, please use your best estimate. Avoid multiple answers or responses that require clarification unless absolutely necessary.

THANK YOU FOR YOUR ASSISTANCE

Stephen M. Shortell, Ph.D.
Principal Investigator

Ellen M. Morrison, M.A.
Project Director

Name of Person Completing This Page _____
(If Different Than for Previous Page)
Title _____
Phone Number (_____) _____

Section I. MARKET SHARE OF SELECTED SERVICES

INSTRUCTIONS: For each service listed below, please circle the most appropriate response. Your response should indicate your hospital's **current market share** (percentage of patients seen or services provided relative to other providers) in your **primary service area.**

Service	We do not offer this service	Much less than other providers (at least one other provider has 1.5 times or greater market share than we have)	Somewhat less than other providers (at least one other provider has up to 1.5 times as much market share as we have)	The same as other providers	Somewhat more than other providers (we have up to 1.5 times more market share than any other providers)	Much more than other providers (we have 1.5 times or greater market share than any other providers)
1. General Inpatient Medical Care	8	1	2	3	4	5
2. General Inpatient Surgical Care	8	1	2	3	4	5
3. General Inpatient Pediatric Care	8	1	2	3	4	5
4. General Inpatient Obstetrics Care	8	1	2	3	4	5
5. General Inpatient Psychiatric Care	8	1	2	3	4	5
6. Outpatient Renal Dialysis	8	1	2	3	4	5
7. Outpatient Diagnostic Services (e.g. Radiology, Laboratory)	8	1	2	3	4	5
8. Home Health Care	8	1	2	3	4	5
9. Long Term Care Programs/Services*	8	1	2	3	4	5
10. Outpatient Alcoholism Treatment Program	8	1	2	3	4	5
11. Inpatient Alcoholism Treatment Program	8	1	2	3	4	5
12. Urgent Care Center	8	1	2	3	4	5
13. Ambulatory Surgery Center**	8	1	2	3	4	5
14. Inpatient or Outpatient Rehabilitation Unit	8	1	2	3	4	5
15. Health Promotion/ Wellness Clinic/ Holistic Health Center	8	1	2	3	4	5

* Includes skilled and intermediate nursing care, hospice care and adult day health services.
** Includes freestanding center, a center on hospital grounds, or a segregated program within the hospital.

Name of Person Completing This Page _____
(If Different Than for Previous Page)
Title _____
Phone Number (_____) _____

Section II. MARKET GROWTH POTENTIAL OF SELECTED SERVICES

INSTRUCTIONS: For each service below, please circle the most appropriate response. Your response should indicate each service's **market growth potential** (potential percentage growth in volume of patients seen or services provided) in your **primary service area.**

Service	We do not offer this service	No growth potential (service may actually be declining)	Low growth potential (1% — 10% per year)	Moderate growth potential (11% — 50% per year)	High growth potential (50% + per year)
1. General Inpatient Medical Care	8	1	2	3	4
2. General Inpatient Surgical Care	8	1	2	3	4
3. General Inpatient Pediatric Care	8	1	2	3	4
4. General Inpatient Obstetrics Care	8	1	2	3	4
5. General Inpatient Psychiatric Care	8	1	2	3	4
6. Outpatient Renal Dialysis	8	1	2	3	4
7. Outpatient Diagnostic Services (e.g., Radiology, Laboratory)	8	1	2	3	4
8. Home Health Care	8	1	2	3	4
9. Long Term Care Programs/Services*	8	1	2	3	4
10. Outpatient Alcoholism Treatment Program	8	1	2	3	4
11. Inpatient Alcoholism Treatment Program	8	1	2	3	4
12. Urgent Care Center	8	1	2	3	4
13. Ambulatory Surgery Center**	8	1	2	3	4
14. Inpatient or Outpatient Rehabilitation Unit	8	1	2	3	4
15. Health Promotion/ Wellness Clinic/ Holistic Health Center	8	1	2	3	4

* Includes skilled and intermediate nursing care, hospice care and adult day health services.
** Includes freestanding center, a center on hospital grounds, or a segregated program within the hospital.

Name of Person Completing This Page _____

(If Different Than for Previous Page)

Title _____

Phone Number (_____)

Section III. PROFITABILITY OF SELECTED SERVICES

For each service below, please circle the most appropriate response(s). Your response should indicate both:

1. Whether the service has been offered for less than two years, and
2. The service's current profitability (net revenues minus direct operating costs, including capital costs and administrative overhead, before taxes if applicable.)

For services that are jointly offered with another provider, indicate the profitability of the service before the profits are distributed.

Service	We do not offer this service	Has service been offered for less than two years? Yes	No	Not currently profitable	In the past 6 months, operating revenues exceeded operating expenses by 1% to 10%	In the past 6 months, operating revenues exceeded operating expenses by more than 10%
1. General Inpatient Medical Care	8	1	0	1	2	3
2. General Inpatient Surgical Care	8	1	0	1	2	3
3. General Inpatient Pediatric Care	8	1	0	1	2	3
4. General Inpatient Obstetrics Care	8	1	0	1	2	3
5. General Inpatient Psychiatric Care	8	1	0	1	2	3
6. Outpatient Renal Dialysis	8	1	0	1	2	3
7. Outpatient Diagnostic Services (e.g., Radiology, Laboratory)	8	1	0	1	2	3
8. Home Health Care	8	1	0	1	2	3
9. Long Term Care Programs/Services*	8	1	0	1	2	3
10. Outpatient Alcoholism Treatment Program	8	1	0	1	2	3
11. Inpatient Alcoholism Treatment Program	8	1	0	1	2	3
12. Urgent Care Center	8	1	0	1	2	3
13. Ambulatory Surgery Center**	8	1	0	1	2	3
14. Inpatient or Outpatient Rehabilitation Unit	8	1	0	1	2	3
15. Health Promotion/ Wellness Clinic/ Holistic Health Center	8	1	0	1	2	3

* Includes skilled and intermediate nursing care, hospice care and adult day health services.

** Includes freestanding center, a center on hospital grounds, or a segregated program within the hospital.

NOTE: THIS SECTION SHOULD BE COMPLETED ONLY BY THE CEO.

PART A. INSTRUCTIONS: From the services listed below, please circle the numbers corresponding to the FIVE SERVICES that are currently MOST IMPORTANT to your hospital's overall goals and strategic plans.

1. General Inpatient Medical Care
2. General Inpatient Surgical Care
3. General Inpatient Pediatric Care
4. General Inpatient Obstetrics
5. General Inpatient Psychiatric Care

6. Outpatient Renal Dialysis
7. Outpatient Diagnostic Services (e.g., Radiology Laboratory)
8. Home Health Care
9. Long Term Care Programs/Services
10. Outpatient Alcoholism Treatment Program

11. Inpatient Alcoholism Treatment Program
12. Urgent Care Center
13. Ambulatory Surgery Center
14. Inpatient or Outpatient Rehabilitation Unit
15. Health Protection/ Wellness Clinic/ Holistic Health Center

PART B. INSTRUCTIONS:

1. For each service listed below that is offered by your hospital, please assign percentage points (from 0 to 100) reflecting the primary strategies which your hospital uses at the present time. Use the following definitions:

A. Market Strategies

Further Penetrate Current Markets — Attempt to attract a greater number of patients from markets which you currently serve with the service.

Develop New Markets — Develop new markets for the service which you currently offer; going beyond the markets which you currently serve.

B. Service Strategies

Refine Current Services — Improve or in some way modify the characteristics of the services which you currently offer; for example, upgrading staffing or updating equipment.

Develop New Services — Start new programs or services which your hospital did not previously provide.

EXAMPLE 1 If you give about equal emphasis to both service refinement and new service development, you might assign the points as follows:

Refine Current Services	Develop New Services	Total
50	50	100

EXAMPLE 2 If the primary strategy used for a given service is to penetrate current markets rather than new market development, you might assign the points as follows:

Further Penetrate Current Markets	Develop New Markets	Total
70	30	100

PLEASE MAKE SURE THAT IN EACH CASE THE TOTAL POINTS ASSIGNED EQUAL 100.

MARKET STRATEGIES

Service	Circle if your hospital does not offer this service	Further penetrate current markets (Attract more patients from geographic markets which you currently serve)	Develop new markets (Attract more patients from markets which you do not currently serve)	Total
1. General Inpatient Medical Care	-8			= 100
2. General Inpatient Surgical Care	-8			= 100
3. General Inpatient Pediatric Care	-8			= 100
4. General Inpatient Obstetrics Care	-8			= 100
5. General Inpatient Psychiatric Care	-8			= 100
6. Outpatient Renal Dialysis	-8			= 100
7. Outpatient Diagnostic Services (e.g., Radiology, Laboratory)	-8			= 100
8. Home Health Care	-8			= 100
9. Long Term Care Programs/Services*	-8			= 100
10. Outpatient Alcoholism Treatment Program	-8			= 100
11. Inpatient Alcoholism Treatment Program	-8			= 100
12. Urgent Care Center	-8			= 100
13. Ambulatory Surgery Center**	-8			= 100
14. Inpatient or Outpatient Rehabilitation Unit	-8			= 100
15. Health Promotion/ Wellness Clinic/ Holistic Health Center	-8			= 100

* Includes skilled and intermediate nursing care, hospice care and adult day health services.
** Includes freestanding center, a center on hospital grounds, or a segregated program within the hospital.

SERVICE STRATEGIES

Refine current services (Change or upgrade current services through changes in staffing technology, etc.)	Develop new services (Start new programs or services which you did not provide previously)	Total
		= 100
		= 100
		= 100
		= 100
		= 100
		= 100
		= 100
		= 100
		= 100
		= 100
		= 100
		= 100
		= 100
		= 100
		= 100

Section V. ORGANIZATIONAL DECISION MAKING

NOTE: THIS SECTION SHOULD BE COMPLETED ONLY BY THE CEO.

INSTRUCTIONS:
1. For the decisions listed below, please designate who has the authority to make the decision **without first checking** with the next higher level person or group in the organization. (NOTE: This decision may **eventually** need to be approved by another individual or group, but the person or group in question can make the decision without **first** having to obtain approval from others.)

The decision maker choices are:

6 = Corporate Board   3 = Hospital Board
5 = Corporate Management   2 = Hospital CEO
4 = Divisional/Regional Board or Management   1 = Individuals below Hospital CEO level

2. Please also rate (on a scale of 1 to 5) the **risk** involved in the decision. Risk includes both the **uncertainty** of the decision in terms of outcome and its **importance** to the organization. The more uncertain the outcome of a decision and the greater its importance, the greater the degree of risk involved. (Low risk decisions would score a "1" and high risk decisions a "5".)

EXAMPLE:

DECISION	WHO HAS THE AUTHORITY TO MAKE THIS DECISION WITHOUT FIRST CHECKING WITH THE NEXT HIGHER LEVEL IN THE ORGANIZATION?						RISK TAKING (UNCERTAINTY AND IMPORTANCE) LOW HIGH				
	6	5	4	3	2	①	①	2	3	4	5
Choosing a laundry service vendor for an individual hospital.											

The response to the decision above indicates that someone below the Hospital CEO chooses the vendor for the hospital laundry service and that it is a low risk decision.

CIRCLE THE MOST APPROPRIATE RESPONSE FOR EACH OF THESE TWO QUESTIONS.

Decision	1. Who has the authority to make this decision without first checking with the next higher level in the organization?						2. Risk Rating (Uncertainty and Importance)				
	Corporate Board	Corporate Management	Divisional/ Regional Board or Management	Hospital Board	Hospital CEO	Individual Below Hospital CEO	Low				High
1. Choosing a marketing plan for a new outpatient service at an individual hospital	6	5	4	3	2	1	1	2	3	4	5
2. Deciding to enter into a joint venture with a system of a different ownership type.	6	5	4	3	2	1	1	2	3	4	5
3. Appointing an individual hospital CEO.	6	5	4	3	2	1	1	2	3	4	5
4. Deciding to decrease the number of nursing hours provided per patient day at an individual hospital.	6	5	4	3	2	1	1	2	3	4	5
5. Determining individual hospital budget levels.	6	5	4	3	2	1	1	2	3	4	5
6. Evaluating individual hospital CEO performance.	6	5	4	3	2	1	1	2	3	4	5
7. Deciding to involve more physicians in individual hospital governance.	6	5	4	3	2	1	1	2	3	4	5
8. Determining when individual hospital budget variances are significant enough for corrective action to be taken.	6	5	4	3	2	1	1	2	3	4	5
9. Acquiring a new hospital.	6	5	4	3	2	1	1	2	3	4	5
10. Filling vacancies which may occur at the individual hospital board of trustees level.	6	5	4	3	2	1	1	2	3	4	5
11. Changing a priority in the hospital's strategic plan in mid year.	6	5	4	3	2	1	1	2	3	4	5
12. Deciding to add an ambulatory surgery center at an individual hospital.	6	5	4	3	2	1	1	2	3	4	5

Section VI. CLASSIFYING YOUR HOSPITAL'S MARKET RESPONSE

NOTE: THIS SECTION SHOULD BE COMPLETED ONLY BY THE CEO.

Below are descriptions of how four hospitals respond to market changes by altering their mix of products, services and markets served. Three of the hospitals are easily classified; the fourth contains elements of the other three. None of the hospital strategies described is inherently "good" or "bad". While none of the hospitals described may be exactly like your hospital, please look for similarities.

Hospital A occupies a "niche" in the health care system by offering a relatively stable set of services to defined markets. Generally Hospital A is not at the forefront of new services or market developments in health care. It tends to ignore changes that have no direct impact on current areas of operation and concentrates instead on doing the best job possible in its existing arena.

Hospital B maintains a relatively stable base of services while at the same time developing selected, promising new services and markets. The hospital is seldom first to provide new services or expand into new markets. However, by carefully monitoring the actions of institutions like Hospital C (below), Hospital B attempts to follow with a more cost-effective or well-conceived service.

Hospital C makes relatively frequent changes in and additions to its set of services and markets served. It consistently attempts to be first to provide new services or develop new markets, even if not all of these efforts ultimately prove to be successful. Hospital C responds rapidly to early signals of market needs or opportunities.

Hospital D operates like all three hospitals above (A, B and C) at different times, and therefore cannot be clearly classified in terms of its approach to changing its services or markets. It does not have a consistent response to market changes. At times, the hospital will not make service/market changes unless forced to by external events (like Hospital A); at times, it will move into new fields only after considerable evidence of potential success (like Hospital B); and at times, it will be an early entrant into new fields of opportunity (like Hospital C).

Hospitals A, B and C might be placed on a hypothetical 7-point continuum of "service/market change" as follows:

	HOSPITAL A		HOSPITAL B		HOSPITAL C	
"Low Change"	1	2	3	4	5	6	7 "High Change"

1. Please circle the number which best reflects how your hospital **now operates** along the 7-point continuum (or circle "Hospital D" if your hospital cannot be characterized by A, B or C).

	HOSPITAL A		HOSPITAL B		HOSPITAL C		HOSPITAL D
"Low Change"	1	2	3	4	5	6	7 "High Change"	D

2. Please rate your hospital as it operated **two years ago.**

	HOSPITAL A		HOSPITAL B		HOSPITAL C		HOSPITAL D
"Low Change"	1	2	3	4	5	6	7 "High Change"	D

3. Please rate your hospital as you predict it will operate **two years from now.**

	HOSPITAL A		HOSPITAL B		HOSPITAL C		HOSPITAL D
"Low Change"	1	2	3	4	5	6	7 "High Change"	D

4. NEW SERVICE AND PRODUCT DEVELOPMENT

Please indicate the extent to which each of the statements below describes your hospital as it is now, as it was 2 years ago, and as you anticipate it will be two years from now by assigning points between 0 and 100 in each of the categories listed below. In each case, the total number of points in each column should be 100.

	Now	Two years ago	Two years from now
We offer new services/products independently.			
We offer new services/products through acquisitions or by joint ventures with others involving **inpatient** services.			
We offer new services/products through acquisitions or by joint ventures with others involving **out-of-hospital** services.			
Total	100	100	100

Section VII. Strategic Planning Process

NOTE: THIS SECTION SHOULD BE COMPLETED ONLY BY THE CEO.

1. INSTRUCTIONS: The following statements reflect stages in the strategic planning process. For each statement below, please rank, in **order of** involvement both the system level participants and the hospital participants in that stage of strategic planning. Use the following ranking schemes:

SYSTEM LEVEL

3 = most involved
2 = second most involved
1 = third most involved
0 = not involved

HOSPITAL LEVEL

4 = most involved
3 = second most involved
2 = third most involved
1 = fourth most involved
0 = not involved

EXAMPLE   Rank from 1 to 3 (0 = not involved)

	SYSTEM LEVEL		
	Corporate Office	Region	Your Hospital
Responsible for Initiating Strategic Planning Process at Your Hospital	3	2	1

Rank from 1 to 4 (0 = not involved)

	HOSPITAL LEVEL		
	CEO	Hospital Board	Hospital Management (Other than CEO)	Physician Leaders
	3	4	2	0

The example above indicates that, of system level participants, your system's corporate office is most involved in initiating the strategic planning process at your hospital. At the hospital level, the hospital board is most involved at this stage and the hospital's physician leaders are not at all involved.

IF YOU HAVE NO FORMAL STRATEGIC PLANNING PROCESS AT YOUR HOSPITAL, PLEASE CHECK HERE AND SKIP TO QUESTION 2 _____

SYSTEM LEVEL

3 = most involved
2 = second most involved
1 = third most involved
0 = not involved

	SYSTEM LEVEL		
	Corporate Office	Region	Your Hospital
Responsible for Initiating Strategic Planning Process at Your Hospital			
Responsible for Formulating the Strategic Plan at Your Hospital			
Responsible for Final Approval of Your Hospital's Strategic Plan			

HOSPITAL LEVEL

4 = most involved
3 = second most involved
2 = third most involved
1 = fourth most involved
0 = not involved

	HOSPITAL LEVEL		
CEO	Hospital Board	Hospital Management (Other than CEO)	Physician Leaders

2. Who is **primarily responsible** for each of the following tasks?

	No One	Corporate Office	Regions/ Divisions	Individual Hospital	Other
a. Assessing national trends	8	3	2	1	6
b. Assessing local demographics and trends	8	3	2	1	6
c. Analyzing your competition	8	3	2	1	6
d. Assessing your hospital's strengths and weaknesses	8	3	2	1	6
e. Providing market research for your hospital	8	3	2	1	6
f. Providing information system support for your strategic plans	8	3	2	1	6
g. Designing compensation and incentive systems to support the plans	8	3	2	1	6
h. Developing specific business plans for your hospital	8	3	2	1	6
i. Monitoring performance against the strategic plan	8	3	2	1	6

3a. Do you use **standardized forms and formats** in developing your strategic plans, (e.g., for recording competitive and environmental analysis, strengths and weaknesses, financial projection for new programs, etc.)?

    2 — Yes, for almost all elements

    1 — Yes, for some elements of the planning process, but not all

    0 — No, standardized forms or formats are rarely used

3b. **If you answer yes above**: Who primarily defines what forms and formats will be used?

    3 — Corporate office

    2 — Regions/Divisions

    1 — Individual hospitals

4. Please indicate your agreement or disagreement with each of the following statements in reference to your hospital. Circle the number which best reflects your judgement regarding each statement.

Statement	Strongly Disagree		Neither Agree Nor Disagree		Strongly Agree
a. Our ability to perform or obtain market research is good	1	2	3	4	5
b. Our information systems are good	1	2	3	4	5
c. Financial data need to be more systematically linked with planning and program data	1	2	3	4	5
d. Our board members are appropriately involved in the strategic planning process	1	2	3	4	5
e. Our strategy implementation plans are well-developed	1	2	3	4	5
f. We lack sufficient agreement on the goals we are pursuing	1	2	3	4	5
g. Our ability to perform or obtain market research needs to be strengthened	1	2	3	4	5
h. Our system's corporate office staff provide useful assistance to us in our strategic planning process	1	2	3	4	5
i. Our system's regional/divisional staff provide useful assistance to us in our strategic planning process	1	2	3	4	5
j. Our hospital strategic planning needs to become more formalized and disciplined	1	2	3	4	5
k. Our information systems need to be strengthened	1	2	3	4	5
l. Our hospital has sufficient physician involvement in the strategic planning process	1	2	3	4	5
m. Our performance appraisal and compensation systems are appropriately linked to our strategic priorities	1	2	3	4	5
n. Our quality assurance program needs improvement	1	2	3	4	5
o. We do a good job assessing and anticipating the responses of our competitors	1	2	3	4	5
p. Our hospital strategic planning process would benefit from more involvement of the department directors/heads	1	2	3	4	5
q. Our current strategies are innovative compared to our past strategies	1	2	3	4	5
r. Our current strategies are innovative compared to those of our competitors	1	2	3	4	5
s. Corporate/regional office staff provide useful assistance to us in our quality assurance activities	1	2	3	4	5

5. Since the introduction of Medicare Prospective Payment (October, 1983), to what degree have you implemented the following **cost containment activities**? Circle the number for each which best applies.

	Not At All 1	2	Somewhat 3	4	A Great Deal 5
a. Upgraded our cost-accounting system	1	2	3	4	5
b. Reduced FTE's in non-medical support areas (e.g., housekeeping, maintenance, dietary)	1	2	3	4	5
c. Reduced FTE's in medical support areas (e.g., laboratory, radiology, pharmacy, etc.)	1	2	3	4	5
d. Reduced FTE's in nursing	1	2	3	4	5
e. Increased use of part-time staff	1	2	3	4	5
f. Reduced FTE's in administration	1	2	3	4	5
g. Consolidated or merged two or more departments or programs	1	2	3	4	5
h. Consolidated or merged two or more functions	1	2	3	4	5
i. Eliminated a non-medical support department, service or function	1	2	3	4	5
j. Eliminated a medical support department, service or function	1	2	3	4	5
k. Contracted out for services that can be provided more efficiently by others	1	2	3	4	5
l. Upgraded our inventory control system	1	2	3	4	5
m. Increased our involvement in discount bulk purchasing programs	1	2	3	4	5
n. Established more stringent criteria for detailed review of new technology and equipment	1	2	3	4	5
o. Initiated zero-based budgeting	1	2	3	4	5
p. Developed incentive compensation linking pay to cost containment and/or improved productivity	1	2	3	4	5
q. Initiated an employee suggestion program for cost containment and/or improved productivity	1	2	3	4	5
r. Strengthened the discharge planning and utilization review process	1	2	3	4	5
s. Reduced inpatient length of stay	1	2	3	4	5
t. Strengthened pre-admission screening criteria	1	2	3	4	5
u. Developed cost containment education programs for physicians	1	2	3	4	5
v. Developed more programs to treat patients on an outpatient basis	1	2	3	4	5
w. Instituted or upgraded industrial engineering and methods improvement programs	1	2	3	4	5

x. Other — List any additional significant efforts which you have undertaken to contain costs and/or improve productivity.

_____

_____

_____

_____

_____

6. How intense is the competition which your hospital faces at the current time? (By intense, we mean the extent to which rival organizations actively attempt to take away your market share and/or pre-empt you from gaining additional market share.

Not At All Intense		Somewhat Intense		Very Intense
1	2	3	4	5

7. Please circle the number which best reflects your judgement regarding each statement below.

	We do not use this strategy	This statement describes our hospital's strategy with respect to **selected** services	This statement describes our hospital's strategy with respect to **all** services
a. We try to provide services at a lower cost than our competitors.	8	1	2
b. We try to differentiate our services based on their superior technical quality.	8	1	2
c. We try to differentiate our services based on their greater convenience and access.	8	1	2
d. We try to differentiate our services based on how well they are managed.	8	1	2

8. Please think about how important **you** believe each of the following factors is for the continued viability of your hospital. Rate each factor by circling the appropriate number on each of the five-point scales shown below. If you do not know the importance of a particular factor, please circle "Don't Know" (7).

Factor	Less Important		Important	Importance	Essential	Don't Know
a. Reducing number of beds	1	2	3	4	5	7
b. Increasing marketing activities	1	2	3	4	5	7
c. Developing more specialized services	1	2	3	4	5	7
d. Gaining access to capital	1	2	3	4	5	7
e. Updating accounting and information systems	1	2	3	4	5	7
f. Improving physician/administrative relations	1	2	3	4	5	7
g. Maintaining/upgrading physical plant	1	2	3	4	5	7
h. Acquiring latest medical technology	1	2	3	4	5	7
i. Controlling costs	1	2	3	4	5	7
j. Enhancing revenues	1	2	3	4	5	7
k. Recruiting and retaining physicians	1	2	3	4	5	7
l. Developing joint ventures with physicians	1	2	3	4	5	7
m. Assuring quality of care	1	2	3	4	5	7
n. Improving community relations	1	2	3	4	5	7
o. Gaining greater impatient market share	1	2	3	4	5	7
p. Attracting and retaining effective administrators	1	2	3	4	5	7
q. Maintaining multi-institutional system affiliation	1	2	3	4	5	7
r. Gaining political influence	1	2	3	4	5	7
s. Diversifying into related health care activities	1	2	3	4	5	7
t. Developing volume-based contractual relations with insurance companies	1	2	3	4	5	7

The following questions refer to your hospital's **formally organized** quality assurance program. (By "formally organized", we mean that a designated person is in charge and that there **are** standard operating protocols for review of physician performance and patient care practices.)

9a. Does a separate identifiable budget exist for the quality assurance program?

    1 Yes

    0 No

9b. **If yes: What is the amount of the budget for the current fiscal year?**

    $ _____

9c. What is the number of full-time equivalent personnel devoted to the quality assurance program? _____ FTE

10. DEMOGRAPHIC INFORMATION

    a. Your age (Please circle appropriate number)

        1. Under 35
        2. 36—45
        3. 46—55
        4. 56—65
        5. Over 65

    b. Sex

        1. Female
        2. Male

    c. Number of years in your current position

        _____ yrs

    d. Number of years you have worked for this system

        _____ yrs

    e. Please indicate your highest level of education completed

        1. High school
        2. College
        3. MBA or equivalent
        4. MPH or equivalent
        5. MHA or equivalent
        6. M.D.
        7. Other graduate degree

Resource B

Interview Questionnaires

Interview Protocol: Vice-President for Strategic Planning

A. Introduction
1. How long have you been employed by
   _____[Name of System]_____ ?

2. How long have you been in your current position?
   _____

3. Could you *briefly* describe your scope of responsibility?
4. In what ways is [Name of System] different from other systems? What makes you unique? What makes you distinctive?
5. a. In regard to your system's strategic plans for the coming year, what are the top three priorities for achievement?

Note: Nearly identical protocols were used for the president and CEO, chief operating officer of the hospital division, vice-presidents for finance, marketing, human resources, information systems, and related positions.

       b.   For each of the above, why are you pursuing this strategy? (For example: in response to competition, what we do best, in response to prospective payment, consistent with our mission, etc.)

B. Specific Areas of Activity

Now I'd like to ask you about four specific areas of activity of your system: inpatient services; ambulatory care services; long-term care services; and nonhealth lines of business. For each of these areas of activity I'm going to ask you the same set of questions.

    1.   What are your plans in the next year or two in regard to each of the above four activities? Do you plan to expand, maintain them as they are, or cut back? In what specific areas?

       a.   What criteria or guidelines do you use in making this decision? (For example: profiitability, market share, market growth potential, return on investment, available skills, community need, etc.)

       b.   How different are your plans in this area from what you have done in the past (e.g., within the past five years)?

Choose one example given above.

Give respondent card.

       c.   What impact will your plans in this area have on.

          1.   other services that you offer?

          2.   your competitors?

          3.   the number and types of health professionals you employ?

          4.   your physicians?

          5.   your productivity?

          6.   your costs?

          7.   your operating margin (direct and indirect costs)?

          8.   your debt/equity ratio?

          9.   your quality of care?

       d.   For your hospitals overall, where are your "hot markets" for these services? Who are your main competitors in those markets?

e. What factors might constrain your ability to implement your plans in this area? (For example: legal barriers, regulatory barriers, lack of capital, lack of human resources, etc.)

2. What other *important plans* do you have over the next year or two which we should discuss? (For example, in the international overseas area.)

a. What criteria or guidelines do you use in making this decision? (For example: profitability, market share, market growth potential, return on investment, available skills, community need, etc.)

b. How different are your plans in this area from what you have done in the past (e.g., within the past five years)?

Choose one example given above.
Give respondent card.

c. What impact will your plans in this area have on:
    1. other services you offer?
    2. your competitors?
    3. the number and types of health professionals you employ?
    4. your physicians?
    5. your productivity?
    6. your costs?
    7. your operating margin (direct and indirect costs)?
    8. your debt/equity ratio?
    9. your quality of care?

d. For your hospitals overall, where are your "hot markets" for these services? Who are your main competitors in those markets?

e. What factors might constrain your ability to implement your plans in this area? (For example: legal barriers, regulatory barriers, lack of capital, lack of human resources, etc.)

3. Do your strategies differ for the hospitals you own

versus those you lease or manage? If so, in what ways?

4. What priority does the hospital division have in relation to other lines of business in your system? Has this changed? Do you foresee change?

5. What do you perceive to be your system's primary strengths and what areas do you primarily need to work on to improve?

C. Strategic Planning Process

1. Please describe your strategic planning process in regard to the following issues: *(Probe for examples in all cases.)*

   a. How long have you had a formal strategic planning process? How formal is the process? What formats do you use?

   b. Is there a strategic planning group? If yes, who are the members? If no, who is most involved in the process?

   c. How is environmental assessment conducted? What methods are used and who gets involved?

   d. How is competitive analysis conducted? What methods are used and who gets involved?

   e. How are the system's strengths and weaknesses assessed? What methods are used and who gets involved?

   f. What are your special strengths and what are the areas you need to work on?

   g. What role do individual hospitals play in the strategic planning process? Do they have their own strategic plans and how do these articulate with the system's overall plans?

2. What elements of your strategic planning process do you believe are different from other systems of which you are aware?

3. What changes or improvements would you like to see in your strategic planning process?

4. How do you communicate new strategic plans to individual hospitals?

Second-Wave Phone Interview: CEO Hospital Division

I. *Overall Mission and Strategic Priorities*
   A. Mission
      1a. Have any changes been made in your system's *mission statement* over the past two years?
      1b. *If yes:* Please describe those changes. Why were the changes made?
   B. Strategies
      1. At present, what are the *strategic priorities* of your system? (List at least three.)
      2. How are you planning to *implement* those priorities? (Ask for the top three strategic priorities and record plans for each one.)
         a. Priority one implementation
         b. Priority two implementation
         c. Priority three implementation
      3. Review the attached list of priorities from two years ago. Ask respondent about the *current status* of each of these (probe about those that have not been accomplished or have been abandoned).
         Priority strategy: _____
         Current status:
         Priority strategy: _____
         Current status:
         Priority strategy: _____
         Current status:
         Priority strategy: _____
         Current status:
         Priority strategy: _____
         Current status:
      4a. Which of your *current* businesses and services are you planning to *expand?*
      4b. Which of your *current* businesses and services are you planning to *deemphasize* or even *delete?*
      4c. What *new* businesses and services are you planning to *develop?*

Note: Identical questions were asked of the vice-presidents for human resources, marketing, and planning.

II. *Organizational Changes*

    1. What are the most significant organizational changes your system has made over the past two years?

    2. What organizational changes are you thinking of making within the next year or two?

    3a. What do you think are the *major strengths* of your system?

    3b. What do you think are major *weaknesses* of your system?

    4a. What is the single biggest *threat* to your system's success?

    4b. What do you see as the most significant *opportunity* available to your system?

III. *Special Topics*

    A. *Physicians*

        1a. In what ways are physicians involved in the *governance* of your individual hospitals?

        1b. In what way are physicians involved in the *management* of your individual hospitals?

        1c. What *changes* do you foresee in the way physicians are involved in the governance and management of your hospitals?

        2a. In what ways are physicians involved at the *regional and divisional levels* of your system's activities?

        2b. What *changes* do you foresee in the nature of physician involvement at the *regional and divisional* levels?

        3a. In what ways are physicians involved at the *corporate* level of your system?

        3b. What *changes* do you foresee in the nature of physician involvement at the *corporate level?*

        4. Please describe the kind of *joint venture activities* with which you are currently involved with your physicians.

    B. *Strategic Planning*

        1a. What kinds of changes have been made over the *past two years* in the way your system does *strategic planning* (formality of the process, who gets involved, kinds of assessments done, how the process is organized, etc.)?

1b.   What kinds of changes do you foresee making within the next year or so?

C.   *Financial Management*

1a.   What kinds of changes have you made over the *past two years* in your system's financial management practices and policies (investment criteria, allocation of corporate overhead costs, depreciation practices, budgeting, financial targets, etc.)?

1b.   What *changes* do you anticipate making in your system's financial management practices and policies within the next year or two?

1c.   What are your current financial targets for:

a)   Profit margin?_____

b)   Revenue growth?_____

c)   Return on equity?_____

d)   Debt/equity ratio?_____

D.   *Marketing* (ask only of the vice-president for marketing)

1a.   What kinds of changes have been made over the *past two years* in your system's approach to *marketing and the organization of the marketing function* (centralization versus decentralization of marketing activities, process of doing market research, use of marketing data, development of product-line management, marketing of physician practices, etc.)?

1b.   What *changes* in your *marketing* plans, policies, and organization do you foresee making over the next year or two?

E.   *Human Resources* (ask only of the vice-president for human resources)

1a.   What kinds of changes have been made over the *past two years* in your system's human resource management policies and practices

and the organization of the human resources
function (recruitment, performance appraisal,
management development, compensation,
etc.)?

1b.   What kinds of *changes* do you foresee making
in your system's human resources area over the
next year or two?

Resource C

Research Variables and Measures

Table C.1. Computation of Environmental Measures:
Principal Components Analysis Using Varimax Rotation.

Market Demand Factor[a]	
Variables	*Factor Loading*
Percent of population below the poverty line	− 0.86
Median family income adjusted by area wage index	0.83
Median home value	0.75
Years of schooling for those over 25	0.74

Resource Supply Factor[b]	
Variables	*Factor Loading*
Actively practicing physicians per 1.000 population	0.86
Central-city location	0.79
Percent white-collar and health professionals in labor force	0.74

[a]Eigenvalue = 4.27; cumulative percent variance explained = 42.7
[b]Eigenvalue = 1.38; cumulative percent variance explained = 56.5

Certificate-of-Need Measurement
(Theoretical Range = 0 to 22)

Percentage of applications approved
  84 percent and above = 1
  70 to 83 percent = 2
  69 percent and below = 3
State certificate-of-need budget per hospital
  None = 0
  Up to $2,200 = 1
  $2,201 to $3,700 = 2
  $3,701 and above = 3
Years since first enactment
  0 to 9 = 1
  10 to 14 = 2
  15 and above = 3
Proposed capital expenditure threshold level
  Not applicable = 0
  $1,000,000 or more = 1
  $550,000 to $999,999 = 2
  Less than $550,000 = 3
Institutional health services threshold level
  Not applicable = 0
  $1,000,000 or more = 1
  $250,000 to $999,999 = 2
  Less than $250,000 = 3
Major medical equipment threshold
  Not applicable = 0
  $400,000 and above = 1
  Less than $400,000 = 2
*Has a moratorium on new expenditures or services development
ever existed?*
  Yes = 1
  No = 0
Has a ceiling or cap on capital expenditures ever existed?
  Yes = 1
  No = 0

Is the program in compliance with federal law?
  Yes = 1
  No = 0
Are there plans to continue the certificate-of-need program?
  Yes = 1
  No = 0
Has there been a bed restriction strategy?
  Yes = 1
  No or don't know = 0

Rate-Review Measurement
(Theoretical Range = 0 to 14)

Type of program
  No program = 0
  Disclosure only = 1
  Voluntary = 2
  Mandatory = 3

Basis for rate setting
  No program = 0
  Disclosure = 1
  Negotiated = 2
  Budget review = 3
  Prospective budget = 4

Years since program started
  No program = 0
  1 to 12 years = 1
  13 to 15 years = 2
  16 years plus = 3

Number of different payors covered
  No program = 0
  One = 1
  Two = 2
  Three = 3
  All payors = 4

The Sixteen Conditions or Procedures

A. *Nonoperative*   *ICDA-9 Codes*
    Acute MI   410 through 410.9

    Acute kidney (tubular) necrosis   584.5

    Congestive heart failure   428.0

    Cholecystitis and cholangitis
        without mention of calculus   575.0
                                                           575.1
                                                           576.1

    Pulmonary embolism   415.1

B. *Operative*
    Lens procedure primary   13.1
                                                           13.11
                                                           13.19
                                                           13.59
                                                           13.71
                                                           13.72

    Cholecystectomy   51.22

    Transurethral resection of prostate   60.2

    Repair of inguinal hernia   53.00
                                                           53.01
                                                           53.02

    Mastectomy   85.41
                                                           85.43

    Excision/destruction of local   57.49
        lesion of bladder

Coronary bypass surgery · · · · · · · · · · 36.11
36.12
36.13
36.14

Laminectomies · · · · · · · · · · 80.5

Total hip replacement · · · · · · · · · · 81.51
81.59

Total knee replacement · · · · · · · · · · 81.41

C. *Complications and Misadventures*
Preventable intraoperative · · · · · · · · · · 998.2
complications · · · · · · · · · · 998.4
998.6

Potentially preventable intra- · · · · · · · · · · 998.0
operative and postoperative · · · · · · · · · · 998.1
complications · · · · · · · · · · 998.3
998.5

Other complications · · · · · · · · · · 998.9

Misadventures in medical care · · · · · · · · · · 999.0

Complications of surgical
procedures · · · · · · · · · · 997.0

Other complications · · · · · · · · · · 995.2
995.3
995.4

Resource D

Availability and Profitability of Hospital Services

Most Frequently Reported Profitable Services
(Profitable = More than 75 percent of all respondents
reported service as profitable)

Outpatient chemotherapy or radiation treatment
Mammography
Coordinated outpatient rehabilitation program
Ultrasound
CT scan
Cardiovascular/pulmonary diagnostic services
Nuclear medicine
Durable medical equipment or medical supplies for home
use

Most Frequently Reported Unprofitable Services
(Unprofitable = more than 50 percent of all respondents
reported service as unprofitable)

Crisis intervention
School health exams
Outpatient services to AIDS patients

Fitness center(s)
Geriatric assessment, consultation, case management
Geriatric day care
Disease- or condition-specific education and counseling
Community health lectures and classes
Home-delivered meals to seniors
Family planning or preparation lectures and classes
Health screening
Hospice
Immunizations

Most Frequently Planned Services

	N
NMR or MRI	110
Durable medical equipment for home use	73
Executive or industrial health services	66
CT scan	58
In-home respiratory therapy	56
In-home infusion therapy	52
Fitness center	50
Sports medicine or orthopedic clinic	49
Community health centers and classes	44
Birthing center	42
Health screening	41
Geriatric assessment, consultation, or case management	40
Freestanding skilled nursing facility or intermediate care facility	40

Most Frequently Discontinued Services

	N
Durable medical equipment	21
Urgent or immediate care centers	19
In-home skilled nursing	15
Home-delivered meals to seniors	13
In-home physical therapy	13
Executive or industrial health services	12
In-home respiratory therapy	12

Resource E

Analyses of Performance: Profitability and Market Share

**Table E.1. Profitability Equations
(Percentage of Diversified Services Profitable).**

	(1)	(2)	(3)	(4)
Resource supply	1.56	.82	− 1.37	− 1.39
	(1.11)	(1.40)	(1.45)	(1.44)
Market demand	3.52[a]	2.71[b]	1.82	1.54
	(1.09)	(1.20)	(1.19)	(1.19)
Stringency of certificate of need		− .034	− .056	− .005
		(.25)	(.25)	(.25)
Stringency of rate review		.461	.50[b]	.56[b]
		(.25)	(.25)	(.25)
Intensity of competition		1.75	1.66	1.32
		(1.01)	(.98)	(.98)
Two or more competitors		− .42	− .84	− .57
		(2.85)	(2.76)	(2.74)
Investor-owned versus not-for-profit			− 2.49	− 3.39
			(3.05)	(3.05)
Bed size			.052[a]	.050[a]
			(.01)	(.011)
Strategic orientation				1.83[a]
				(.75)
$\hat{R}^2 =$	.03	.04	.10	.11
F =	6.55	3.25	5.95	6.02
P =	≤ .001	≤ .004	≤ .001	≤ .001

[a]$p \leq .001$.
[b]$p \leq .05$.

365

Table E.2. Market Share Equation.
(Market share greater than competitors
adjusted for number of competitors.)

	(1)	(2)	(3)	(4)
Resource supply	1.64[a]	.67[a]	.61[a]	.61[a]
	(.13)	(.14)	(.14)	(.14)
Market demand	.81[a]	.31[a]	.24[b]	.20
	(.12)	(.12)	(.12)	(.12)
Stringency of certificate of need		.026	.037	.04
		(.024)	(.025)	(.025)
Stringency of rate review		.000	.011	.019
		(.024)	(.025)	(.024)
Intensity of competition		− .008	− .001	− .04
		(.099)	(.098)	(.098)
Two or more competitors		3.16[a]	3.18[a]	3.21[a]
		(.28)	(.28)	(.27)
Investor-owned versus not-for-profit			− .66[b]	− .77[b]
			(.306)	(.304)
Bed size			.002[b]	.001
			(.001)	(.001)
Strategic orientation				.24[b]
				(.07)
$\hat{R}^2 =$	.38	.54	.55	.57
F =	110.9	73.6	57.7	53.7
p =	≤ .0001	≤ .0001	≤ .0001	≤ .001

[a]$P \le .001$.
[b]$P \le .05$.

Resource F

Related Study Publications

Friedman, B. S., and Shortell, S. M. "The Financial Performance of Selected Investor-Owned and Not-For-Profit System Hospitals Before and After Medicare Prospective Payment." *Health Services Research,* 1988, *23* (2), 237–267.

Golden, B. "Business Strategy as a Critical Contingency for the Corporate-Division Relationship." Unpublished doctoral dissertation, Department of Organization Behavior, J. L. Kellogg Graduate School of Management, Northwestern University, June 1989.

Shortell, S. M. "The Evolution of Hospital Systems: Unfulfilled Promises and Self-Fulfilling Prophesies." *Medical Care Review,* 1988, *45* (2), 177–214.

Shortell, S. M. "New Directions in Hospital Governance." *Journal of Hospital and Health Services Administration,* 1989, *34* (1), 7–23.

Shortell, S. M., and Hughes, E.F.X. "The Effects of Regulation, Competition, and Ownership on Mortality Rates Among Hospital Inpatients." *The New England Journal of Medicine,* 1988, *318,* 1100–1107.

Shortell, S. M., and others. "Hospital Ownership and Nontraditional Services." *Health Affairs,* 1986, *5,* 97–111.

Shortell, S. M., and others. "Diversification of Health Care Services: The Effects of Ownership, Environment, and Strategy." In L. Rossiter and R. Scheffler (eds.), *Advances in Health Economics and Health Services Research.* Vol. 7. Greenwich, Conn.: JAI Press, 1987.

Shortell, S. M., Morrison, E. M., and Hughes, S. L. "The Keys to Successful Diversification: Lessons from Leading Hospital Systems." *Hospital and Health Services Administration. 39,* Fall 1989.

Shortell, S. M., Morrison, E. M., and Robbins, S. R. "Strategy-Making in Health Care Organizations: A Framework and Agenda for Research." *Medical Care Review,* 1985, *42* (2), 219–266.

Shortell, S. M. and Zajac, E. J. "Assessing the Reliability and Validity of Miles and Snows's Strategic Types." Discussion Paper No. 22, General Motors Center for Strategy in Management, J. L. Kellogg Graduate School of Management, Northwestern University, Evanston, Ill., May, 1989.

Zajac, E. J., and Shortell, S. M. "Changing Generic Strategies: Likelihood, Direction, and Performance Implications." *Strategic Management Journal,* 1989.

References

Albert, S. "A Delete Design Model for Successful Transitions." In J. R. Kimberly and R. E. Quinn (eds.), *New Futures: The Challenge of Managing Corporate Transitions.* Homewood, Ill.: Dow Jones-Irwin, 1984.

Aldrich, H. *Organization and Environments.* Englewood Cliffs, N.J.: Prentice-Hall, 1979.

Aldrich, H., and Whetten, D. A. "Organization-Sets, Action-Sets and Networks: Making the Most of Simplicity." In P. C. Nystrom and W. H. Starbuck (eds.), *Handbook of Organizational Design.* New York: Oxford University Press, 1981.

Alexander, J. A., Morlock, L. L., and Gifford, B. D. "The Effects of Corporate Restructuring on Hospital Policymaking." *Health Services Research,* 1988, *23,* 311–337.

American College of Health Care Executives, American Hospital Association, and Heidrick and Struggles. *CEO Turnover Report.* Chicago: American Hospital Association, 1988.

American Hospital Association. *Ameriplan: A Proposal for the Delivery and Financing of Health Services in the United States.* Report of a Special Committee on the Provision of Health Services. Chicago: American Hospital Association, 1970.

American Hospital Association. *U.S. Hospital Closures: 1980–1987.* Chicago: American Hospital Association, 1988.

Anderson, C. R., and Zeithaml, C. D. "Stages of the Product Life Cycle, Business Strategy, and Business Performance." *Academy of Management Journal,* 1984, *27,* 5–24.

Argyris, C., and Schön, D. A. *Organizational Learning.* Reading, Mass.: Addison-Wesley, 1978.

Armour, H. O., and Teece, D. J. "Organizational Structure and Economic Performance: A Test of the Multi-divisional Hypothesis." *Bell Journal of Economics,* 1978, *9* (1), 106–122.

Arthur Andersen & Co. and the American College of Hospital Administrators. *Health Care in the 1990s: Trends and Strategies.* Chicago: Arthur Andersen & Co. and the American College of Hospital Administrators, 1984.

Arthur Andersen & Co. and the American Hospital Association. *Multi-Hospital Systems: Perspectives and Trends.* Chicago: American Hospital Association, 1987.

Astley, W. G., and Fombrun, C. J. "Collective Strategy: The Social Ecology of Organizational Environments." *Academy of Management Review,* 1983, *8,* 576–587.

Astley, W. G., and Van de Ven, A. H. "Central Perspectives and Debates in Organization Theory." *Administrative Science Quarterly,* 1983, *28,* 245–273.

Barney, J. B. "The Context of Formal Strategic Planning and the Economic Performance of Firms." Strategy Group Working Paper Series, no. 88-005. College Station: Department of Management, Texas A & M University, Apr. 1988.

Barney, J. B., and Ouchi, W. G. (eds.). *Organizational Economics: Toward a New Paradigm for Understanding and Studying Organizations.* San Francisco: Jossey-Bass, 1986.

Bernstein, S. C., and Associates. *The Future of Health Care Delivery in America.* New York: Sanford C. Bernstein & Co., 1985.

Bhambri, A., and Greiner, L. "Types, Conditions, Processes of Strategic Change." Paper presented at meeting of the Strategic Management Society, Boston, Oct. 1987.

Bice, M. D. "Corporate Culture and Business Strategy: A Health Management Company Perspective." *Hospital and Health Services Administration,* 1984, *29* (4), 64–78.

Binns, G. "The Inter-Relationship Among Quality Indicators, Profitability, and Market Share for Hospitals Treating Medicare Beneficiaries." Paper presented at Center for Health Administration Studies Workshop Seminar, University of Chicago, Jan. 12, 1989.

Blendon, R. J. "The Public's View of the Future of Health Care." *Journal of The American Medical Association,* 1988, *259,* 3587–3593.

Blendon, R. J. "Polls Show Discontent with Health Care." *New York Times,* Feb. 15, 1989a, p. 8.

Blendon, R. J. "Three Systems: A Comparative Survey." *Health Management Quarterly,* 1989b, *11* (1), 2–10.

Blumberg, M. "Risk-Adjusting Health Care Outcomes: A Methodological Review." *Medical Care Review,* 1986, *43,* 351–396.

Boeker, W. "The Permanence of Organizational Strategy." *Proceedings of the Academy of Management,* Aug. 10, 1988, pp. 2–5.

Brook, R. "The Public's Role in Assuring the Quality of Health Care." The John H. Hollister Memorial Lecture, Northwestern University, Evanston, Ill., Feb. 22, 1989.

Brook, R. H., and Lohr, K. N. "Efficacy, Effectiveness, and Quality: Boundary-Crossing Research." *Medical Care,* May 1985, 710–722.

Brown, L. D. "The Managerial Imperative and Organizational Innovation in Health Services." In E. Ginzberg (ed.), *The U.S. Health Care System: A Look to the 1990's.* Totowa, N.J.: Rowman and Allanheld, 1985.

Burgelman, R. A. "A Model of the Interaction of Strategic Behavior, Corporate Context, and the Concept of Strategy." *Academy of Management Review,* 1983, *8* (1), 61–70.

Burgelman, R. A. "The Intra-Organizational Ecology of Strategy Making and Organizational Adaptation: A Conceptual Integration." Working paper, Strategic Management Program, Graduate School of Business, Stanford University, Nov. 1987.

Buzzell, R., and Gale, B. *The PIMS Principles: Linking Strategy to Performance.* New York: Free Press, 1987.

Cameron, K. S., and Whetten, D. *Organizational Effectiveness:*

A Comparison of Multiple Models. Orlando, Fla.: Academic Press, 1983.

Camillus, J. C. *Strategic Planning and Management Control.* New York: Lexington Press, 1986.

Carper, W. B., and Litschert, R. J. "Strategic Power Relationships in Contemporary Profit and Nonprofit Hospitals." *Academy of Management Journal,* 1983, *26,* 311–320.

Chakravarthy, B. S. "Measuring Strategic Performance." *Strategic Management Journal,* 1986, *7,* 437–458.

Chandler, A. *The Visible Hand: The Managerial Revolution in American Business.* Cambridge, Mass.: Harvard University Press, 1977.

Chandler, A. D., Jr. *Strategy and Structure: Chapters in the History of the Industrial Enterprise.* Cambridge, Mass.: MIT Press, 1962.

Chapko, M., and others. "Development of a Multi-Dimensional Measure of Capital Expenditure and Rate Regulation for Hospitals." Working paper, Department of Health Services, University of Washington, June 1984.

Cheng, J. C., and Kesner, I. F. "Responsiveness to Environmental Change: The Interactive Effects of Organizational Slack and Strategic Orientation." *Proceedings of the Academy of Management,* Aug. 10, 1988, pp. 165–169.

Child, J. "Organizational Structure, Environment, and Performance—The Role of Strategic Choice." *Sociology,* 1972, *6,* 2–22.

Child, J., and Kieser, A. "Development of Organizations Over Time." In P. C. Nystrom and W. H. Starbuck (eds.), *Handbook of Organizational Design.* New York: Oxford University Press, 1981.

Christensen, H. K., and Montgomery, C. A. "Corporate Economic Performance: Diversification Strategy vs. Market Structure." *Strategic Management Journal,* 1981, *2,* 328–343.

Clement, J. P. "Does Hospital Diversification Improve Financial Outcomes?" *Medical Care,* 1987, *25,* 988–1001.

Coile, R. "Health Care 1989: Top 10 Market and Management Trends." *Hospital Strategy Report,* 1988, *1* (2), 1–8.

Cook, K., Shortell, S. M., Conrad, D., and Morrisey, M. A. "A Theory of Organizational Response to Regulation: The

Case of Hospitals." *Academy of Management Review,* 1983, *8,* 193–205.

Covin, J. G., and Slevin, D. P. "Strategic Management of Small Firms in Hostile and Benign Environments." *Strategic Management Journal,* 1989, *10,* 75–88.

Coyne, J. S., and Cobbs, D. L. *Financial Growth and Diversification of Hospitals and Multi-Hospital Systems.* Chicago: American Hospital Association, 1988.

Cresap. *The Effective Head Office.* Northants, England: British Institute of Management, 1988.

Daft, R., Sormunen, J., and Parks, D. "Chief Executive Scanning, Environmental Characteristics, and Company Performance: An Empirical Study." *Strategic Management Journal,* 1988, *9,* 123–139.

Deal, T. E., and Kennedy, A. A. *Corporate Cultures: The Rites and Rituals of Corporate Life.* Reading, Mass.: Addison-Wesley, 1982.

Delbecq, A., and Gill, S. L. "Developing Strategic Direction for Governing Boards." *Hospital and Health Services Administration,* 1988, *33,* 25–36.

Denzin, N. *Sociological Methods: A Source Book.* New York: McGraw-Hill, 1970.

Dess, G. G., and Beard, D. W. "Dimensions of Organizational Task Environments." *Administrative Science Quarterly,* 1984, *29,* 52–73.

Dess, G. G., and Davis, P. S. "Porter's (1980) Generic Strategies as Determinants of Strategic Group Membership and Organization Performance." *Academy of Management Journal,* 1984, *27,* 467–488.

Dess, G. G., and Robinson, R. B., Jr. "Measuring Organizational Performance in the Absence of Objective Measures: The Case of the Privately Held Firm and the Conglomerate Business Unit." *Strategic Management Journal,* 1984, *5,* 265–273.

Dill, W. "Environment as an Influence on Managerial Autonomy." *Administrative Science Quarterly,* 1958, *3,* 409–443.

DiMaggio, P., and Powell, W. W. "The Iron Cage Revisited: Institutional Isomorphism and Collective Rationality in Organizational Fields." *American Sociological Review,* 1983, *48,* 147–160.

Doz, Y., and Prahalad, C. K. *The Multinational Mission: Balancing Local Demands and Global Vision.* New York: Free Press, 1987.

Dranove, D., and Cone, K. "Do State Rate Setting Regulations Really Lower Hospital Expenses?" *Journal of Health Economics,* 1985, *4,* 159–165.

Drazin, R., and Van de Ven, A. H. "Alternative Forms of Fit in Contingency Theory." *Administrative Science Quarterly,* 1985, *30,* 514–539.

Duncan, R. B. "Characteristics of Organizational Environments and Perceived Environmental Uncertainty." *Administrative Science Quarterly,* 1972, *17,* 313–327.

Duncan, R. B. "What Is the Right Structure?" *Organizational Dynamics,* 1979, *7,* 59–80.

Dutton, J. E., and Duncan, R. B. "The Creation of Momentum for Change Through the Process of Strategic Issue Diagnosis." *Strategic Management Journal,* 1987, *8,* 279–295.

Ellwood, P. M. "Shattuck Lecture — Outcomes Management: A Technology of Patient Experience." *New England Journal of Medicine,* 1988, *318,* 1549–1556.

Ellwood, P. M. "Outcomes Management: The Next Step Beyond Quality Assurance." *Hospital Strategy Report,* 1989, *1,* 1–5.

Enthoven, A., and Kronich, R. "A Consumer-Choice Health Plan for the 1990's: Universal Health Insurance in a System Designed to Promote Quality and Economy." *New England Journal of Medicine,* 1989, *320,* 29–37.

Fahey, L., and Christensen, H. "Evaluating the Research on Strategy Content." *Journal of Management,* 1986, *12* (2), 167–183.

Feder, J., Hadley, J., and Zuckerman, S. "How Did Medicare's Prospective Payment System Affect Hospitals?" *New England Journal of Medicine,* 1987, *317* (14), 867–873.

Fiol, C. M., and Lyles, M. A. "Organizational Learning." *Academy of Management Review,* 1985, 803–813.

Foley, H. A. "Health Planning — Demise or Reformation?" *New England Journal of Medicine,* 1981, *304* (16), 969–972.

Fombrun, C. J., and Zajac, E. J. "Structural and Perceptual Influences on Intraindustry Stratification." *Academy of Management Journal,* 1987, *30,* 33–50.

Fox, R. C. "Reflections and Opportunities in the Sociology of Medicine." *Journal of Health and Social Behavior,* 1985, *26,* 6–14.

Freeman, E. *Stakeholder Management.* Marshfield, Mass.: Pitman, 1984.

Friedman, B., and Shortell, S. M. "The Financial Performance of Selected Investor-Owned and Not-for-Profit System Hospitals Before and After Medicare Prospective Payment." *Health Services Research,* 1988, *23* (2), 237–267.

Friedman, G. "Another Pennsylvania Hospital Prevails in Tax-Exemption Battle." *Healthweek News,* Jan. 9, 1989, p. 5.

Galbraith, J. R. *Designing Complex Organizations.* Reading, Mass.: Addison-Wesley, 1973.

Garnick, D. W., Luft, H. S., Robinson, J. C., and Tetreault, J. "Appropriate Measures of Hospital Market Areas." *Health Services Research,* 1987, *22,* 69–89.

Ghemawat, P. "Building Strategy on the Experience Curve." *Harvard Business Review,* 1985, *63,* 143–149.

Gilbert, X., and Strebel, P. "Strategies to Outpace the Competition." *Journal of Business Strategy,* 1987, *8,* 28–36.

Ginn, G. O., and McDaniel, R. R. "Strategic Adaptation in the Hospital Industry." *Proceedings of the Academy of Management,* Aug. 1987, pp. 87–90.

Ginsberg, A., and Grant, J. H. "Research on Strategic Change: Theoretical and Methodological Issues." *Proceedings of the Academy of Management,* Aug. 1985.

Ginsberg, A., and Venkatraman, J. "Contingency Perspectives of Organizational Strategy: A Critical Review of the Empirical Research." *Academy of Management Review,* 1985, *10,* 421–434.

Golden, B. "Business Strategy as a Critical Contingency for the Corporate-Division Relationship." Unpublished doctoral dissertation, Department of Organization Behavior, J. L. Kellogg Graduate School of Management, Northwestern University, June 1989.

Goldsmith, J. A. "A Radical Prescription for Hospitals." *Harvard Business Review,* 1989, *67,* 104–111.

Goodman, P. S., Pennings, J. M., and Associates. *New Perspectives on Organizational Effectiveness.* San Francisco: Jossey-Bass, 1977.

Goold, M., and Campbell, A. "Many Best Ways to Make Strategy." *Harvard Business Review,* 1987, *65,* 70–76.

Govindarajan, V. "Decentralization, Strategy, and Effectiveness of Strategic Business Units in Multi-Business Organizations." *Academy of Management Review,* 1986, *11,* 844–856.

Govindarajan, V. "A Contingency Approach to Strategy Implementation at the Business-Unit Level: Integrating Administrative Mechanisms with Strategy." *Academy of Management Journal,* 1988, *31,* 828–853.

Grant, J. H. (ed.) *Frontiers of Strategic Management.* Greenwich, Conn.: JAI Press, 1988.

Gray, B. H. *Profit, Corporate Change, and Accountability in American Health Care.* New York: 20th Century Fund, forthcoming.

Gray, B. H., and Ariss, S. S. "Politics and Strategic Change Across Organizational Life Cycles." *Academy of Management Review,* 1985, *10,* 707–723.

Green, A. "Comments on the Evolution of Hospital Systems." Paper presented at Rush–Presbyterian–St. Luke's Eighth Annual Symposium on Health Care Affairs, Chicago, Feb. 13, 1989.

Greiner, L. E., and Bhambri, A. "New CEO Intervention and Dynamics of Deliberate Strategic Change." *Strategic Management Journal,* 1989.

Griffith, J. *The Well Managed Community Hospital.* Ann Arbor, Mich.: Health Administration Press, 1987.

Guncheon, K. "Mission Control." *Multi's,* Sept. 1984, p. M84.

Gupta, A. "SBU Strategies, Corporate-SBU Relations, and SBU Effectiveness in Strategy Implementation." *Academy of Management Journal,* 1987, *30* (3), 477–500.

Guterman, S., and Dobson, A. "Impact of the Medicare Prospective Payment System for Hospitals." *Health Care Financing Review,* 1986, *7* (3), 97–114.

Hambrick, D. C. "Environment, Strategy, and Power Within Top Management Teams." *Administrative Science Quarterly,* 1981, *26,* 253–276.

Hambrick, D. C. "Some Tests of the Effectiveness and Functional Attributes of Miles and Snow's Strategic Types." *Academy of Management Journal,* 1983, *26,* 5–26.

Hambrick, D. C. "Turnaround Strategies." In W. H. Guth (ed.), _Handbook of Business Strategy._ Boston: Warren, Gorham, and Lamont, 1985.

Hambrick, D. C. _The Executive Effect: Concepts and Methods for Studying Top Managers._ Greenwich, Conn.: JAI Press, 1988.

Hambrick, D. C., and Finkelstein, S. "Managerial Discretion: A Bridge Between Polar Views and Organizational Outcomes." In B. Staw and L. L. Cummings (eds.), _Research in Organizational Behavior._ Vol. 7. Greenwich, Conn.: JAI Press, 1987.

Hambrick, D. C., and Mason, P. A. "Upper Echelons: The Organization as a Reflection of Its Top Managers." _Academy of Management Review,_ 1984, _9,_ 193–206.

Hannan, M., and Freeman, J. "The Population Ecology of Organizations." _American Journal of Sociology,_ 1977, _82,_ 929–964.

Hannan, M. T., and Freeman, J. "Structural Inertia and Organizational Change." _American Sociological Review,_ 1984, _49,_ 149–164.

Hansmann, H. G. "The Role of Not-for-Profit Enterprise." _Yale Law Journal,_ 1980, _89_ (5), 835–901.

Hartman, S. E., and Mukamel, D. B. "How Might a Low-Cost Hospital System Look?" _Medical Care,_ 1989, _27,_ 234–243.

Health Care Financial Management Association. "Hospital Industry Financial Report." _Modern Health Care,_ 1988, _18,_ 92.

Health Care Financing Administration. _Impact of Medicare Prospective Payment on the Quality of Medical Care: A Research Agenda._ Santa Monica, Calif.: Rand, 1985.

Henderson, B. D. _The Experience Curve Reviewed IV: The Growth Share Matrix of the Product Portfolio._ Boston: Boston Consulting Group, 1973.

Herzlinger, R. E., and Krasker, W. S. "Who Profits from Non-Profits?" _Harvard Business Review,_ 1987, _65,_ 93–106.

Hill, C.W.L., and Hoskisson, R. E. "Strategy and Structure in the Multiproduct Firm." _Academy of Management Review,_ 1987, _12_ (2), 331–341.

Hirsch, P. M. "Organizational Effectiveness and the Institutional Environment." _Administrative Science Quarterly,_ 1975, _20,_ 327–344.

Hirsch, P. M. "The Study of Industries." In S. B. Bacharach (ed.), *Research in the Sociology of Organizations.* Vol. 3. Greenwich, Conn.: JAI Press, 1984.

Hofer, C. W., and Schendel, D. E. *Strategy Formulation: Analytical Concepts.* St. Paul, Minn.: West, 1978.

Hoskisson, R. E. "Multidivisional Structure and Performance: The Contingency of Diversification Strategy." *Academy of Management Journal,* 1987, *30* (4), 625–644.

Hrebiniak, L. G., and Joyce, W. F. "Organizational Adaptation: Strategic Choice and Environmental Determinism." *Administrative Science Quarterly,* 1985, *30,* 336–349.

Huff, A. S., and Reger, R K. "A Review of Strategic Process Research." *Journal of Management,* 1987, *13* (2), 211–236.

Institute of Medicine. *For-Profit Enterprise in Health Care.* (B. Gray, ed.) Washington, D.C.: National Academy Press, 1986.

Interstudy. *HMO Report.* Minneapolis, Minn.: Interstudy, 1988.

Jarillo, C. J. "On Strategic Networks." *Strategic Management Journal,* 1988, *9,* 31–41.

Johnson, G., and Thomas, H. "The Industry Context of Strategy, Structure, and Performance: The U.K. Brewing Industry." *Strategic Management Journal,* 1987, *8,* 343–361.

Jones, G. R., and Hill, C. "Transaction Cost Analysis of Strategy-Structure Choice." *Strategic Management Journal,* 1988, *9,* 159–172.

Kane, R. L. "The U.S. Health Care System: Basic Goals." In Public Policy Institute, American Association of Retired Persons, *Changing America's Health Care System: Proposals For Legislative Action.* Glenview, Ill.: Scott, Foresman, 1989.

Kanter, R. M. *The Change Masters.* New York: Simon & Schuster, 1984.

Kanter, R. M., and Brinkerhoff, D. "Organizational Performance: Recent Developments in Measurement." *Annual Review of Sociology,* 1981, *7,* 321–349.

Karnani, A. "Generic Competitive Strategies — An Analytical Approach." *Strategic Management Journal,* 1984, *5,* 367–380.

Kazanjian, R. K., and Drazin, R. "Implementing Internal Diversification: Contingency Factors for Organization Design Choices." *Academy of Management Review,* 1987, *12,* 342–354.

Keats, B. W., Conant, J. S., and Mokwa, M. P., "Strategic Orientation and Relative Effectiveness Among Health Maintenance Organizations." Paper presented at meeting of the Academy of Management, Anaheim, Calif., Aug. 1988.

Kimberly, J. R., Miles, R. H., and Associates. *The Organizational Life Cycle: Issues in the Creation, Transformation, and Decline of Organizations.* San Francisco: Jossey-Bass, 1980.

Kinzer, D. M. "The Potential for New Regulatory Strategies." *Frontiers of Health Services Management,* 1988, *5,* 3–40.

Kirkman-Liff, B. L., Lapre, R., and Kirkman-Liff, T. L. "The Metamorphosis of Health Planning in the Netherlands and the U.S.A." *International Journal of Health Planning and Management,* 1988, *3,* 89–110.

Kovner, A. R. "Improving the Effectiveness of Hospital Governing Boards." *Frontiers of Health Services Management,* 1985, *2,* 4–23.

Kralewski, J., Gifford, G., and Porter, J. "Profit vs. Public Welfare Goals in Investor-Owned and Not-for-Profit Hospitals." *Hospital and Health Services Administration,* 1988, *33,* 311–329.

Lambkin, M. "Order of Entry and Performance in New Markets." *Strategic Management Journal,* 1988, *9,* 127–140.

Lawrence, P. R., and Dyer, D. *Renewing American Industry.* New York: Free Press, 1983.

Lawrence, P. R., and Lorsch, J. W. *Organization and Environment: Managing Differentiation and Integration.* Boston: Graduate School of Business Administration, Harvard University, 1967.

Leatt, P., Shortell, S. M., and Kimberly, J. R. "Organization Design." In S. M. Shortell and A. D. Kaluzny (eds.), *Health Care Management: A Text in Organization Theory and Behavior.* (2nd ed.) New York: Wiley, 1988.

Lenz, R. T., and Engledow, J. L. "Environmental Analysis: The Applicability of Current Theory." *Strategic Management Journal,* 1986, *7,* 329–346.

Lewin, L. S., Eckels, T. J., and Miller, C. B. "Setting the Record Straight: The Provision of Uncompensated Care by Not-for-Profit Hospitals." *New England Journal of Medicine,* 1988, *318,* 1212–1215.

Lewis, B. L., and Alexander, J. A. "A Taxonomic Analysis of Multi-Hospital Systems." *Health Services Research,* 1986, *21,* 29–56.

Lieberman, M. B., and Montgomery, D. B. "First-Mover Advantages." *Strategic Management Journal,* 1988, *9,* 41–58.

Light, D. W. "Social Control and the American Health Care System." In H. E. Freeman and S. Levine (eds.), *Handbook of Medical Sociology.* (4th ed.) Englewood Cliffs, N.J.: Prentice-Hall, 1987–88.

Lohr, K. N. (ed.). "Advances in Health Status: Conference Proceedings." *Medical Care,* Supplement, 1989, *27* (3), S2–S294.

Lohr, K. N., and others. *Conceptualization and Measurement of Physiologic Health for Adults: Overview of Chronic Disease in a General Adult Population.* Santa Monica, Calif.: Rand, 1986.

Lorange, P. "Formal Planning Systems: Their Role in Strategy Implementation." In D. E. Schendel and C. W. Hofer (eds.), *Strategic Management: A New View of Business Policy and Planning.* Boston: Little, Brown, 1979.

Lorange, P., Scott-Morton, M. F., and Ghoshal, S. *Strategic Control Systems.* St. Paul, Minn.: West, 1986.

Luft, H., and Robinson, J. *Hospital Competition, Nursing Wages, and the Cost of Care.* PB88-181045/AS. Springfield, Va.: National Technical Information Service, U.S. Department of Commerce, 1988.

Luft, H., Robinson, J., Garnick, D., Maerki, S., and McPhee, S. "The Role of Specialized Clinical Services in Competition Among Hospitals." *Inquiry,* 1987, *23,* 83–94.

Luft, H. S., and others. "Hospital Behavior in a Local Market Context." *Medical Care Review,* 1986, *43* (2), 218–251.

Luke, R. D., and Begun, J. W. "Strategic Orientations of Small Multihospital Systems." *Health Services Research,* 1988, *23* (5), 597–618.

Luke, R. D., Begun, J. W., and Pointer, D. D. "Quasi Firms: Strategic Interorganizational Forms in the Health Care Industry." *Academy of Management Review,* 1989, *14* (1), 9–19.

MacMillan, I. C. "Preemptive Strategies." *Journal of Business Strategy,* 1983, *3,* 16–22.

McNerney, W. *The Health Policy Agenda for the 1990's: Unfinished Business.* Chicago: Governance Institute, Illinois Hospital

Association, J. L. Kellogg Graduate School of Management, Northwestern University, and Ernst & Whinney, 1988.

Melnick, G. A., and Zwanziger, J. "Hospital Behavior Under Competition and Cost Containment Policies." *Journal of the American Medical Association,* 1988, *260,* 2669–2675.

Meyer, A. "Adapting to Environmental Jolts." *Administrative Science Quarterly,* 1982, *27,* 515–537.

Michael, S. R. "Feedforward Versus Feedback Controls in Planning." *Management Planning,* 1980, *29,* 34–48.

Mick, S. S., and Conrad, D. A. "The Decision to Integrate Vertically in Health Care Organizations." *Journal of Hospital and Health Services Administration,* 1988, *33,* 345–360.

Miles, R., and Cameron, K. *Coffin Nails and Corporate Strategies.* Englewood Cliffs, N.J.: Prentice-Hall, 1982.

Miles, R. E., and Snow, C. C. *Organizational Strategy, Structure, and Process.* New York: McGraw-Hill, 1978.

Miller, D. "Configurations of Strategy and Structure: Towards a Synthesis." *Strategic Management Journal,* 1986, *7* (3), 233–249.

Miller, D., and Friesen, P. H. *Organizations: A Quantum View.* Englewood Cliffs, N.J.: Prentice-Hall, 1984.

Mintzberg, H. "Patterns in Strategy Formation." *Management Science,* 1978, *24,* 934–948.

Mintzberg, H., and McHugh, A. "Strategy Formation and Adhocracy." *Administrative Science Quarterly,* 1985, *30,* 160–197.

Mohr, L. B. *Explaining Organizational Behavior: The Limits and Possibilities of Theory and Research.* San Francisco: Jossey-Bass, 1982.

Montgomery, C. A. "The Measurement of Related Diversification: Some New Empirical Evidence." *Academy of Management Journal,* 1982, *25,* 299–307.

Morrisey, M. A., Conrad, A. A., Shortell, S. M., and Cook, K. "Hospital Rate Review; A Theoretical and Empirical Review." *Journal of Health Economics,* 1984, *3,* 25–47.

Nielsen, R. P. "Cooperative Strategies." *Strategic Management Journal,* 1988, *9,* 475–492.

Office of Technology Assessment. *Medicare's Prospective Payment System.* Washington, D.C.: U.S. Government Printing Office, 1985.

Oster, S. "Intra-Industry Structure and the Ease of Strategic Change." *Review of Economics and Statistics,* 1982, *64,* 376–383.

Pearson, A. "Tough-Minded Ways to Get Innovative." *Harvard Business Review,* 1988, *66,* 99–106.

Peters, J. P., and Tseng, S. *Managing Strategic Change in Hospitals: Ten Success Stories.* Chicago: American Hospital Association, 1983.

Pettigrew, A. M. (ed.). *The Management of Strategic Change.* Oxford, England: Basil Blackwell, 1987.

Pfeffer, J., and Salancik, G. *The External Control of Organizations: A Resource Dependence Perspective.* New York: Harper & Row, 1978.

Physician Payment Review Commission. *Annual Report to Congress.* Washington, D.C.: Physician Payment Review Commission, 1989.

Porter, M. E. *Competitive Strategy.* New York: Free Press, 1980.

Porter, M. E. *Competitive Advantage.* New York: Free Press, 1985.

Prescott, J. E. "Competitive Environments, Strategic Types, and Business Performance: An Empirical Analysis." Unpublished doctoral dissertation, Pennsylvania State University, 1983.

Prospective Payment Assessment Commission. *Report and Recommendations to the Secretary.* Washington, D.C.: Prospective Payment Assessment Commission, 1987.

Quinn, J. B. *Strategies for Change: Logical Incrementalism.* Homewood, Ill.: Irwin, 1980.

Ragin, C. C. *The Comparative Method: Moving Beyond Qualitative and Quantitative Strategies.* Berkeley: University of California Press, 1987.

Ramanujam, V., and Venkatraman, N. "Planning System Characteristics and Planning Effectiveness." *Strategic Management Journal,* 1987, *8* (5), 453–468.

Ramanujam, V., Venkatraman, N., and Camillus, J. "Multi-Objective Assessment of Effectiveness of Strategic Planning: A Discriminant Analysis Approach." *Academy of Management Journal,* 1986, *29* (2), 347–372.

Rappaport, A. *Creating Shareholder Value: The New Standard for Business Performance.* New York: Free Press, 1986.

Rasheed, A., and Prescott, J. "Dimensions of Organizational Task Environments Revisited." Paper presented at the Academy of Management Meeting, New Orleans, Aug. 1987.

Reep, J. "Managing the Information Explosion." Paper presented at Digital Health Care Corporate Leaders' Forum, Tucson, Ariz., Nov. 14, 1988.

Relman, A. S. "The New Medical-Industrial Complex." *New England Journal of Medicine*, 1980, *303*, 963–970.

Roberts, E. B., and Berry, C. A. "Entering New Businesses: Selecting Strategies for Success." *Sloan Management Review*, 1985, *26*, 3–17.

Robinson, J., Garnick, D., and McPhee, S. "Market and Regulatory Influences on the Availability of Coronary Angioplasty and By-Pass Surgery in U.S. Hospitals." *New England Journal of Medicine*, 1987, *317*, 85–90.

Robinson, J., and Luft, H. "The Impact of Hospital Market Structure on Patient Volume, Average Length of Stay, and the Cost of Care." *Journal of Health Economics*, 1985, *4*, 333–356.

Robinson, J., Luft, H., McPhee, S., and Hunt, S. "Hospital Competition and Surgical Length of Stay." *Journal of the American Medical Association*, 1988, *5* (260), 696–700.

Romanelli, E. "Organization Persistence and Adaptation: A Comparison of Alternative Theoretical Models." Working paper, Fuqua School of Business, Duke University, July 1988.

Rumelt, R. P. *Strategy, Structure, and Economic Performance.* Boston: Graduate School of Business Administration, Harvard University, 1974.

Rumelt, R. P. "Diversification Strategy and Profitability." *Strategic Management Journal*, 1982, *3*, 359–369.

Schendel, D., and Hofer, C. *Strategic Management: A New View of Business Policy and Planning.* Boston: Little, Brown, 1979.

Schlesinger, M., and Dorwart, R. "Ownership and Mental Health Services: A Reappraisal of the Shift Toward Privately Owned Facilities." *New England Journal of Medicine*, 1984, *311*, 959–965.

Schlesinger, M., and others. "Multi-Hospital Systems and Access to Healthcare." In R. Scheffler and L. Rossiter (eds.),

Advances in Health Economics and Health Services Research. Vol. 7. Greenwich, Conn.: JAI Press, 1987.

Schramm, C. J., and Gabel, J. "Prospective Payment: Some Retrospective Observations." *New England Journal of Medicine,* 1988, *318, 1681*–1683.

Schreyogg, G., and Steinmann, H. "Strategic Control: A New Perspective." *Academy of Management Review,* 1987, *12* (1), 91–103.

Scott, W. R. "The Adolescence of Institutional Theory." *Administrative Science Quarterly,* 1987, *32,* 493–511.

Seay, J. D., and Sigmond, R. M. "Community Benefits Standards for Hospitals: Perceptions and Performance." *Frontiers of Health Services Management,* 1989, *5,* 3–39.

Severance, D. G., and Passino, J. H. *Senior Management Attitudes Toward Strategic Change in U.S. Manufacturing Companies.* Ann Arbor: University of Michigan Press, 1986.

Shank, J. K., Niblock, E. G., and Sandall, S. W. "Balance Creativity and Practicality in Formal Planning." *Harvard Business Review,* 1973, *51,* 87–95.

Shortell, S. M. "The Medical Staff of the Future: Replanting the Garden." *Frontiers of Health Services Management,* 1985, *1,* 3–48.

Shortell, S. M. "The Evolution of Hospital Systems: Unfulfilled Promises and Self-Fulfilling Prophesies." *Medical Care Review,* 1988, *45* (2), 177–214.

Shortell, S. M. "New Directions in Hospital Governance." *Journal of Hospital and Health Services Administration,* 1989, *34* (1), 7–23.

Shortell, S. M., Morrisey, M. A., and Conrad, D. A. "Economic Regulation and Hospital Behavior: The Effects on Medical Staff Organization and Hospital-Physician Relationships." *Health Services Research,* 1985, *20* (5), 597–628.

Shortell, S. M., Morrison, E. M., and Hughes, S. L. "The Keys to Successful Diversification: Lessons from Leading Hospital Systems." *Hospital and Health Services Administration. 39,* Fall 1989.

Shortell, S. M., Morrison, E. M., and Robbins, S. "Strategy Making in Health Care Organizations: A Framework and Agenda for Research." *Medical Care Review,* 1985, *42,* 219–265.

Shortell, S. M., and Zajac, E. J. "Internal Corporate Joint Ventures: Development Process and Performance Outcomes." *Strategic Management Journal,* 1988, *9,* 527–542.

Shortell, S. M., and others. "The Effects of Hospital Ownership on Nontraditional Services." *Health Affairs,* 1986, *5,* 97–120.

Shortell, S. M., and others. "Diversification of Health Care Services: The Effects of Ownership, Environment, and Strategy." In R. M. Scheffler and L. F. Rossiter (eds.), *Advances in Health Economics and Health Services Research.* Vol. 7. Greenwich, Conn.: JAI Press, 1987.

Shrader, C. B., Taylor, L., and Dalton, D. R. "Strategic Planning and Organizational Performance: A Critical Appraisal." *Journal of Management,* 1984, *10,* 149–171.

Simons, R. "Accounting Control Systems and Business Strategy: An Empirical Analysis." *Accounting Organizations and Society,* 1987, *12,* 357–374.

Singh, J. V., Tucker, D. J., and House, R. J. "Organizational Legitimacy and the Liability of Newness." *Administrative Science Quarterly,* 1986, *31,* 171–193.

Sloan, F. A., Morrisey, M. A., and Valvona, J. "Medicare Prospective Payment and the Use of Medical Technologies In Hospitals." *Medical Care,* 1988, *26,* 837–853.

Smart, C., and Vertinsky, I. "Strategy and the Environment: A Study of Corporate Responses to Crisis." *Strategic Management Journal,* 1984, *5,* 199–213.

Smith, K. G., and Grimm, C. M. "Environmental Variation, Strategic Change, and Firm Performance: A Study of Railroad Deregulation." *Strategic Management Journal,* 1987, *8,* 363–376.

Smith, K. G., Guthrie, J. P., and Chen, M. J. "Miles and Snow's Typology of Strategy, Organizational Size, and Organizational Performance." *Academy of Management Best Papers Proceedings,* 1986, pp. 45–59.

Snow, C. C., and Hrebiniak, L. G. "Strategy, Distinctive Competence, and Organizational Performance." *Administrative Science Quarterly,* 1980, *25,* 317–336.

Starkweather, D. B., and Carman, J. M. "Horizontal and Vertical Concentrations in the Evolution of Hospital Competition." In R. M. Scheffler and L. F. Rossiter (eds.), *Advances in Health Economics and Health Services Research.* Vol. 7. Greenwich, Conn.: JAI Press, 1987.

Starr, P. *The Social Transformation of American Medicine.* New York: Basic Books, 1982.

Staw, B. M. "Knee Deep in the Big Muddy: A Study of Escalating Commitment to a Chosen Course of Action." *Organizational Behavior and Human Performance,* 1976, *16,* 27–44.

Teece, D. J. (ed.). *The Competitive Challenge: Strategies for Industrial Innovation and Renewal.* Cambridge, Mass.: Ballinger, 1987.

Thompson, A., Pettigrew, A. M., and Rubashow, N. "British Management and Strategic Change." *European Management Journal,* 1985, *3* (165), 173.

Thompson, J. D. *Organizations in Action: Social Science Bases of Administrative Theory.* New York: McGraw-Hill, 1967.

Tichy, N. *The Transformational Leader.* New York: Wiley, 1986.

Tushman, M. L., Newman, W. H., and Romanelli, E. "Convergence and Upheaval: Managing the Unsteady Pace of Organizational Evolution." *California Management Review,* 1987, *29* (1), 1–16.

Varadarajan, P. R., and Ramanujam, V. "Diversification and Performance: A Re-Examination Using a Two-Dimensional Conceptualization of Diversity in Firms." *Academy of Management Journal,* 1987, *30* (2), 380–393.

Veliyath, R. "Choice Determinants in Strategic Control: A Structural Equation Modeling Approach." Working paper PS-86-4, Virginia Polytechnic Institute, Apr. 1987.

Venkatraman, N. *Performance Implications of Strategic Co-Alignment. Sloan Working Paper Series,* no. 1753. Cambridge, Mass.: MIT Press, 1986.

Venkatraman, N. "The Concept of Fit in Strategy Research: Towards Verbal and Statistical Correspondence." In *Academy of Management Review,* 1989, *14* (3), 423–444.

Walker, D. C., and Ruekert, R. W. "Marketing's Role in the Implementation of Business Strategies: A Critical Review and Conceptual Framework." *Journal of Marketing,* 1987, *51,* 15–33.

Walton, R. E. *Innovating to Compete: Lessons for Diffusing and*

Managing Change in the Workplace. San Francisco: Jossey-Bass, 1987.

Wegmiller, D. C. "Boards Must Address Regional Issues." *Health Management Quarterly,* 1988, Third Quarter, pp. 3–5.

Weick, K. E. *The Social Psychology of Organizing.* Reading, Mass.: Addison-Wesley, 1979.

Wennberg, J. E. "Dealing with Medical Practice Variations: A Proposal for Action." *Health Affairs,* 1984, *3* (2), 6–32.

White, R. E. "Generic Business Strategies, Organizational Context and Performance: An Empirical Investigation." *Strategic Management Journal,* 1986, *7,* 217–231.

Williamson, O. E. *Markets and Hierarchies: Analysis and Anti-Trust Implications.* New York: Free Press, 1975.

Williamson, O. E. "Transaction-Cost Economics: The Governance of Contractual Relations." *Journal of Law and Economics,* 1979, *22,* 233–261.

Williamson, O. E., and Ouchi, W. G. "The Markets and Hierarchies Perspective: Origins, Implications, Prospects." In A. Van de Ven and W. F. Joyce (eds.), *Assessing Organization Design and Performance.* New York: Wiley, 1981.

Wrigley, L. "Divisional Autonomy and Diversification." Unpublished doctoral thesis, Harvard Business School, 1970.

Yoder, C. G. "Economic Theories of For-Profit and Not-for-Profit Organizations." In B. Gray (ed.), *For-Profit Enterprise in Health Care.* Washington, D.C.: National Academy Press, 1986.

Zahra, S. "Corporate Strategic Types, Environmental Perceptions, Managerial Philosophies and Goals: An Empirical Study." *Akron Business and Economic Review,* 1987, *18,* 64–77.

Zahra, S. "Research Evidence on the Miles and Snow Typology." *Journal of Management,* 1989.

Zajac, E. J., and Bowman, E. H. "Perspectives and Choices in Strategy Research." Paper presented at the Academy of Management Meetings, Boston, 1986.

Zajac, E. J., and Shortell, S. M. "Changing Generic Strategies: Likelihood, Direction, and Performance Implications." *Strategic Management Journal,* 1989.

Zaltman, G., Duncan, R., and Holbek, J. *Innovations and Organizations.* New York: Wiley, 1973.

Index

A

Accountability, 323; fiscal and clinical, 319–321

Adaptation. *See* Strategic adaptation

Administrative domain, 283–285

Aldrich, H., 15, 27, 33, 287, 296

Alexander, J. A., 11, 278

Altamore Hospital, 200–201

American College of Health Care Executives, 10

American College of Hospital Administrators, 8

American Hospital Association, 6, 9, 10, 257, 267, 274, 321

American Medical International (AMI), 12, 56, 57, 59, 60; organizational structure of, 91, 92, 93–95; overview of, 61–64; profile of, 46–47

Analyzers, 16–19; background of, 113–114, 115–116; challenge for, 186–190; creating synergy in, 193–196; developing new skills in, 198–203; environment of, 114, 117–120; examples of, 183–186; future of, 130–131; guidelines for managing, 205–206; lessons for, 241–242; managing complexity in, 190–193; maximizing learning in, 196–198; and new services, 193–196; and ownership, 127–130; performance of, 120–124, 186, 187, 188, 189; and physicians, 203–205; planning and control in, 124–127. *See also* Strategic orientation(s)

Anderson, C. R., 287

Angston Hospital, 251

Archetype. *See* Strategic archetype

Argyris, C., 196, 234

Ariss, S. S., 287

Armour, H. O., 40

Arthur Andersen & Co., 8, 257, 267, 274

Astley, W. G., 28

Austerly Memorial Hospital, 198

B

Baker General Hospital, 208–209

Barney, J. B., 291, 294

389

Beard, D. W., 14, 33
Begun, J. W., 8, 35, 296
Bernstein, S. C., 6
Berry, C. A., 142
Bevan Hospital, 197
Bhambri, A., 30, 294
Bice, M. D., 145, 251, 268
Binns, G., 277
Blendon, R. J., 257, 303, 304
Blue Cross, 6
Blue Shield, 6
Blumberg, M., 304, 325
Boards, development of, 278–279
Boeker, W., 29, 33
Bonner Hospital, 201
Brinkerhoff, D., 43
Brook, R., 304, 323
Brook, R. H., 325
Brown, L. D., 302, 315, 323
Burgelman, R. A., 289, 292, 294
Buzzell, R., 277

C

Cameron, K., 29, 36, 43, 141
Camillus, J. C., 41
Carman, J. M., 310
Carper, W. B., 270
Carswell Medical Center, 216–217
Catastrophic Health Care Act, 257
Centralization: in defenders, 177–179;
    of planning, 91, 124. See also Orga-
    nizational structure
CEOs: measures by, 17; turnover of,
    10
Chakravarthy, B. S., 23
Chandler, A., 261
Chandler, A. D., Jr., 28
Change: ability to, 38–39; frame-break-
    ing, 7–11; hospital position on,
    281–282; managing, 40–44, 274;
    need to, 31–37. See also Strategic
    change
Chapko, M., 13–14, 15
Cheng, J. C., 33, 138, 283
Child, J., 28, 29
Christensen, H., 23, 43, 294
Chrysler, 6
Clement, J. P., 141

Cobbs, D. L., 8
Coile, R., 260
Common provider entities (CPEs),
    269
Community Memorial Hospital, 161–
    163
Complexity, in analyzers, 190–193; and
    new strategy selection, 39
Conant, J. S., 35, 114
Cone, K., 4
Conrad, A. A., 4
Conrad, D., 36
Conrad, D. A., 14, 15, 261, 296
Consumer Price Index, and medical
    care inflation, 5
Control. See Strategic planning and
    control
Continuums of care, 260–262
Contract management, 107
Cook, K., 4, 36
Cost(s), health care, 3–4; for auto com-
    panies, 6; defender management of,
    168–173; for insurance companies, 6
Cost containment: findings on, 58–59;
    in future, 255–256; measure of, 21;
    in reactors, 219–220; of strategic
    orientations, 127
Covin, J. G., 123, 283
Coyne, J. S., 8
Cresap, 265

D

Daft, R., 293
Data, sources of, 13–14
Decker Hills Hospital, 195
Defenders, 16–19; background of, 113–
    114, 115–116; centralization for,
    177–179; challenge for, 167–168;
    cost management for, 168–173;
    differentiation for, 173–174; diver-
    sification for, 174–176; environment
    of, 114, 117–120; examples of, 161–
    163; future of, 130–131; guidelines
    for managing, 181–182; lessons for,
    240–241; and ownership, 127–130;
    performance of, 120–124, 163–167;
    and physicians, 179–181; planning
    and control in, 124–127; resources

for, 176–177. *See also* Strategic orientation(s)

Delbecq, A., 278

Denzin, N., 13

Designs. *See* Organizational designs

Dess, G. G., 14, 33

Development: of leadership, 274–279; stages of, 53–54

Differentiation: and defenders, 173–174; and prospectors, 144–147

DiMaggio, P., 33

Diversification: constant, 144–147; of defenders, 174–176; lessons on, 230–232; measure of, 19–20; of prospectors, 137–144; of reactors, 216–218

Diversity, 39

Divisibility, 39

Divisional designs, 91–93

Dobson, A., 7

"Doing good" measure, 22, 120–121, 123; for analyzer, 187; for defender, 164; for prospector, 135; for reactor, 210

"Doing well" measure, 22–23, 122, 123; for analyzer, 188; for defender, 165; for prospector, 136; for reactor, 211

Dorwart, R., 23

Doz, Y., 30

Dranove, D., 4

Duncan, R., 39

Duncan, R. B., 34, 43, 90

Dutton, J. E., 34, 43

E

Eastwood Hospital, 214–215

Eckels, T. J., 23

Ellwood, P. M., 304

Engledow, J. L., 33

Enthoven, A., 321, 324

Entrepreneurial problem, 16–17

Environment: future, 254–260; institutional, 33; of strategic orientations, 114, 117–120; task, 33

Environmental jolt, 44–45; Prospective Payment System as, 4–11

Evangelical Health System, 12, 56, 57, 59, 60; organizational structure of,

91, 92, 98–100; overview of, 71–74; profile of, 49

Experience curve, and prospectors, 147–150

F

Fahey, L., 23, 43, 294

Feder, J., 7

Finkelstein, S., 28, 34, 293

Fiol, C. M., 196, 234

Foley, H. A., 302

Fombrun, C. J., 28, 296

For-profit systems. *See* Investor-owned systems

Ford Motor Company, 6

Forrest Falls Hospital, 194

Freeman, E., 43

Freeman, J., 27, 287

Friedman, B., 14, 130, 310

Friesen, P. H., 35, 36

Functional designs, 90–91

Functional strategies, and prospectors, 153–154

Future: environment in, 254–260; health policy themes of, 302–305; managing strategic adaptation in, 260–279; and Porter's framework, 308–311

G

Gabel, J., 7

Galbraith, J. R., 90

Gale, B., 277

Garnick, D., 15, 310

Garnick, D. W., 312

Gateway Hospital, 215

General Motors, 6

Ghemawat, P., 148

Ghoshal, S., 41

Gifford, B. D., 278

Gifford, G., 128

Gilbert, X., 153

Gill, S. L., 278

Ginn, G. O., 30, 35, 114

Ginsberg, A., 29, 31, 287

Glen Oaks Hospital, 194–195

Golden, B., 296

Goldsmith, J. A., 327
Goodman, P. S., 43
Government, federal: health care expenditures by, 4; and health policy, 301–305; and industry interface, 315–317. *See also* Health policy
Govindarajan, V., 40, 108, 236, 295
Grant, J. H., 29, 31, 287
Gray, B. H., 24, 287
Green, A., 268
Greiner, L., 30
Greiner, L. E., 294
Griffith, J., 278
Grimm, C. M., 30, 285
Guncheon, K., 191, 200
Gupta, A., 40, 294
Guterman, S., 7

H

Hadley, J., 7
Halston Community Hospital, 223–224
Hambrick, D. C., 28, 34, 38, 123, 282, 293
Hannan, M. T., 27, 287
Hansmann, H. G., 23
Hartman, S. E., 321
Health care: expenditures for, 3, 6; future environment for, 254–260
Health Care Financing Administration, 4, 7
Health Central (Health One), 12, 56, 57, 59, 60; organizational structure of, 91, 92, 100–102; overview of, 74–77; profile of, 50
Health Insurance Association of America, 4, 7
Health maintenance organizations (HMOs), 6, 308
Health Planning and Resource Development Act, 4
Health policy, 301–302; for government/industry interface, 315–317; and health industry, 305–311; proposal for, 317–319; and strategic orientations, 311–315; themes for, 302–305; for year 2000, 319–327
Health professionals, future conflict among, 258–260

Health status, 277
Health Care Financial Management Association, 5
Heidrick, 10
Herzlinger, R. E., 23
Hill, C., 294
Hill, C.W.L., 40, 294
Hofer, C., 28, 41
Holbek, J., 39
Hortonville Memorial Hospital, 215
Hoskisson, R. E., 40, 294
Hospital Corporation of America (HCA), 12, 56, 57, 59, 60; organizational structure of, 91, 92, 95–97; overview of, 64–68; profile of, 47–48
Hospitals: expenditures for, 4; ownership of, 23–24; and physicians, 268–274; and Prospective Payment System, 4–11. *See also* Systems
Hostility, 15
House, R. J., 28
Hrebiniak, L. G., 28, 212, 224
Huff, A. S., 294
Hughes, S. L., 154, 230
Hunt, S., 310

I

Independent practice associations (IPAs), 269
Inertia, 27–28
Institute of Medicine, 24
Institutional environment, 33
Insurance companies, 6
Intermountain Health Care, 12, 56, 57, 59, 60; organizational structure of, 91, 92, 102–104; overview of, 78–81; profile of, 50–51
Interstudy, 6
Investor-owned systems, 23–24; structuring in, 90–93, 107–109; in study, 11–12. *See also* Ownership; Systems

J

Jarillo, C. J., 28, 296
Jones, G. R., 294
Joyce, W. F., 28

K

Kane, R. L., 323
Kanter, R. M., 43, 145
Keats, B. W., 35, 114
Kemper Union Hospital, 221, 222
Kesner, I. F., 33, 138, 283
Kieser, A., 29
Kimberly, J. R., 90, 287
Kinzer, D. M., 317
Kirkman-Liff, B. L., 302
Kirkman-Liff, T. L., 302
Kovner, A. R., 278
Kralewski, J., 128
Krasker, W. S., 23
Kronich, R., 321, 324

L

Lapre, R., 302
Lawrence, P. R., 28
Leadership: development of strategic, 274–279; for reactors, 214–216. See also Management
Learning: in analyzers, 196–198; lessons on, 233–234; in reactors, 221–222
Leatt, P., 90
Lenz, R. T., 33
Lewin, L. S., 23
Lewis, B. L., 11
Lieberman, M. B., 147
Light, D. W., 304
Litschert, R. J., 270
Lohr, K. N., 325
Lorange, P., 41
Lorsch, J. W., 28
Luft, H., 15, 310
Luft, H. S., 310, 312
Luke, R. D., 8, 35, 296
Lyles, M. A., 196, 234

M

McDaniel, R. R., 30, 35, 114
McKinley Memorial Hospital, 249
MacMillan, I. C., 170
McNerney, W., 302

McNerney, W. J., 301
McPhee, S., 15, 310
Maerki, S., 15
"Managed care" programs, 6
Management: of analyzers, 205–206; and change feasibility, 38; of defenders, 181–182; in model, 33–34; processes of, 40–42; of prospectors, 159–160; of reactors, 224–225. See also Administrative domain; Leadership
Management team, 293–294
Market biographies, 311–312
Marketing, necessity of, 9–10
Mason, P. A., 34
Matrix designs, 93
Maturation stage, 53
Measures, in study, 14–23, 24–25. See also "Doing good" measure; "Doing well" measure
Medicaid, 3, 4
Medicare, 3, 4. See also Prospective Payment System (PPS)
Melnick, G. A., 310
Meyer, A., 27, 44, 287
Michael, S. R., 41
Mick, S. S., 261, 296
Miles and Snow typology, 15–18
Miles, R., 29, 36, 141
Miles, R. E., 15–16, 35, 36, 37, 123, 167, 282, 283, 285, 381; typology of, 15–18
Miles, R. H., 287
Miller, C. B., 23
Miller, D., 35, 36
Mintzberg, H., 17, 220, 238, 289
Mission, 34
Mohr, L. B., 13
Mokwa, M. P., 35, 114
Montgomery, C. A., 141
Montgomery, D. B., 147
Morietto Hospital, 224
Morlock, L. L., 278
Morrisey, M. A., 4, 7, 14, 15, 36
Morrison, E. M., 29, 154, 230
Moston General Hospital, 195
Mukamel, D. B., 321
Munificence, 14–15

N

Nartan Memorial Hospital, 219
National Medical Enterprises (NME),
    12, 56, 57, 59, 60; organizational
    structure of, 91, 92, 97–98; overview
    of, 68–71; profile of, 48–49
Networks: future research on, 296–297;
    managing, 275
Neuhauser, 260
Newman, W. H., 7
Niblock, E. G., 186
Nielsen, R. P., 28, 296
Not-for-profit systems, 23–24; structur-
    ing in, 90–93, 107–109; in study,
    11–12. See also Ownership; Systems

O

Office of Technology Assessment, 4
Organizational designs, 90–93, 107;
    divisional, 91–93; functional, 90–91;
    matrix, 93
Organizational structure, 90–93, 107–
    109; of American Medical Interna-
    tional, 93–95; of Evangelical Health
    System, 98–100; of Health Central,
    100–102; of Hospital Corporation of
    America, 95–97; of Intermountain
    Health Care, 102–104; of National
    Medical Enterprises, 97–98; of Sis-
    ters of Mercy Health Corporation,
    104–105; of Southwest Community
    Health Services, 105–107
Organizations, multidivisional, 40;
    future research on, 294–296; report-
    ing structures for, 92
Orientation. See Strategic orientation(s)
Ouchi, W. G., 40, 294
Ownership, 23–24; of hospitals in study,
    12; and strategic orientation, 127–
    130, 286–287

P

Pangor Hospital Corporation, 219
Parks, D., 293
Passino, J. H., 30
Passmore Hospital, 245

Pearson, A., 39
Peer review organizations (PROs), 6
Pennings, J. M., 43
Performance: of analyzers, 186, 187,
    188, 189; of defenders, 163–167;
    measure of, 22–23; past, 33; of pros-
    pectors, 134–137; of reactors, 209–
    213; and resource allocation, 321–
    322, 323; and strategic adaptation
    model, 42–44; and strategic comfort
    zones, 123–124; of strategic orien-
    tations, 120–123
Peters, J. P., 38, 250, 293
Pettigrew, A. M., 29
Pfeffer, J., 28, 34
Physician Payment Review Commis-
    sion, 255
Physicians: and analyzers, 203–205;
    and defenders, 179–181; and future
    conflict, 258–260; and hospitals,
    268–274; lessons on, 236–238; after
    Prospective Payment System, 9–10;
    and prospectors, 154–159; and reac-
    tors, 222–224
Physician-hospital organizations
    (PHOs), 269
Planning. See Strategic planning and
    control
Pointer, D. D., 8, 296
Policy. See Health policy
Porter, J., 128
Porter, M. E., 33, 35, 36, 305, 306
Powell, W. W., 33
PPS. See Prospective Payment System
    (PPS)
Prahalad, C. K., 30
Preferred provider organizations
    (PPOs), 6
Prescott, J., 14
Professional practice associations
    (PPAs), 269
Prospective Payment Assessment Com-
    mission, 7
Prospective Payment System (PPS), as
    environmental jolt, 4–11
Prospectors, 15–19; background of,
    113–114, 115–116; challenge for,
    137–139; and differentiation, 144–
    147; and diversification, 137–144;

environment of, 114, 117–120; example of, 133–134; and experience curve, 147–150; functional strategies in, 153–154; future of, 130–131; guidelines for managing, 159–160; lessons for, 239–240; and local market synergies, 150–153; and ownership, 127–130; performance of, 120–124, 134–137; and physicians, 154–159; planning and control in, 124–127. *See also* Strategic orientation(s)
Prosser Medical Center, 250

Q

Quinn, J. B., 27, 36

R

Ragin, C. C., 25, 298
Ramanujam, V., 21
Rappaport, A., 43
Rasheed, A., 14
Reactors, 16–19; background of, 113–114, 115–116; challenge for, 213–214; cost containment in, 219–220; and diversification, 216–218; environment of, 114, 117–120; examples of, 207–209; future of, 130–131; guidelines for managing, 224–225; leadership for, 214–216; learning in, 221–222; lessons for, 242–243; and new services, 218–219; and ownership, 127–130; performance of, 120–124, 209–213; and physicians, 222–224; planning and control in, 124–127, 220–221. *See also* Strategic orientation(s)
Reep, J., 233
Refocusing, 54, 305
Reger, R. K., 294
Relman, A. S., 8
Renewal, 54, 305
Research: existing strategic change, 29–31; further, 287–297; market, 233–234. *See also* Study
Resources: allocation of, 321–322; and defenders, 176–177; slack, 232–233

Reversibility, and new strategy selection, 39
Rinaldo Medical Center, 220
River Glen Hospital, 194
Robbins, S., 29
Roberts, E. B., 142
Robinson, J., 15, 310
Robinson, J. C., 312
Romanelli, E., 7, 292
Rubashow, N., 29
Ruekert, R. W., 141
Rumelt, R. P., 30, 36, 40, 141

S

Salancik, G., 28, 34
Sandall, S. W., 186
Schendel, D., 28, 41
Schlesinger, M., 23
Schön, D. A., 196, 234
Schramm, C. J., 7
Schreyogg, G., 295
Scott, W. R., 33
Scott-Morton, M. F., 41
Seay, J. D., 10, 23, 277
Services, new: of analyzers, 193–196; of reactors, 218–219
Severance, D. G., 30
Shank, J. K., 186
Shortell, S. M., 4, 8, 14, 15, 17, 29, 30, 31, 35, 36, 55, 90, 130, 143, 154, 230, 262, 264, 269, 278, 309, 310
Sigmond, R. M., 10, 23, 277
Silverado Memorial Hospital, 195
Simons, R., 295
Singh, J. V., 28
Sisters of Mercy Health Corporation (SMHC), 12, 56, 57, 59, 60; organizational structure of, 91, 92, 104–105; overview of, 81–84; profile of, 51–52
Skills, new, in analyzers, 198–203
Slevin, D. P., 123, 283
Sloan, F. A., 7
Smart, C., 36
Smith, K. G., 30, 285
Snow, C. C., 15–16, 35, 36, 37, 123, 167, 212, 224, 282, 283, 285, 293; typology of, 15–18

Sormunen, J., 293
Southwest Community Health Services, 12, 56, 57, 59, 60; organizational structure of, 91, 92, 105–107; overview of, 84–88; profile of, 52–53
Starkweather, D. B., 310
Starr, P., 8
Startup phase, 53
Staw, B. M., 39
Steinmann, H., 295
Strategic adaptation, xix, 27–29; future research on, 287–300; managing, 260–279; model of, 31–44; structuring for, 90–93, 107–109; study findings on, 88–89. See also Strategic change
Strategic archetype, xix; background of, 115–116; environment of, 117–118. See also Strategic orientation(s)
Strategic change, xix; existing research on, 29–31; findings on, 54–55; measurement of, 15–18. See also Strategic adaptation
Strategic choice, 28
Strategic comfort zones, 18–19, 36–37; lessons on, 238–239; and performance, 123–124
Strategic control system, 41–42
Strategic leadership, development of, 274–279
Strategic orientation(s), xix, 35; of American Medical International, 61–62; background of, 113–114, 115–116; changes in, 56; current, 35–36, 38–39; environment of, 114, 117, 120; future for, 130–131; of Health Central, 74–76; and health policy, 311–315; of Hospital Corporation of America, 65; increasing understanding of, 311–315; of Intermountain Health Care, 78–79; lessons for all, 229–239; measurement of, 15–18; of National Medical Enterprises, 68–69; and ownership, 127–130, 286–287; performance of, 120–124; planning and control in, 124–127; of Sisters of Mercy Health Corporation, 81–82; of Southwest Community Health Services, 85–

86; switching, 243–253. See also Analyzers; Defenders; Prospectors; Reactors; Strategic archetype
Strategic planning and control: at American Medical International, 62–63; for analyzer, 189; for defender, 166; at Evangelical Health System, 73; flexible, 234–236; at Health Central, 76–77; at Hospital Corporation of America, 66; at Intermountain Health Care, 79; measure of, 20–21; at National Medical Enterprises, 69–70; for prospector, 137; quality of, 55–58; at Sisters of Mercy Health Corporation, 83; at Southwest Community Health Services, 86–87; of strategic orientations, 124–127; structuring for, 90–93, 107–109
Strategy(ies), 29; better, 282–283; functional, 153–154; selection of new, 39; switching of, 243–253, 285–286
Strebel, P., 153
Structure. See Organizational structure
Struggles, 10
Study: data sources for, 13–14; interviews for, 25–26; measures in, 14–23, 24–25; ownership issue in, 23–24; sample for, 11–13. See also Research
Synergy(ies): creating, 193–196; local market, 150–153
Systemness, 262–268
Systems: findings on, 54–61; future behavior as, 262–268; growth of, 8; individual, 61–88; profiles of, 46–54; in study, 12. See also Investor-owned systems; Not-for-profit systems

T

Task environment, 33
Teece, D. J., 40, 294
Tetreault, J., 312
Thompson, A., 29
Tseng, S., 38, 250, 293
Tucker, D. J., 28
Tushman, M. L., 7, 28, 287

V

Valvona, J., 7
Van de Ven, A. H., 28
Veliyath, R., 41
Venkatraman, N., 21, 283, 287
Vertinsky, I., 36
Viability: findings on, 59–61; measure of, 22

W

Walden Memorial Hospital, 207–208
Walker, D. C., 141
Walton, R. E., 39
Weick, K. E., 34
Wells Fargo Memorial Hospital, 133–134
Wennberg, J. E., 304

Westview Memorial Hospital, 215
Whetten, D., 43
Whetten, D. A., 296
Williamson, O. E., 40, 142, 294
Wrigley, L., 267

Y

Yoder, C. G., 23

Z

Zahra, S., 120
Zajac, E. J., 17, 28, 30, 31, 35, 55, 143, 296
Zaltman, G., 39
Zeithaml, C. D., 287
Zuckerman, S., 7
Zwanziger, J., 310